Bleed, Blist

A History of Medicine on the American Frontier

Volney Steele, M.D.

Mountain Press Publishing Company
Missoula, Montana
2005

Fourth Printing, January 2009

Cover art: *The Doctor* by Sir Luke Fildes (1891)
Courtesy Tate Gallery, London, and Art Resource, New York

Library of Congress Cataloging-in-Publication Data

Steele, Volney.
    Bleed, blister, and purge : a history of medicine on the American
frontier / Volney Steele.
        p. cm.
    Includes bibliographical references and index.
    ISBN 0-87842-505-5 (paper : alk. paper)
    1. Medicine—West (U.S.)—History. 2. Frontier and pioneer life—
West (U.S.) I. Title.
R154.5.W47S74 2005
610'.978—dc22
                                2005002325

MOUNTAIN PRESS PUBLISHING COMPANY
P.O. Box 2399 ✦ Missoula, Montana 59806
406-728-1900

To my great-grandfather Marion DeKalb Steele, M.D.,
and my father, Raphael William Steele, M.D.,
who were frontier physicians

CONTENTS

ACKNOWLEDGMENTS

My book owes much to many. I am indebted to those people across the country and on the Internet who responded generously to my inquiries or who directed me to someone who could answer them. To the surviving family members of physicians, nurses, and Native Americans, I am especially indebted, for they shared unstintingly their correspondence, memorabilia, home videos, and precious recollections. Like all authors, I have benefited from the faithful service of librarians at universities and historical societies across the country, and especially from the staff of the Montana Historical Society in Helena and the Montana State University Library in Bozeman. Many friends and colleagues, knowing about this project, gave me tips, sent clippings, and offered suggestions. Now, they can see for themselves where those items lodged in the fabric of the book. I am especially grateful to my friend Ann, who helped edit the final version of this book during a period of painful and stressful hospitalization. And last but not least to Gwen McKenna and others at the Mountain Press in Missoula for their patience and wisdom, as well as close family and friends who have suffered through my frustrations. Thanks.

Special thanks to:

Ed Amberg, Grace Balice, Lindsey Baskett, Art Coffin, Deane Epler, Ray B. Farnsworth, Burton D. Firehammer, Timothy Gordon, Mari Graña, E. R. Grigg, Ruth Hall, Bernard John Heetderks Sr., Harry L. Helton, Gary Hettrick, Ann Huffine, Stillman Jones, Martha Kohl, Ronald Loge, Ron Losee, Alfred Lueck, Stan Lynde, Pierce Mullen, Joseph Mussulman, Roxanne Neagle, Phil Pallister, Charles Rankin, Jodi Rasker, William A. Reynolds, Todd Savitt, Wilfred P. Schoenberg, S. J. "Clem" Seerley, Roy E. Seitz, Theodora J. Smith, Anton Sohn, Connie Staudohar, Katarzyna (Kasia) Steele, Dave Walter, Meg Watson, Starr Wheelan, John H. Whelan, Malcolm and Beth Winter, and Margaret Woods.

The Country Doctor

May the family doctor never be completely eliminated.

—Montana Medical Association, *First One Hundred Years*[i]

FRONTIER LIFE didn't end all at once. Well into the mid-twentieth century, especially in the West, there were still physicians who were practicing with little help and scarce resources. The isolated country doctor faced daily responsibilities beyond the comprehension of most modern people, physicians included. Few know how difficult that kind of medical practice was. The "buck stopped" with the rural doctor. The patient, whatever the complaint, depended on him or her to diagnose and treat the problem, usually right then and there. Only the strongest and most courageous physicians could endure such demands.

My father and great-grandfather were frontier doctors. And, for a short time and on a lesser level, so was I. My interest in medical history began a long time before I understood the Krebs cycle or memorized Koch's Postulates. As a young boy, my nickname was "Little Doc." I was going into medicine "no matter what." In my family there was no higher calling than medicine. My paternal great-grandfather, Marion D. Steele, M.D., was also an ordained Methodist minister. I was raised to believe that there was something spiritual about doctoring.

Ralph, my father, graduated from the medical department of the University of Arkansas on May 11, 1916. Soon afterward, he became a lieutenant in the Army Medical Corps, attached to the First New York Division, and was sent to France. When he returned in 1918, young Dr. Ralph Steele settled near his home and extended family in Arkansas. Here, by horseback, buggy, and Model T, he practiced medicine. He had no access to a hospital, a laboratory, or X-ray equipment. His doctor's bag held a stethoscope, a blood-pressure cuff, a thermometer, a percussion hammer, maybe a stomach tube, assorted catheters, a syringe, a needle and sutures, scissors and clamps, a tracheostomy tube for that rare case of diphtheria, rubbing alcohol, and miscellaneous drugs like morphine, laudanum, chloroform, and, oh yes, those old-time cure-alls calomel and castor oil.

I must admit I questioned my own admiration for medicine all too often when my father prescribed a "round" of calomel and a dose of castor oil, administered in orange juice, for my stomachaches. In time I learned never to tell anyone about an upset stomach. As most readers know, these strong purges, useless and toxic, were for ages considered a panacea, and they were employed well into the twentieth century until safer and more scientifically sound medicines replaced them. Ferrol Sams, in his novel *Run with the Horsemen*, described those days just as I remember them. His character Dr. Witherspoon "was hardly ever in his office. . . . If someone wanted the doctor, he could be found on the street and would treat the patient on the spot for everything except surgical procedures. He had one vest pocket full of powdered calomel, and a good-sized pinch between his thumb and forefinger was a dose for an adult. . . . He never forgot to caution that the calomel should be followed with a dose of castor oil."[ii] All of which goes to support that things were different then.

In the few years I was privileged to know my dad, I learned a great deal about the profession I would join years later. Dad suffered from severe, debilitating rheumatoid arthritis, a disease of the joints and collagen of the body that had no known cause or cure then. Arthritis of the kind that my father had was very common. One of the first remedies an arthritic often tried was a total dental extraction, on the mistaken premise that the cause of this debilitating illness lurked in the mouth. Dad was no exception and attempted this cure. It didn't help, nor did the injections of gold that some claimed were beneficial. There was some evidence in the medical literature that bee stings could improve the lot of an arthritic, and I remember driving my father to visit a beekeeper so he might try this unusual and painful therapy. After Dad convinced the skeptical beekeeper that he wasn't psychotic in making his request, the man captured a few bees in a fruit jar and held the open end of the container against Dad's bare arm. I don't know how many stings Dad endured, but it was painful even to watch. He never uttered a sound, but there were tears in his eyes. I'll never forget the look on that beekeeper's face as we drove away. It was like the countenance of one who had just participated in some satanic ritual. Dad's condition stayed the same, and we never went back.

As early as I can remember, Dad was confined to a wheelchair and could walk only short distances on crutches. To help him get from place to place, I was given a special driver's license at an early age—never mind that I needed to sit on a stack of books to see over the Ford's steering wheel. One of my uncles said that one of the books must have been a Bible because we never had a wreck. The most important skill a chauffeur could have in those days—the 1930s—was knowing how to rapidly and efficiently change a flat tire. On even the shortest drive over the crude gravel roads and rickety bridges of northwest Arkansas, one could expect at least one or two flats.

On our drives into and around the hill country, Dad had time to talk about his experiences as a doctor. He was a good storyteller and my personal hero. By the time I was ready for college and Dad was resting alongside his mother and father in the family plot in Gentry, Arkansas, I had a feel for what it was to be a country doctor. My respect for him and for his peers persists to this day.

At that time and place, seeing patients meant making house calls. Sometimes, especially in the spring, rivers and streams had to be forded, so the trips could be wet and cold. On several occasions Dad was stranded in the middle of a river in his partially flooded car until some farmer with a team of horses came along to pull him out. House calls were often overnight trips, and on some miserable Ozark nights the young doctor, already beginning to suffer from swollen, painful joints, slept cramped in a backseat or in a mountaineer's bedbug-infested cabin.

In the country, especially during the Depression, commodities such as meat, livestock, and bushels of wheat were used to settle a bill. Most rural doctors gladly accepted payment in any form. For years, one grateful little old lady who lived far back in the hills paid Dad with a turkey whenever he treated her family. One Montana doctor took a pair of workhorses in payment for an appendectomy. According to the story, he hired a trucker to take the horses to Billings for sale. The trucker's fee was five dollars more than what the horses sold for.[iii]

One of Dad's first patients after he opened his office in Decatur, Arkansas, was the teenage daughter of the turkey lady. The time was 1919, and the world was just beginning to breathe again after the great scourge of flu had finally subsided and the War to End All Wars was over. The aftermath of the flu brought complications, among them encephalitis, known as "sleeping sickness." Dad had driven the muddy spring roads to visit the girl, who, he was told, could not stay awake, "not even for a little while." Dad was young at the time, just starting practice, and no doubt was unsure of himself. The girl had no fever, and Dad couldn't find anything physical to explain why she slept all the time. According to her parents, she had been well until a few days before. Though there was no history of flu, the family suspected "sleeping sickness."

Not sure what he was dealing with, Dad returned to town and called Dr. John Smiley, an older physician (later Dad's partner) who lived in Siloam Springs, more than a few bumpy and rutted miles away. Dr. Smiley returned with Dad to the home of the sick girl. Dr. Smiley was a large, whiskered man, complete with a three-piece suit and gold watch chain, and with all the convincing doctorly mannerisms. He, too, examined the young woman carefully and methodically. He used a safety pin to check nerve distribution on both the lower and upper extremities, and looked for nuchal rigidity. He stroked the soles of her feet for a Babinski reflex and used his rubber hammer to check her other reflexes. He even looked into her eyeballs with his new ophthalmoscope, which had only recently been purchased in Little Rock.

A quiet, contemplative man, Dr. Smiley sat and observed his patient for a long time while my dad and the girl's parents stood by quietly, hardly breathing. Then Dr. Smiley stood up and quietly asked the girl's father to bring him a bucket of well water. When the bucket arrived, without so much as a word of explanation, Dr. Smiley dumped the water on the sleepy girl, bringing her screaming to her feet. Dad and the girl's parents were nearly as shocked as she was. Her mother found dry bedding and another nightgown for the shivering girl. She settled back into her now dry bed and to all appearances fell sound asleep again. Dr. Smiley asked the father for another bucket of water. Before the father could respond, the girl cried out, "Oh God, no, Doc! This is my last clean nightgown! I'm awake now, for sure."

Dr. Smiley and Dad took the parents into the next room, still within earshot of the young lady, and Dr. Smiley said, "I am sure she will be all right now. I have found that this kind of shock treatment works nearly all the time. If not," he added, "it is something you folks can use if needed." The girl was able to fool her parents and my dad, but not wise old Dr. Smiley.

There were a lot of snakes in this part of Arkansas, and snakebites were not uncommon. Most likely to cause trouble was the cottonmouth, an aggressive, poisonous viper with a nasty bite that was often followed by a severe infection. Most of the time, the homegrown emergency treatments people used, according to Dad, were deplorable and made the condition worse. A freshly killed chicken applied to the bite caused little trouble, but fresh cow manure was messy. The biggest problem was the tourniquet. It was believed that poison from a bite could spread to the heart and cause death, and that a tourniquet applied very tightly would slow the movement of the toxin up the extremity. Sometimes people used something like a shoestring, obstructing the blood flow—if the "treatment" was prolonged, it could result in gangrene. In such cases a doctor often had to operate to remove the deeply buried tourniquet. One of my father's patients was the victim of a tight homemade tourniquet, and several hours elapsed before Dad was called. The man lost much of his forearm.

When I was very young, about three or four, I slipped in the bathtub and fell down very hard on my bottom. Soon thereafter my mother discovered that I had a small inguinal hernia on the left side. After trusses and other suspensory methods were applied to the rupture, it was obvious that the little protuberance was not going away. The next thing I knew I was in the Siloam Springs "hospital"—a small area upstairs from the local fire department—being prepared for surgery. The safest anesthesia at the time was "open drop" ether. My father, without ceremony, covered my nose and mouth with a "mask" soaked in this acrid, volatile anesthetic, and the panic I felt at the sensation of suffocation is as vivid today as it was at that moment. During my later career as a family physician, I was often called upon to administer an anesthetic using the same archaic technique, and each time my own memory was painfully reawakened.

Dr. Smiley and my dad repaired the hernia. When I awoke, I was alone with a large woman dressed in white. Like someone out of *One Flew Over the Cuckoo's Nest*, she was very stern. I was not allowed out of bed. At the end of the week, I had to relearn how to walk.

My own medical practice began in Meeker, Colorado, in 1951. With an internship, a few years of residency, and the U.S. Navy experience behind me, I settled down, essentially penniless, with my young family in this small ranching community. Injuries from horses, tractors, and livestock kept me constantly busy, and during the summer, rodeo mishaps brought me additional business. I practiced in Meeker for two years. Although I had some training in surgery, I refused to do major procedures, always referring these cases to the most competent doctors available.

My office was in a cold and drafty building formerly occupied by the O.K. Saloon, near the city square. One of my first cases was memorable and tragic. One day I was called to the Meeker Memorial Hospital, a brand-new institution, to see an emergency patient. When I arrived, a young rancher named Truman Caldwell was still crumpled in the backseat of the car in which a neighbor had driven him into town. Truman had been crushed beneath a large, heavy haystacker while towing it across a field by tractor. He was in extreme pain and totally paralyzed from the waist down. Extracting his six-foot frame from the car was a difficult procedure, made somewhat easier by an injection of morphine.

A portable X-ray revealed a crushed vertebra in Truman's lower thoracic region. As soon as possible, I was on the phone with a neurosurgeon in Denver. He agreed that the patient needed immediate surgery to relieve the pressure on his spinal cord, and a plane was dispatched to pick Truman up and take him to Denver. Just then, a freak October blizzard struck Rio Blanco County with a vengeance. New to the area, I was totally amazed to see how quickly the visibility disappeared. Within a short time, a foot of snow had accumulated. Nevertheless the valiant pilot made several attempts at a landing on our small airstrip. We on the ground could hear his engine zoom each time he neared the runway. Finally the pilot was forced to give up and return to Denver.

I called an orthopedic surgeon in Grand Junction who agreed to see Truman as soon as we could get him there. Hours had passed, and it was nearly midnight when the ambulance (which doubled as a hearse when needed), with Truman and me in the back and driven by the owner of the local sporting-goods store, left for Grand Junction. We arrived in the early morning hours, and the surgeon operated. Sadly, it did no good. The spinal cord was mashed, and Truman was never able to walk again without braces and support.

Hunting season in Meeker sometimes resembled a war zone. Gunshot and knife wounds were common. I remember a young man shot in both thighs by his father. The two were walking up a hill in the dark, following the scent of elk. The father mistook his son for an elk and shot. The bullet tore the skin and some muscle from the front of both thighs, and the femoral artery and vein were exposed on both sides. I patched him up the best I could and sent him by air to Denver. He recovered.

In my two years of general practice in Meeker, I also delivered numerous babies and treated a number of complications. My last delivery—as it turned out, my last obstetrical case of any kind—was an arm presentation that required internal manipulation, the first and last such delivery I ever performed. In fact, it never should have happened. Since I was leaving practice, I wanted to refer the young woman, whose due date was still a couple of weeks away, to another doctor, but she wanted me to deliver her. Against my better judgment, I induced labor by stripping and rupturing the membranes. Immediately her labor pains became intense. A few minutes later her labor began in earnest, and I was stunned to see an arm protruding from the incompletely dilated cervix. The delivery required anesthesia and the complete rotation of the fetus, followed by a breech extraction. With a good deal of luck, I was able to complete the delivery. I am glad to say that both mother and infant did well afterward.

Having a solitary country practice is a deeply lonely experience. Secluded from one's peers by many lonely miles, the rural doctor might have to confront a "croupy" child with a laryngeal obstruction, a youngster unconscious from a fall from his father's pickup truck, a young woman with vaginal bleeding in the third trimester of pregnancy, or any number of illnesses and injuries. The day-to-day challenges may seem stimulating at first, but only the most self-confident and self-sufficient could stick it out for the long haul. From my small country practice in Meeker, I returned to postgraduate training. Upon being certified in pathology, I returned to the West as soon as I could. One cold January day in 1959, I entered the last phase of my career, the practice of pathology and laboratory medicine in Bozeman, Montana.

This book is about those doctors who stayed in practice on the frontier. They didn't do it for money—there isn't enough money in the world to compensate for the prolonged anxiety, disturbed sleep, and long, exhausting days. Today's small-town doctors are less isolated and have more resources, and the wild West has been civilized. Still, for those who choose medicine as a profession, there will always be a frontier.

The Past
Enlightens the Future

It's better to have a future than a past.

—Anonymous quote from *A Century of American Medicine, 1776–1876*[iv]

SIR WILLIAM OSLER (1875–1919), the great physician-teacher of his time, said, "A look at the past will show that the philosophies of one age become the absurdities of the next, and the foolishness of yesterday becomes the wisdom of tomorrow." The nineteenth and twentieth centuries were an age of discovery in medicine. This book, in spite of what the title suggests, is not intended to be a criticism of doctors reluctant to relinquish old habits and prejudices. Rather it is meant to be a sympathetic tribute to physicians and nurses laboring in isolation and difficult circumstances, who struggled to heal and comfort without modern knowledge or technology, and who, above all, respected the patient as a human being deserving conscientious and sensitive care.

This book is an account, often anecdotal, of health care on the American frontier. Who were the first western doctors? How were they educated? Who were the other caregivers, the midwives, the nurses and housewives and herbalists who did the best they could without formal training? My purpose is to shed light on and celebrate the dedication and humanitarianism of those many physicians, nurses, shamans, and people of sound practical sense who saw their patients—often friends and family—through the adversities that bedeviled them.

The American frontier was not a large block of virgin territory inhabited first by homeless adventurers and later settled by cultivators of the soil. It was an ephemeral line of occupation that progressed westward to the Pacific. As Frederick Jackson Turner noted in 1893, "The fall line marked the frontier of the seventeenth century; the Alleghenies that of the eighteenth; the Mississippi that of the first quarter of the nineteenth;

the Missouri that of the middle of this century (omitting the California movement); and the belt of the Rocky Mountains and the arid tract, the present frontier."[v] The West did not become completely developed until well into the twentieth century.

The first practitioners of healing on the western plains and in the Rocky Mountains were Native Americans, and this is where this book begins. At first, the aborigines' health was essentially stable. Not in one thrust, but gradually over the major part of a century, immigrants came into their home territory in what appeared to be a never-ending queue of explorers, trappers, gold seekers, railroad builders, bison killers, cattlemen, and homesteaders. The white man's civilization and devastating disease arrived together, and Indian culture was forever altered. In this book, although much knowledge has been lost, I attempt to analyze the medicine of that culture, which disappears a little more with each generation.

Meriwether Lewis and William Clark were among the first healers to come to the West from the so-called civilized world. They spent a great deal of time exploring the land and visiting with the natives along the great waterways they followed toward the setting sun. Although the two captains were not sanctioned as physicians by any authority, their worldly experience and military service had arguably prepared them to practice on a par with most early American doctors. Their skills and knowledge were challenged daily during the arduous "Voyage of Discovery." The small contingent of men, a woman, and a child underwent extreme hardship, danger, and exposure to disease, yet returned having lost only one man. Along the way they also administered to many Native Americans competently and compassionately. The student of Lewis and Clark will see that much of the expedition's success was due to the leadership and medical skills of the captains, who were physicians in the fullest sense of the word. The medical aspects of their trip, although reported before, warrant repeating with a fresh perspective.

Subsequent chapters of this book follow more or less chronologically the progression of western settlement. The fur traders and restless mountain men were generally the first white people to occupy a region, and they moved on as soon as cattlemen, miners, or pioneer farmers arrived. As restless and searching immigrants settled further and further into the wilderness looking for places to call their own, medical practitioners followed. It took a long time for well-trained physicians, medical innovations, and hospitals to find the less-populated reaches of thousands of square miles of mountains and prairies and desert. For instance, Montana, the

"Treasure State" as its promoters called it, retained its frontier character for several decades into the twentieth century, long after other places had shed that status. Indeed today, except for Billings and Miles City, the eastern half of Montana is less peopled than it was when Turner spoke in 1893. No one announced the beginning of "frontier life" in the West, but it is easier to mark its inception than to determine its end.

Throughout the West, there were remote places that remained "frontier" until well after World War II. Clusters of people lived where transportation was difficult. It might take a family with a sick loved one hours to travel by a cantankerous automobile to a place where a doctor was available. If the problem was beyond the resources of the physician in residence, more travel might be required to get the patient to the nearest community with a hospital. Even after cars became commonplace, storms and inadequate roads could make them useless.

Today, it is hard to imagine a time and place where medical care was so inaccessible. Yet there are people now who remember living in such circumstances. A ranch woman in northern Montana told me of witnessing her mother's death in the early 1940s from hemorrhage following a self-induced abortion. It was her mother's eighth pregnancy; she had never seen a doctor. Their remote ranch was fifty wagon miles from the nearest physician. Another woman, who grew up on the north bank of the Missouri River, miles from any type of medical care, related how her father gave her and her brothers shots of penicillin each time they complained of any kind of illness—using the same needles and syringes that he treated his livestock with. One of her brothers is totally deaf from recurrent ear infections (could it be, as we are left to surmise, the result of the streptomycin in the veterinarian-grade antibiotic, which is known to cause deafness?).

The story of those who suffered and those who helped them may never be completely told. Between the pages of diaries kept in attics, in the local histories of western communities, and in the fading recollections of those survivors who participated in the great settlement lie undiscovered dramas,° both wonderful and tragic. This book describes only a small part of the picture. Though it may be better to have a future than a past, it is that extraordinary past upon which the future will be founded.

Milestones of Medical Progress

Science knows no country, because knowledge belongs to humanity, and is the torch which illuminates the world.

—Louis Pasteur

THE ACCUMULATION OF medical knowledge began in antiquity. Techniques for inoculating against smallpox, for instance, originated in India and China more than a thousand years ago. In Euro-American culture, Edward Jenner (1749-1823) is generally credited with founding immunology by introducing pustular fluid from cowpox lesions into the skin of healthy people to create immunity against the related disease of smallpox. By the twentieth century, the simple procedure of vaccination had eliminated that terrible scourge from the face of the earth. The same principles have been applied over the years to dozens of other diseases, and we now have vaccines for polio, measles, whooping cough, diphtheria, Rocky Mountain spotted fever, rabies, tetanus, and many others.

Medical science as we now know it began with some fundamental discoveries. Andreas Vesalius (1514-1564) was a great anatomist who changed the course of medicine in 1543 when he wrote and illustrated *De Humani Corporis Fabrica libri Septem* ("Seven Books on the Structure of the Human Body"). Building on this knowledge, William Harvey (1578-1657) established that blood circulates within a closed system, with the heart serving as a pump. To the modern reader this seems so simple, yet at that time it was a momentous discovery and changed the direction of medical thought.

Sometime later, microscopic anatomy was born when Antoni van Leeuwenhoek (1632-1723), using only a hand lens, saw "animalcules." These little microscopic "animals" were probably bacteria and protozoa.

Later he manufactured compound lenses and built microscopes capable of magnifying objects hundreds of times. With this instrument he and other scientists unveiled the complex inner structure of animals and plants. Later scientists observed microscopic changes in tissues and organs, leading to a better understanding of disease.

Some medical advances were based on strict scientific achievement, such as Avogadro's Law, proposed in 1811. This principle allowed chemists to calculate atomic weights and led to the ability to determine molecular structure. Based on this knowledge, twentieth-century scientists expanded their understanding of physiology and developed untold numbers of drugs and enzymes. Many other scientific discoveries were serendipitous. For example, Dr. James Lind discovered in 1747 that citrus fruits could prevent the terrible consequences of scurvy. He didn't know why, however. We now know that these fruits are loaded with vitamin C, a deficiency of which was the cause of scurvy. His observations, although not accepted by all his contemporaries, saved thousands of lives.

Some medical discoveries were the result of a combination of research and luck. In 1854 John Snow traced the epidemic of cholera that London was facing at the time to contaminated water at the Broad Street Pump in the city's Golden Square. His solution was simple. He had the pump handle removed, forcing citizens to get their water elsewhere. The epidemic ended, and the value of public health was permanently established.

The work of Louis Pasteur (1822-1895) was another watershed in medical progress and forever changed the way doctors looked at disease. For hundreds of years, infectious illnesses had been thought to be caused by miasmas (toxic vapors from decomposing organic matter), rather than by microscopic organisms. Pasteur, studying the process of fermentation in the 1860s, was the first to recognize that microscopic organisms transformed wine to vinegar. His insight was the beginning of microbiology. He further discovered that heat stopped the fermentation process by killing the organisms. This led to the process of pasteurization to control contamination.

Baron Joseph Lister (1827-1912), an English surgeon, inspired by Pasteur's research, introduced practical antisepsis for medical procedures. Using carbolic spray to kill bacteria allowed surgeons to enter body cavities with less fear of infection. Over time, scientists identified the bacteria that cause diseases that have plagued mankind for thousands of years.

The antibiotic era began with Sir Alexander Fleming's chance observation in 1928 that colonies of *Staphylococcus aureus* on culture media were inhibited by a contaminant mold (*Penicillium notatum*). Because penicillin was unstable, its value against bacterial infections wasn't appreciated until ten years later. As a medical student in the 1940s, I was among the fortunate few who saw the tremendous influence of penicillin on the practice of medicine. At that time a chemical called sulfanilamide ("sulfa") and its derivatives were known to have a limited value in slowing down the action of some bacteria. Emergency rooms and military doctors sprinkled sulfa powder into wounds as an antiseptic. It helped but was far from infallible. Then came penicillin, and the results were almost miraculous. What previously would have been fatal cases of bacterial endocarditis were cured, as were many other streptococcal infections. Moreover, thousands of syphilis sufferers were rescued from a life of gummas, Charcot joints, aortic aneurysms, and insanity.

Building on this foundation of discoveries about sanitation, immunization, antibiotics, and other advances, many infectious diseases were eventually prevented or cured. Today, because of astounding anesthetic methods, technological devices, and supportive techniques, surgical procedures, even on vital organs such as the heart or the brain, are daily routines in many institutions. Dreaded mortal malignancies are often curbed if not eliminated with pharmaceuticals, radiation, and hormones. Organ transplants, battery-operated electronic devices, even mechanical hearts allow thousands of men and women to live nearly normal lives.

Some students of medical history believe that modern medicine began with the discovery of penicillin. This is arguable in view of the other great medical discoveries of the last two hundred years. Many bright lights have illuminated the medical profession's journey through recent centuries and are guiding us into the next one.

The Metamorphosis of American Medicine in the Nineteenth Century

When people's ill, they comes to I,
I physics, bleeds, and sweats 'em;
Sometimes they live, sometimes they die
What's that to I? I lets 'em.
—Dr. J. C. Lettsom[1]

THE PROFESSION OF MEDICINE in America got off to a bad start. Early doctors were marooned in beliefs and techniques centered around the humors of the body—blood, phlegm, yellow bile, and black bile—and whether the illness was "cold" or "hot." There were no curative drugs or methods. If purging, blistering, sweating, or bleeding didn't work, there were no alternatives. Sporadically, epidemics wiped out thousands, and no one knew why some survived and others didn't. Solving this question led to the science of medicine.

Until after the Civil War, medical practice in America was in the dark ages. But the latter part of the nineteenth century brought progress. The discovery of bacteria as a cause of infection in the 1880s literally revolutionized public health. Antisepsis and the emergence of anesthetic agents opened broad vistas to the surgeon. By the 1900s medical advances had relieved society of some of its burden of disease and suffering. In the meantime, however, certain dogmas, whose roots arrived with the colonists, prevailed.

"Heroic" Medicine: Treatments in Early America

From the 1790s to about the middle of the 1800s was essentially the age of "heroic" medicine (allopathy), and a few allopathic physicians in

1

the United States dominated medical philosophy and education. One famous physician of the era, Benjamin Rush, told his students that there was only one disease, which he called "morbid excitement induced by capillary tension."[2] Whatever he meant by this claim, which cannot be translated into modern terms, he asserted that this sole disease had a sole remedy: bloodletting and the purging of the stomach and bowels. Doctors who were taught to follow these rigid prescripts became known as "sanguinary physicians," or more derisively as "leeches."[3]

The harsh treatments punished sick people and could even shorten life. To practice allopathic medicine, a doctor needed only a sharp lancet to slice into a vein or leeches to suck blood from his patient, suction cups to enhance blood flow from small incisions or to withdraw "toxins" from an inflamed part of the body, ipecac to produce vomiting, calomel to empty the bowels, and mustard to make a plaster to burn blisters on the skin. These ancient therapies were based on the premise that toxins could

Bleeding patients was an ancient form of treatment for many ailments. Employing leeches to draw blood was just one of many methods. The leech is still used, though rarely, in certain kinds of injuries to reduce hematoma formation. —Courtesy National Library of Medicine, History of Medicine Division

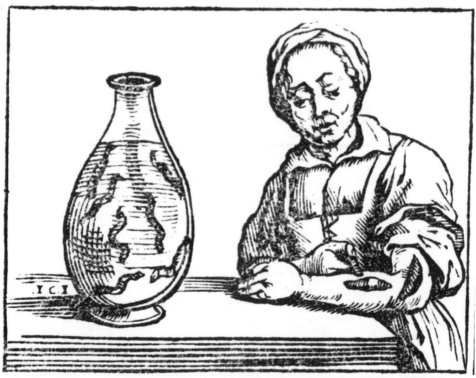

be extracted from a sick body via bodily fluids. Even after allopathy began to lose its luster, many frontier doctors still insisted that clysters (enemas), cathartics, and sometimes cupping were the answer to most complaints.

Despite the fact that these "heroic" methods of treatment date back to antiquity, some medical historians blame Dr. Rush for their popularity in American medicine.[4] When someone as politically important as Dr. Benjamin Rush, patriot and close friend of President Thomas Jefferson and other leaders, spoke, people listened. Though some of his contemporaries differed with him, theirs was like a voice in the wilderness.

Rush perfected his theories during the yellow fever epidemic of 1793 in Philadelphia. During that period of pestilence, he kept his lancet busy draining blood from one and all, sometimes in massive amounts.[5] Many of the sick he treated and "cured" probably didn't have yellow fever at all, and he ascribed his failures to belated treatment.

One of Rush's most effective critics wasn't a doctor, but a vitriolic journalist named William Cobbett, who attacked Rush viciously in the press. He wrote, "The times are ominous indeed, when quack to quack cries, 'Purge and bleed! . . . Blood, blood, still they cry, more blood!'"[6] The writer launched abuse daily until the good doctor's lawyers shut him up with court action.

It is very easy to look back and see Rush's flaws, but there are other things about him that deserve to be remembered as well. He believed in the education of women. He also urged his contemporaries to follow his example and treat the "virtuous poor" with respect. A vocal medical reformer, Rush criticized the military and the colonial government for the terrible conditions of soldiers' hospitals during the Revolutionary War. He saw the "putrid fever" that spread rapidly in the hospitals for what it was, a poisoning directly related to crowding and filth. As an early proponent for public health, he deplored the condition of Philadelphia's Dock Creek, which was used as a dump for "animal and vegetable offal matters," and urged the city assembly to stop the dumping.[7]

Nevertheless, as part of Rush's mixed legacy, his tenets extended the use of therapeutic bleeding, purging, and blistering. These harsh and often harmful methods of treatment were not based on any science but were as ancient as Hippocrates. The death of George Washington in 1799 shows how heroic methods were applied to the detriment of the patient. Washington was dying of a throat infection that obstructed his airway (most medical historians believe he suffered from a form of severe tonsillitis with abscess formation). Washington began the bleeding process himself before the doctors arrived by having a servant open a vein in his arm. When the doctors came, they continued the process, and he was bled four more times. On the fourth bloodletting, one of the doctors noted that "the blood ran very slowly—appeared very thick."[8] Probably this was an indication of anoxia and dehydration and perhaps beginning shock.

One of Washington's doctors, Elisha Cullen Dick, argued against further bleeding, saying, "He needs all his strength—bleeding will diminish it."[9] Dr. Dick pleaded with the other two physicians to operate to open an airway into the general's larynx (a tracheotomy) to bypass the point of obstruction. His sensible arguments suggest that some physicians were challenging the formulaic practices of the time. That the challenge was ignored suggests how entrenched the orthodoxy was. During the hours before Washington died, the doctors applied blistering poultices and gave him doses of calomel and other purges. Years later, one of Washington's physicians, Dr. Gustavus Richard Brown, admitted that they should have heeded Dr. Dick, and that had they "taken no more blood from him, our good friend might have been alive now. But we were governed by the best light we had, we thought we were right, and so we are justified."[10]

A powerful critic of medical practice and education during this period was Thomas Jefferson, who wrote, "the inexperienced and presumptuous band of medical tyros let loose on the world, destroys more of human life in one year, than all the Robinhoods, Cartouches, and Macheaths do in a century."[11] To aspiring medical students, Jefferson advised, "His mind must be strong indeed if . . . it can maintain a wise infidelity against the authority of his instructors."[12] The increasing pressure of such intellectual critics and high-profile failures like Washington's case contributed to a loss of respect for doctors. Physicians would have to make changes.

What kind of changes should be made, however, was a subject of great debate among doctors, and reforms were not uniform. Bitter disputes developed among physicians and within medical school faculties. For example, Dr. Benjamin Dudley, a medical instructor in the early decades of the 1800s, long before germs were discovered, implored his colleagues to boil their surgical instruments to prevent infection, a practice he followed. As often happened, the new idea was greeted with derision and hostility by his colleagues, in part because Dudley had a cantankerous personality.[13] One can only speculate how many lives might have been saved during the Civil War if physicians had followed the grouchy Dr. Dudley's advice.

Another physician of the era, Dr. J. Crawford of Baltimore, wrote several articles pronouncing that mosquitoes were the source of malaria and yellow fever. Unfortunately, it was a viewpoint that contradicted the theories of the time, and he was rewarded by ridicule and nearly lost his practice. But Crawford's hypothesis inspired Dr. Walter Reed and the others who, years later, finally proved the transmission of yellow fever by mosquitoes. The heroic work of Dr. Stubbins Ffirth also contributed to the finding. In 1804 this young physician proved that yellow fever was not contagious from person to person. He verified his theory by exposing himself to direct and intimate contact with those suffering from the disease. In one experiment, he cut the skin of his arm and introduced fresh black vomit from infected people into the wounds, repeating the procedure twenty times. He also vaporized the liquid vomit and breathed the steam, and he even swallowed fresh vomit. Still the intrepid doctor did not develop yellow fever.[14] Although this kind of scientific study appears foolhardy, it is only one of hundreds of such stories. Physicians throughout the history of the profession, and especially during the nineteenth century, proved their points with self-experimentation.

"Irregular" Doctors: Homeopathy and Other Alternatives

By the 1830s "regular" doctors, or allopaths, and their "heroic" therapies of bloodletting, purging, and blistering faced significant competition by practitioners known as homeopaths. No love was lost between them. From the modern viewpoint, it is hard to understand why people ever tolerated the harsh methods of the early allopaths, but apparently some sufferers believed that "the more bitter the taste, the better the medicine." After paying for a professional call, some patients expected more than "time and nature" to heal them.

Homeopaths, or "irregular" doctors, avoided all "heroic" measures. Calomel, a toxic mercurial purge to treat syphilis, and other severe purges were seen as poison, and homeopaths did not blister the skin or bleed the patient by use of scalpel, cup, or leech. The homeopath "stressed the need for sympathetic attention" and "provided an alternative to the . . . excesses of orthodox physicians."[15] Homeopathy, perhaps understandably, was more popular, and the practice attracted many well-to-do clients who didn't wish to be punished with abrasive methods. Furthermore, allopaths found it difficult to criticize homeopathic results because their results were no better. The homeopathic discipline was certainly less agonizing to the sick, and most homeopaths were equivalent in education to allopaths. As an added bonus, homeopaths usually prescribed whiskey as a diluent for their medicine. The beneficial effects of drugs, they believed, were magnified when diluted with alcohol.

In competition with the homeopaths, "regular" doctors also began prescribing strong alcoholic "tonics." Here they found a "medicine" they knew would uplift their patients' spirits and improve the allopathic image. Undoubtedly, to a degree they were right. It is strange, however, that even though regular doctors were losing ground with their harsh methods, there continued to be more of them than homeopaths.[16]

A myriad of other kinds of "healers" also proclaimed their skill at treating any and all human illness, and the dominant groups judged all others as embracing "false" doctrines. With all the confusion and controversy, it was difficult if not impossible for a sick person to judge which method was superior.[17] Among the choices were hydropaths and botanic doctors who specialized in roots and herbs, as well as vendors of various and sundry nostrums. Midwives delivered most of the babies. Other healers claimed to be bonesetters and inoculators; cancer doctors advertised their cures in local newspapers; and even a few abortionists were available. There were some who pretended to be "Indian doctors" and practiced in a variety of styles meant to emulate what the public perceived as natural, or "Indian," healing. Ironically, even though the Native American culture was looked down on as paganistic by most white people, Indian "healers" were very popular. Various amalgamations of these different factions of medical conduct produced a bewildering array of choices for the sick.[18] As sectarianism and suspicion prevailed, it is no wonder medicine lagged behind other scientific fields.

Some of the theories and practices of the different schools of treatment had merit. Take the "water treatments" recommended by hydropaths, for instance. A considerable number of common medical problems such as rheumatism, arthritis, and skin disorders were relieved by soaking in water, especially if it was hot and smelled of sulphur. At a time when few people bathed regularly, water treatments accompanied by soap may have been even more therapeutic. Hydrotherapy is ancient. Plato in his *Dialogues* wrote, "Limbs of the rustic worn with toil will derive more benefit from warm water than from the prescriptions of a not overwise doctor."[19]

The medical practitioner of any persuasion had some useful drugs, among them laudanum (opium) to ease pain; foxglove (digitalis), used as a stimulant in heart failure; colchicine for gout; and cinchona bark (quinine) against the omnipresent fever, malaria (ague). Regardless of the type of application, medicine and herbs conveyed a certain mystique. Nevertheless, most nineteenth-century Americans seldom saw a physician and took little interest in the various sects. Doctors in general were not altogether trusted, and they were expensive. Much of the populace, living in remote backwoods locations, relied on "folk medicine" to restore their health.

Although few doctors would admit it, much medical knowledge was taken from folk wisdom. Drugs and treatments handed down over hundreds of years augmented the educated physician's know-how. Remedies that performed were kept and others discarded. Foxglove, or digitalis, came from English women of the late 1700s, who discovered the herb's use as a cardiac stimulant. The housewife had used foxglove for heart failure, or "dropsy," for many decades before it was accepted by the medical profession. Colchicine was another herb that "old wives" had used

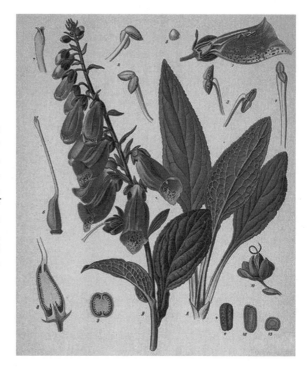

Digitalis purpurea: *From this plant, also known as foxglove, is derived digitalis, a heart stimulant, still in use. Many of today's drugs come from plants.* —From A Modern Herbal by Maud Grieve, 1931

successfully for years in the treatment of gout before doctors adopted it. Both of these drugs are still kept in a modern physician's dispensary.

Folklore about disease and treatments accompanied immigrants to America from Europe and other points of origin. As the pioneers homesteaded in the West, their kitchen shelves were replete with "cures" passed on by word of mouth from mother to daughter and father to son. Though much "old wives" knowledge was sound, some popular therapies were founded in superstition or religious dogma. Seldom, however, were these old remedies harmful. Sometimes soot and cobwebs in a fresh cut or a poultice of fresh manure to stop bleeding may have led to an infection, but in general "old time" treatments were at least innocuous. And families with a grandmother who understood the value of rest, medicinal herbs, and good nutrition were fortunate.

For a long time, the medical profession refused to admit that the body had healing powers of its own and that nature was an ally, not an enemy. Somehow they were able to ignore the fact that many sick people got well on their own. As an example, during an epidemic of diphtheria in the mid-1800s in New York, two out of three patients treated by physicians died, in contrast to only two of nine patients treated only with "ice packs and prayer."[20] In time, even the most stubborn doctors learned what many "old wives" had known for years: that rest, fluids, and tender loving care cured a majority of illnesses.

New Ideas in "Doctoring"

Disagreements among doctors over the theory of medicine and how it should be taught continued to rage through midcentury. Some of these conflicts resulted in lawsuits and even physical battles. In 1856 at a medical school in Cincinnati, a dispute among the faculty became so intense that actual warfare ensued with "knives, pistols, bludgeons and blunderbusses." When one of the opposing factions brought out a loaded six-pound cannon, both sides sensibly dispersed.[21]

As the various factions bickered and battled, leading doctors in the East began to organize, and in 1846 the American Medical Association was formed. About 1858, prominent doctors began to speak out forcefully against "heroic" medicine, and soon many physicians had abandoned some of the deplorable methods of treatment. Within a few years, medical schools quit teaching bloodletting, and by the time of the Civil War, almost all physicians had quit exsanguinating their patients, though venesection (bleeding) still has a minor place in medicine.[22]

STETHOSCOPES.

Early stethoscopes, which evolved into the binaural apparatus that is frequently seen dangling around the necks of today's doctors and nurses —Courtesy National Library of Medicine, History of Medicine Division

Meanwhile, science entered the picture. Some physiologic parameters like blood pressure and temperature could now be measured, and heart, lung, and abdominal sounds could be heard and classified with the stethoscope. Due to the work of Louis Pasteur and others (see Overview), there evolved an appreciation of bacteria as a cause of infections. Furthermore, and of great importance to the profession of medicine, it became apparent that many illnesses were self-limited regardless of treatment.

By 1880 allopaths had to face the fact that their conflict with the homeopaths had been fought to a draw. Regardless of a physician's sect, the practice of medicine became more scientific. Many homeopathic practitioners, forced to admit that science was changing the playing field, adopted some of the allopaths' technical practices.[23] Similarly, as science cast doubt on certain allopathic treatments, regular doctors began to abandon them.

The major schools of medical thought went through the nineteenth century debating the merits of the various philosophies and unconsciously borrowed from one another. While there were still doctors who were true cultists, narrowly focused and arbitrary, many others had open minds and judged on their own what was best for their patients. Gradually, a mainstream of "doctoring" developed in America. At the same time, the profession was gaining a new respect. "Doctoring" had not been viewed very highly up to the late 1800s. Little progress in health care having been made, cynicism prevailed. But publicized scientific discoveries changed the public attitude dramatically. In 1885, after it was reported that French scientist Dr. Louis Pasteur had discovered a treatment to prevent the rare but terribly feared disease called rabies, the public took notice. Previous discoveries had been more or less ignored, but a preventative for rabies was front-page stuff: "Hydrophobia Cured," read the headlines. Suddenly medicine became a popular topic, and enough scientific discoveries followed to keep writers busy for years. The medical profession had turned the corner.[24]

Dr. Joseph C. Hunter administering nitrous oxide in his office in Boulder Hot Springs, Montana, in 1884. By the time this picture was taken, doctors all over the country were using this gas as an anesthetic in addition to ether and chloroform. Nitrous oxide was popularized by dentist Horace Wells in 1844. —Courtesy Montana Historical Society, Helena

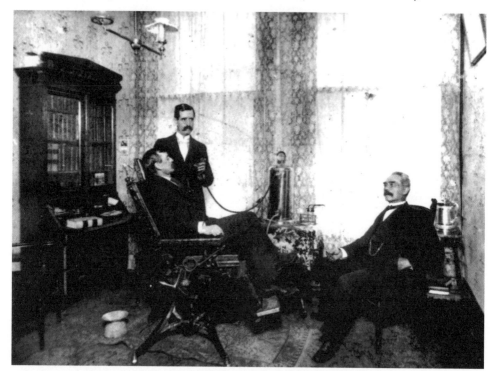

Toward the end of the nineteenth century, there was more scientific progress. An improved understanding of microbes encouraged physicians to accept Joseph Lister's technique of antiseptic surgery that he first described in 1867, and sterilization and aseptic methods took shape as well. In addition, anesthetics—ether, nitrous oxide, and chloroform—which had been available since 1831 but were used mainly as recreational drugs, came into use for surgery, replacing opium and other less effective substances. In 1842 Dr. Crawford W. Long of Georgia had used ether as anesthesia for minor operations, and a few years later Connecticut dentist Dr. Horace Wells used laughing gas (nitrous oxide) for the same purpose. By 1880 the practice had caught on, and surgeons could, with a new degree of assurance, open the abdomen to correct injuries, remove tumors, and perform appendectomies.

During the same period, doctors became expert at differential diagnosis. For example, the two major diarrheal diseases, cholera and typhoid, were differentiated. By careful observation, the rose patches of typhoid were distinguished from the rash of measles or the exanthem of scarlet fever. Now medicine could name many conditions with accuracy, though there wasn't any specific treatment.

New drugs were being developed, however. Medications such as chloral hydrate (a sedative) and salicylates and antipyrine (two analgesics) enlarged the pharmacopoeia of the practicing doctors. Still, as Richard Gordon wrote in *The Alarming History of Medicine*, "Physicians ventured into the twentieth century lightly armed. They bore mercury for syphilis . . . digitalis to strengthen the heart, iodine for goiter, colchicum for gout, chloral for the excitable, a pomegranate alkaloid for tape-worms. Since 1867, they had amyl nitrite for angina . . . iron for anemia."[25] Medical textbooks were thick with diagnoses, but they lacked the "happy endings" of successful treatments.

Nevertheless, doctors of the time were justifiably optimistic. In 1887 Dr. J. M. DaCosta, a leading physician of his time, summarized proudly, "A generation that has witnessed the introduction of the hypodermic syringe, of the bromides, of chloral, of nitro-glycerine, of cocaine, and antiseptics, need not despair of gaining more agents potent for control."[26]

Great strides in preventive medicine were also emerging. Gradually doctors developed a better understanding of sanitation and the transmission of infection. In 1880 the causes of cholera, typhoid, and diphtheria were identified. About 1895 diphtheria antitoxin became available. Another public health milestone was reached when pasteurization all but eliminated milk as a carrier of typhoid, diphtheria, tuberculosis, and brucellosis. As citizens began to recognize and accept public health measures, laws were passed to isolate and quarantine transmissible diseases. It was agreed that outhouses should be placed downstream or away from the water supply, that rotting garbage must be buried at a certain distance from permanent camps, and that dead bodies could transmit disease and contaminate water.

Instruments, too, improved. Laennec's stethoscope, used by most doctors to listen to the beat of the heart and whisper of the lungs, was no longer the physician's only tool. Then came other "scopes." The ophthalmoscope had been improved since Helmholz discovered it in 1851, and the eye grounds (the inside of the eyeball) promised information never before imagined. Some "specialists" were looking into the larynx, and other orifices were being probed and explored. There was even strong support by many, but not all, physicians for the use of the sphygmomanometer for studying pulse pressure (later called blood pressure), and the standardized thermometer was touted as an aid to the diagnosis and prognosis of infectious diseases. Now the doctor could more carefully study the vagaries of the different fevers. "What's next?" doctors seemed to be asking, and they were only looking at the tip of the iceberg. Inexorably, new ideas replaced the old. Wilhelm Röentgen soon discovered the medical use of cathode ray radiation, and in 1888 Madame Marie Curie, studying the element radium, prepared the way for the X-ray, which revolutionized the diagnostic ability of physicians all over the world.

During the last few decades of the century, a few older doctors became concerned, perhaps threatened, by the intrusion of science into the art of medicine. In 1884 the president of the American Medical Association warned against "the innumerable instruments of precision, which promise to substitute mathematical accuracy for vague guesses and which are too often used, not to supplement but to supplant other and valuable methods of investigation." Furthermore he was distressed "by all the 'scopes,' all the 'graphs,' and all the 'meters,'" used by specialists.[27] Stanley Joel Reiser, Harvard physician and historian, wrote in 1978, "The historical experience of medicine thus reveals diagnostic technology to be a double-edged sword. Its use can enlarge the doctor's knowledge of disease, but it also can erode his confidence in his ability to make independent judgments. The doctor can rely too much upon machines and technical experts."[28]

In spite of the fears, the promise of science in the practice of medicine filled doctors with new hope just when they had become pessimistic and discouraged. Most of them had learned that the "old" methods weren't effective, and they welcomed the growing power of experimental science.

By the 1890s doctors also had begun to recognize the value of the hospital as a place to treat people, not just to put them until they died. Many new hospitals were established, and laboratories and X-ray machines were installed. In hospital practice, physicians in America utilized autopsies to more accurately understand the pathogenesis of disease and to apply this information to living patients. Hence the Clinical Pathological Conference, or CPC, became a teaching tool of great value to the advancement of medical understanding of disease, as symptoms in a sick person were correlated with postmortem anatomical findings. Previously, many American doctors had to go to Europe to study cadavers; now pathologists could do so in their own hospitals.

In 1901 Dr. Emil Adolf von Behring received the Nobel Prize. In his acceptance speech he acknowledged a century of progress in medical science. He honored Edward Jenner, Louis Pasteur, and Robert Koch for their work in vaccines and microbiology. He himself was being honored for his work in developing specific serums with which to treat infectious disease, a method thought by many to be the final blow to infections. But it didn't work. Within ten years the euphoria about this new tool turned to frustration.[29] Such are the vagaries of scientific achievement. But overall it had been a great century.

The Evolution of Medical School

In 1889 William Osler, one of America's greatest physicians and teachers of medicine, complained, "It makes one's blood boil to think that there are sent out year by year scores of men called doctors, who have never attended a case of labor, and who are utterly ignorant of the ordinary everyday diseases which they may be called upon to treat. . . . Is it to be wondered . . . that there is a widespread distrust in the public of professional education, and that quacks, charlatans and impostors possess the land?"[30]

In nineteenth-century America, one could become a doctor in three ways: 1) attend a medical school; 2) apprentice himself (or herself) to a practicing physician; or 3) simply purchase a diploma. Diploma mills began a lucrative business sometime around 1853, when states began to issue licenses and require credentials for medical practice. Thousands of people were willing to pay for this "education." In spite of the dubious reputation of the profession, a medical career was unaccountably fashionable and popular. By 1850 there were forty-two medical schools in the United States, and by 1876 there were sixty-four.[31] Many of these were in the economically depressed West, where it was essential that education be inexpensive.

Among the many problems of early medical education were poorly prepared students, short sessions, insufficient compensation of teachers, and lack of adequate buildings and equipment. Most schools had to resort to grave robbing to acquire cadavers for anatomical dissection. At the 1869 convention of the American Medical Association, William O. Baldwin, the organization's president, complained that colleges admitted anyone willing to pay the fee. Standards were so low, he said, that it was "but a short step from the plough-handles to the diploma."[32]

Slowly and fitfully, medical education and practice improved. At most schools during the mid-nineteenth century, the student attended two four-month sessions, a year apart, with lectures in the basic sciences: anatomy, physiology, chemistry, surgery, and midwifery. If the student came back and finished the second year, he was given a diploma. Most aspiring physicians combined this education with an apprenticeship, and some enlightened schools required a preceptorship before issuing a certificate.[33]

The preceptorship was creatively American. An apprentice, or preceptor, "read" and "rode" with a qualified doctor for a variable period. Ideally the physician was a good teacher and the preceptorship lasted for several years. During this time, the trainee had the advantage of practical application of the available wisdom as he assisted and observed his physician instructor in his daily practice. Sometimes the neophyte doctor groomed the horses, kept the office clean, cut firewood, and did other chores to pay for his keep and his education. When the preceptor believed his student to be qualified, he gave the apprentice a document testifying that he or she was qualified to be called "doctor." This form of education was a practical and inexpensive way for even the most poverty-stricken candidates to learn medicine.[34] Still, it had obvious deficiencies and many critics, and education by apprenticeship began to lose support about 1870.

While the practice lasted, apprenticeships provided some very good physicians to rural America. Doctors like Ephraim McDowell, who performed the first abdominal operation in 1809, was a graduate of this informal schooling, as was Dr. Daniel Drake, who played a large part in paving the way to medical education and better health in the West. During his career Drake methodically studied the frontier and wrote

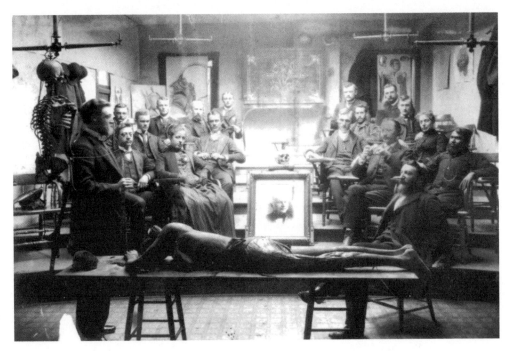

Anatomy class, 1890s. Note that there are only two women in the group.
—Courtesy Arizona Historical Society, Tucson

volumes describing western trails and settlements. In remote places, Drake met pioneer healers, talked with trappers and hunters, and stayed with adventurous families who had already penetrated the wilderness. He became expert in the diseases of the times, and he was the first to see that if malaria (ague) wasn't conquered, America could not expand. He advocated nature's healing processes in fevers and opposed the use of violent drugs such as calomel and other purges. Drake's contributions also included the establishment of a great medical school, which survives today as the University of Cincinnati.[35]

Near the turn of the century, medical schools increased their admission requirements. Courses were lengthened, and the whole system gradually improved. Student doctors witnessed autopsies, performed dissections, and learned more pathology and pathogenesis of disease. Young doctors attended conferences where cases of strange maladies were presented. The medical wards of hospitals became teaching laboratories. Medical journals that included up-to-date information increased in number and were circulated to medical libraries as well as some doctors' offices.

Students were taught to recognize different manifestations of illness, and the skills of physical diagnosis were honed.

Still, doctor training left much to be desired. Early in the twentieth century, educator Abraham Flexner, financed by the Carnegie Foundation, set out to analyze medical education in the United States. His in-depth, two-year analysis, published in 1910, uncovered many egregious practices.[36] The report launched a revolution. After a great public outcry, many schools closed their doors while others attempted to establish various improvements. Over a long period, educational quality waxed and waned, but many medical schools, especially those who added a preceptorship to their didactic courses, produced some excellent doctors. Physicians who had worked as apprentices entered practice in remote areas with practical experience. Many of those areas were in the West.

Part One

OLD WEST
HEALERS AND
HEALING

ONE

Indian Medicine

Native American Health
Before and After the White Man

Our children feel and hear the drum before birth.

—Quoted in *Walking in the Sacred Manner: Healers, Dreamers,
and Pipe Carriers—Medicine Women of the Plains Indians*[37]

SINCE PALEOLITHIC TIMES, when our species began to walk upright and developed a larger brain, humans have held dominion over other animals. Learning to conceptualize and speak gave man an awareness of self, time, and mortality; a sense of history and a concern for the future followed. Through thousands of years of trial and error, with the powers of memory and observation, primitive humans found methods of treatment for wounds and illnesses.[38]

In North America, Native Americans were the first caregivers. By the time the American colonies were settled, the quality of medical practice of the Indian was at least comparable and perhaps even superior to that of the European. Native American men and women had identified scores of herbs to treat common illnesses. They knew about cathartics, antifebriles, tonics, astringents, antiseptics, and numerous other natural remedies. Native healers also understood the value of massage, bandages, splints, suturing, applied heat, and enemas.[39] Sweat lodges and bathing in natural hot springs were used to treat lung disease, skin disorders, and rheumatism. The Indian also valued rest, nutrition, and fluid intake in maintaining good health. Some native healers became specialized and developed skills that gained them a degree of renown among their peers.

Anthropologists have discovered that ancient surgeons knew how to trephine a skull to relieve intracranial pressure from depressed skull fractures, a common injury at that time. The Incas' use of spiked clubs of copper or stone to settle their disagreements gave their surgeons a lot of practice. That this surgery was successful in prolonging some lives is evident from the healing around the trephine cuts. Obsidian knives, copper forceps, suture material of human or animal hair, analgesic substances derived from the coca and other plants, fine-mesh cotton gauze, and crude antiseptics, together with a knowledge of anatomy, allowed these aborigine surgeons to perform amputations, treat fractures, and remove arrows.[40]

In later centuries, Indians did not commonly perform surgery other than the occasional lancing of abscesses and other superficial procedures. Most of the native doctor's methods were noninvasive, but he could on occasion enter the mouth or rectum to treat a problem. With an animal bladder as a syringe and a hollow bone as a tube, enemas were used to cleanse the lower intestine, to instill an herbal concoction, or to give nutrients.

As white explorers and immigrants came west, some of them witnessed and recorded the Indians' medical expertise. According to these reports, medicine men produced some miraculous cures. In 1721 Pierre Charlevois described what he called "admirable results"—a broken bone that was "perfectly solid in eight days." Another account reported the case of a French soldier cured of epilepsy by a "pulverized root."[41] In *Doctors of the American Frontier*, Richard Dunlop describes how a Cheyenne doctor treated William Bent of Bent's Fort for a throat infection, possibly diphtheria: "The medicine man strung a sinew with sandburs and dipped it into hot buffalo tallow. This he forced down Bent's throat with a peeled stick. When the tallow melted, he jerked the string out, pulling the infected membrane with it. Bent survived."[42]

Another observer, Johnathan Carver, witnessed the use of a "plantain" (a plant that has never been identified) as an antidote to venomous snakebites. According to his report, the Indians were even willing to demonstrate its potency by allowing a snake to bite them, then spitting the chewed herb onto the wound.[43] Rattlesnakes abounded on the plains, and bites were common. Another popular treatment was a brew of the root of the rattlesnake weed (*Echinacea angustifolia*) poured into the fang punctures.[44] It wasn't hard to convince the early frontiersmen to use similar methods. Plains people and early white traders used a related species called pale purple coneflower (*Echinacea pallida*) for rattlesnake bites as well as for insect stings.[45]

Modern medicine is skeptical of some stories of Indian healing methods, but we can't be sure. Scientists continue to search for answers to the mystery of Native American medicine, but many tribes have guarded

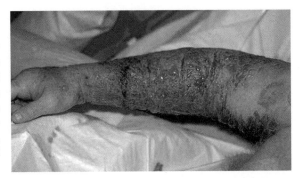

Snakebite was a very common injury on the frontier. Death and debility from snakebite were usually related to secondary infection or gangrene. —Courtesy Centers for Disease Control

specific details from outsiders. One frustrated Seneca elder, a respected medicine man, said to his family when strangers arrived, "Hide the sacred things, the Bigheads are coming!"[46]

Most early Christian observers could not understand the rituals of Native American healers and viewed their practices as paganistic, even sacrilegious. To the few outsiders who looked beyond the medicine man's pageantry, it was obvious that many Indian cures were as effective as those prescribed by European doctors, if not more so. Another thing white culture could not fathom was the way Native Americans viewed mental illness. Indians tolerated insane people and treated them with kindness. Most medicine men understood human nature, and they were uncommonly successful in treating hysteria.[47] Their practices contrast sharply with the brutal way the mentally ill were handled in "civilized" society during the same era. Whites locked many mentally ill people out of sight in filthy insane asylums, often referred to in the twentieth century as "snake pits."

The Native American view of the word *medicine* is totally different from its connotation in the white world. Religion and healing were inseparable; the spiritual and physical were entwined like two vines growing together. These beliefs crossed tribal boundaries, though methods of diagnosis and treatment were diverse. Native American medicine was, and is, based on connectedness and wholeness, and its ultimate source is "the Great Mystery."[48] In the words of John Fire (Lame Deer), a Sioux medicine man born about 1900, quoted in *Lame Deer, Seeker of Visions,* "I am a medicine man. . . . That's a white man's word like squaw, papoose, Sioux, tomahawk—words that don't exist in the Indian language. I wish there were better words to make clear what 'medicine man' stands for, but I can't . . . and you can't either."[49]

Many Indians saw disease as a disturbed relationship between humans and the supernatural world. According to one tribe, dwarf spirits (*nynymbi*) caused disease by shooting invisible arrows into people. There were also many taboos, such as eating food prepared by a menstruating woman or using cruel words or violence against a friend or loved one. Ignoring a taboo could bring on pain, weakness, illness, or injury.[50]

Over thousands of years, Indians developed a combination of health care and religion that was complicated and ritualistic, yet also practical and sensible. The Indian found therapy not only in ceremonial prayer, chanting, and the sounds of a drum or rattle, but also in the laying on of hands and counseling. The "sweat lodge," comparable to a sauna, was important to religion as a place for prayer and purification, but it was also therapeutic. The ritual was conducted in an enclosed, domed space covered by skins. Vapor, sometimes enhanced with aromatic herbs, was produced by pouring water over hot rocks in a pit at the center of the

The erection of a Cheyenne sweat lodge. The sweat lodge could be a place of worship, healing, and purification. A framework of arched willow branches covered with buffalo skins or blankets held in the steam from heated stones sprinkled with water. —Courtesy Montana Historical Society

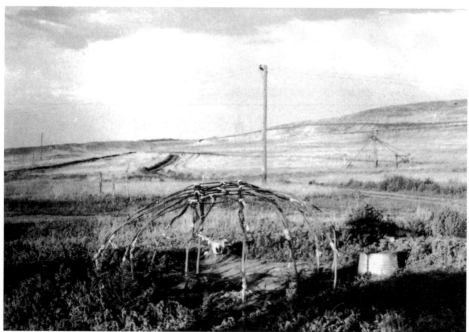

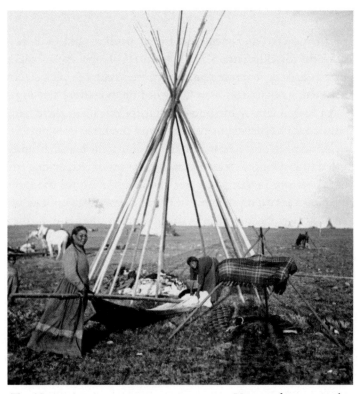

Two Native American women erecting a tepee. Hanging from a tripod is a medicine bundle. The contents of medicine bundles varied according to individual and tribe, and its importance was immense. —Courtesy Montana Historical Society

lodge. Sweat lodges are an ancient form of therapy. Yale scientists studying Mayan ruins in Guatemala found sweatbaths used for "sweating, enema rituals, purgation, and genital blood letting."[51]

To many Indians, "medicine" meant a charm, and each family group kept in its teepee a medicine bundle that contained the spirits of the "helpers" it needed for healthy survival.[52] Bundles contained a variety of articles that were deemed sacred based on a tribe's myths and traditions. Such items might include animal skins, headdresses, shields, knives, pipes, bones, arrowheads, or other things of significance to the tribal history or to the individual. Among the Plains Indians, the medicine bundle and the medicine pipe were called upon to bring health to the people, call in the buffalo, influence the weather, or ensure victory in war. Great powers were attributed to these items, and they were treated in special ways to keep them sacred and protected from outsiders and untrustworthy people. In the Blackfeet tradition, the ritual of opening of the beaver bundle to reveal its contents was one of the most complex ceremonies known. Burning tobacco and the liturgy of the pipe were also important rituals. An Indian who made a solemn pledge on the medicine pipe was the equivalent of a Christian swearing upon the Bible in a court of law.[53]

The Spartan life of the nomadic tribes didn't allow the chronically ill or disabled to live long; it was survival of the fittest. According to Virgil J. Vogel's *American Indian Medicine*, "It was common for the Indians to leave the old to perish on the prairies."[54] The severely injured, adults and children alike, were also regularly abandoned to their fate. In the Crow and other tribes, custom accepted infanticide to control population, especially during drought or famine.[55] This kind of behavior may seem cruel, but it served the common good.

The Medicine Man

In the tribes of North America, the medicine man, or shaman, called "witch doctor" by many white immigrants, was an honored and respected leader, second only to the chief.[56] Sometimes, in fact, he was the chief. Those called upon to be healers needed intelligence, common sense, and a good understanding of human behavior. Sitting Bull was an outstanding example of this kind of medicine man. According to Stephen E. Ambrose in *Crazy Horse and Custer*, this great and well-known Sioux chief was "an orator, a philosopher, an advisor, a propagandist for his cause, a lay preacher, a teacher, a husband and father, a healer of the sick, a psychiatrist, a political leader and a man."[57]

The archetypal medicine man was thought to be in contact with the Great Spirit, and his people relied on him to keep evil away and to heal the sick. A shaman was often called upon to do the virtually impossible. For instance, he might be asked to predict when it would rain. If he had studied past weather patterns carefully, or perhaps observed the behavior of animals, he may have made an educated estimate—close enough to hold on to his reputation.

Although most shamans were men, according to historian Valerie S. Mathes, a few women also answered the call to become healers.[58] In the West, women were allowed to become shamans in the Crow, Gros Ventre, and Assiniboine tribes. In Montana, a Gros Ventre woman was sometimes summoned through a dream to become a medicine woman, or, as the wife of a medicine man, she might learn the healing art from

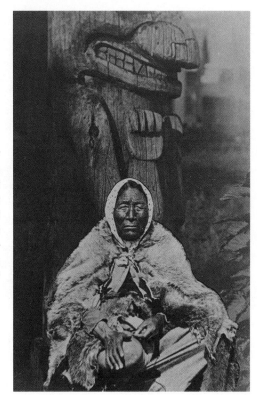

Shaman of the Skeena River (British Columbia) tribe. American Indians had a great deal of medical knowledge when the white man first invaded their territory. The medicine man was an important member of his community.
—Courtesy Library of Congress

her husband. Crow women were the primary caretakers of the medicine bundle, and they played an important part in doctoring the sick. Like most tribes, however, the Crows regarded women as taboo during menstruation. Nevertheless, most tribes found ways to include women in shamanism. Many Indian women took sweat baths and participated in ceremonies such as the Sun Dance.

There was considerable variation in the techniques used by shamans. There were those who were primarily herbalists; others claimed supernatural powers and gained their strength through visions or dreams.[59] Many used drums, rattles, or other noisemakers, and chanting. Some healers were adept at the art of suggestion, and some were tricksters who used sleight of hand, ventriloquism, and other illusions. What was most important was that the shaman's patients trusted him. One Indian said, "Our children feel and hear the drum before birth."[60]

This connection between trust and response to shaman treatment is illustrated by the following story involving Dr. Charles Robinson Hume,

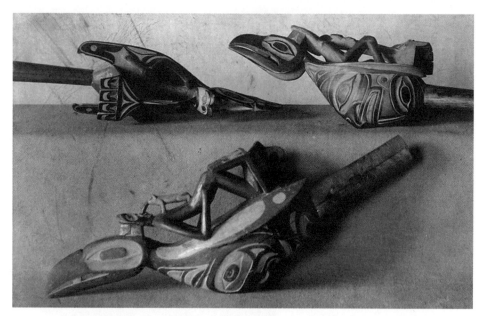

A shaman's rattles. Some Native American healers used rattles, drums, and other noisemakers to drive evil spirits out of the patient. —Courtesy Library of Congress

Agency Physician on the reservation at Anadarko, Oklahoma, in 1890. On one occasion Hume treated a very sick Indian chief using conventional therapy without any improvement. A famous medicine man, Dah-Va-Ca, was called. After much occult ceremony, the shaman moved his hands beneath the cloth that covered the sick chief, pulled out a live possum, and claimed that it came from the chief's body. The chief made an immediate and uninterrupted recovery.[61]

The way to become a shaman varied from tribe to tribe. An aspiring medicine man frequently made a "vision quest" to determine his potential for becoming a shaman. Blackfeet medicine men sometimes selected a successor, usually a young boy or man, and trained him. The schooling was called "the seven tents of medicine," meaning that it took seven years to become a shaman.[62] The Gros Ventre shaman Bull Lodge was visited with seven visions at different mountaintop locations in his tribal lands in north-central Montana, all in preparation for a transition from warrior to healer.[63]

In his study *American Medicine*, Henry Sigerist includes the story of one Blackfeet medicine man's quest. When he was fifteen, living near the

Sweetgrass Hills of northern Montana, the youth went to a shaman and asked him how he could enter the society of healers. The old medicine man sang some songs, prayed to the sun, and said to the spirits, "Look down on this boy. . . . Give him some power. . . . Help him to become a great chief." The boy went to the mountains and fasted for seven days. He was afraid, but he was warned not to run away or he would lose his power. A raven came and took him to a man who told him that arrows or bullets could not harm him, but if anyone struck him with a moccasin, his powers would be lost. Finally, the man said to the boy, "I give you power to doctor men shot by bullets [and] . . . power to take out things sticking in the throat." Thus the student proclaimed, "Now I have this power."[64]

Not all medicine men were good people. One of the worst was a chief named du Gauche, who led a branch of the Assiniboine tribe during the late eighteenth and early nineteenth centuries. Du Gauche, or He Who Holds the Knife, as he was later called, cunningly poisoned those who stood in his way to power. His people were astonished at his "spiritual" ability to predict the death of his enemies.[65]

Healers of all kinds gain respect by predicting the course of disease. An observant physician or shaman can make a reasonably accurate prediction about the outcome of a disease he knows, even though he has no cure. Hippocrates' *Prognostics* told doctors, "a knowledge of prognosis . . . leads the sick to trust in the physician."[66]

And trust is still the first step in patient management. Using mysterious rituals and the power of suggestion, many shamans maintained a good record of results. Most physicians learn that the majority of illnesses are self-limited—patients simply recover on their own. Before modern drugs and treatment methods, seventy percent of people sick with typhoid fever survived after a few weeks, and a few pneumonia patients who appeared close to death suddenly recovered. In cases of spontaneous recovery, the doctor or shaman is often credited with the "cure." Of course, it can work the other way, too. In 1876 and 1877, when epidemics of measles swept through the Paiute tribes in the Owens Valley, dozens of shamans and their sons were put to death for witchcraft.[67]

Herbs

Herbal remedies might be considered the first line of defense in the Native American's armamentaria against illness, and the native caregiver had a large selection of plants to choose from. The Northern Cheyennes alone recognized at least 138 species of plants for both food and medicine. The first United States National Formulary (1888) adopted over two hundred indigenous vegetable drugs from the Indian; some are still listed. People in Europe, thousands of miles away and with no history of contact with the New World, discovered independently some of the same herbs used by Native Americans. Willow bark (*Salix spp.*) is one of these and was used by the ancients to reduce fever and as an analgesic. This plant was similarly employed and prescribed by the Greek physician Dioscorides (ca. A.D. 60). Chemists later discovered that salicin in the bark converted to salicylic acid—a drug similar to the commercial preparation called aspirin. It is still used for arthritic pain and as a febrifuge today.[68]

Herb gatherers prepared medicine from plant stems, flowers, roots, and fruit. Great care and ceremony prevailed in acquiring and preparing each medicine. It was thought to be dangerous not to follow certain spiritual formalities in the collection of materials, and the drugs themselves might be harmful rather than helpful if not properly processed. The herbal material was used in many different ways. It might be pulverized, moistened, applied as a poultice, chewed and mixed with saliva, boiled with grease for a salve, or introduced into the skin with needles or by shallow scratches. Sometimes the drug was mixed with tobacco and smoked, or injected into the rectum as an enema or occasionally vaporized and inhaled in a sweat lodge. Concoctions were drunk in the form of teas, and some preparations were used directly on wounds as antiseptics. Dosages of medications were empirical. There was no science involved, only trial and error.

The Crows, Cheyennes, and Flatheads had many uses for a plant called yarrow (*Achillea millefolium*), which coagulated blood. This Indian discovery was independent from that of the Old World, where the herb had been used for the same purpose—mythology tells us that injured soldiers in the battle of Troy used yarrow on their wounds to stop bleeding. Scientists have extracted from yarrow an alkaloid called achilleine that shortens the clotting time of blood. The Crows also made a poultice and salve from yarrow for burns, and the Flatheads and Cheyennes found it to be a reliable sudorific for fevers.[69]

Indigenous healers understood something of sepsis that followed trauma such as cuts and stabbings, gunshot wounds, imbedded arrows, and burns. Frances Densmore, who studied the Cree Indians early in the twentieth century, reports that "the bark of the Juniper and Canada

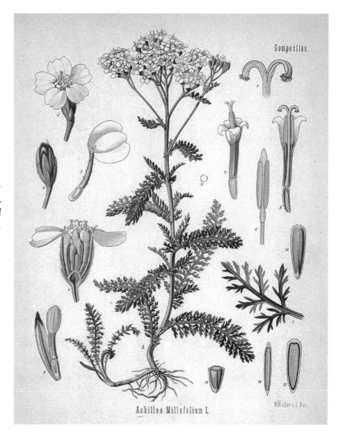

The yarrow plant,
Achillea millefolium.
—From *A Modern Herbal*
by Maud Grieve, 1931

balsam tree are doubtless as good an application to wounds as a people unversed in antiseptic application and ignorant of the existence of bacteria could devise."[70] Certain tribes favored an antiseptic made from the crushed root of the Oregon grape (*Berberis repens*), which was placed directly into wounds. Some Indian herbalists thought the Oregon grape had an additional value as a treatment for venereal disease.[71] Other disinfectants used on the plains were derived from the inner bark of the white pine (*Pinus strobus*), wild cherry (*Prunus serotina*), and wild plum (*Prunus americana*).[72]

Nutrition

Over hundreds of years, tribes discovered the pragmatic use of foods available to them. Empirically they found that some foods were necessary for good health. For example, Native Americans were not as prone to developing scurvy as the white man. While this terrible dietary deficiency was one of the most common illnesses among the early European explorers, settlers, and soldiers on the frontier, the Native American diet included herbaceous plants containing sufficient vitamin C. This essential vitamin is also found in fresh meat, fat, and liver. Many tribes relished not only fresh uncooked liver, fat, and bile, but also the undigested vegetable contents of the rumen (the first stomach) of ruminants such as buffalo—another substance rich in vitamin C.

During periods of scarcity, an Indian preparation called pemmican—jerked meat or fish pounded to a powder, mixed with berries, and fused with melted fat—prevented vitamin deficiency. A nutritionist reported that the Indians of the Yukon prevented scurvy by eating the adrenal glands of the animals they killed. It has been determined that these organs are the richest source of vitamin C in all animal or plant tissues.[73]

The Indian also discovered that eating raw buffalo liver was beneficial to those who had lost a lot of blood. In other words, they were able to treat at least one form of anemia. Liver is rich in both iron and vitamin B12. Rickets, a bone disorder related to a deficiency of vitamin D, was rare, probably because Indian women nursed their children longer than white people, giving the child a good reserve of vitamin D. Nursing was such an important function in native life that several herbs were used to enhance lactation. Cheyenne and Sioux women made tea from a plant they called milkweed (rush skeletonweed, or *Lygodesmia juncea*), which was thought to increase the flow of breast milk.[74] The Nez Perces and Flatheads drank a tea made from the bitterroot (*Lewisia rediviva*), for the same purpose.[75]

Wounds, Fractures, and Broken Bones

Some Native Americans were skilled in treating trauma such as bullet and arrow wounds. After centuries of using the bow and arrow, native healers had more experience with arrow injuries than did U.S. Army surgeons. They opened perforated and contaminated wounds for drainage, keeping them from becoming infected and collecting pus. An army surgeon who witnessed an Indian doctor remove an embedded arrow described the procedure as follows: A willow stick was split, the pith scraped out, and the ends curved. The two-pronged stick was used to probe the arrow track along the shaft until the ends covered the barbs of the arrowhead, whereupon they were securely bound to the shaft, and all were withdrawn together. This method of arrow removal is remarkably similar to that described by the ancient physician Celsus, who practiced in the second century. Celsus dilated the wound entrance, then crushed the arrowhead with pliers or enclosed the head within the grooves of a split reed, and thus extracted the missile without lacerating soft parts.[76]

Indians also understood the concept of immobilization of fractures and dislocations. In splinting bone fractures, they used many different materials as splints, some of which were unique. The Shoshones used rawhide softened with water and molded around the fracture site; when the hide dried, it hardened to form a cast.[77] Eagle Shield, a Sioux sha- man, had forty years of experience in treating fractures and developed an exceptional reputation as a bone healer. He described his system of treatment: First he pulled the injured extremity "until the bone slipped into place." Then he immobilized the fracture with a parfleche case laced together with thongs. He adjusted and tightened the casing daily as the swelling subsided, to keep support above and below the fracture snug. At the same time, he greased his hands with an herbal ointment and mas- saged the skin and muscle around the fracture. Eagle Shield said that the purpose of this was to keep the muscles from becoming stiff. While applying the medicine by massage, he sang a special song four times. The song thanked the "bear" from whom the ointment had come.[78]

Childbirth

Most Native Americans saw pregnancy as a normal life function, and usually the mother had little difficulty in delivery. Full-blooded Indians seemed to have less problem during childbirth than some other groups. Complications such as eclampsia, sepsis, and postpartum hemorrhage were rare. Most of the Plains Indians built special huts for labor, or the mother delivered in her own tepee. This custom exposed her to bacteria to which she was accustomed and probably prevented many postpar- tum infections. At times during prolonged labor, stakes were driven into the dirt for the mother to grasp during her pains. In most instances the woman was on her own and delivered in a squatting position. She was rarely offered aid unless there was a complication.

Most tribes, if they did any intervention, restricted their maneuvers to the outside of the body, such as pressing on the abdomen or manipu- lating the infant through the abdominal wall. For instance, the Sioux sometimes took the woman in labor on their back, belly downward, and bounced her about. The Dakotas occasionally used a "squaw belt" and tightened it over the protruding uterus in an effort to force the infant out.[79] Crow women knelt, leaning against a support while a midwife pressed the lumbar region. The Nez Perces were the only Indians who used intravaginal manipulation of the baby, and the practice was sometimes disastrous, resulting in hemorrhage or infection.[80]

Few drugs were administered to women in labor. Powdered rattles from snakes were used by the Mandans to enhance labor.[81] Sacagawea, we are told, received this concoction just before she delivered Pompey. Some tribes posted a man with a gun near the enclosure where a woman was in labor. On signal, the gun was fired in the hope that the noise would startle the mother into stronger contractions.

Fortunately most tribes used gentle methods to deliver the placenta and membranes. They exerted some traction on the cord with light massage to the uterine fundus, a procedure that is still useful and safe when properly employed. Sometimes the woman was encouraged to sneeze in the belief that this sudden exertion would empty the uterus of the afterbirth. The Flatheads used tea from the roots of Oregon grape to stimulate uterine cramping and to hasten the release of the postpartum placenta. Modern chemists have found an alkaloid in this plant, which they called berberine; in the laboratory, the chemical stimulates contraction of involuntary muscles like those in the female uterus.[82]

After delivery most women received no special treatment. Flathead mothers, for instance, took no rest period. Considering the life of the nomadic Plains Indians, it is doubtful that any of these societies granted new mothers much rest.

Abortion was an option for some Indian women. The practice depended on many factors, including the social structure of the tribe, the presence of disease, or the shortage of food. When women were impregnated by white men, the resulting half-breed infant, according to some medical observers, made delivery more difficult, so this circumstance was considered an indication for abortion.[83] In some tribes, abortions were induced during periods of disease, starvation, or other stressful epochs so the baby would not perish or suffer. Such procedures took place with approval of husbands and knowledge of the entire village. Trader Edwin Thompson Denig estimated that abortion was practiced by two-thirds of married women in the tribes with which he was familiar.[84]

The methods used to perform an abortion were so crude that many young women died in the process. Friends were sometimes recruited to bounce on the woman's abdomen, or she might insert a slippery elm stick into her vagina. Some herbs such as a decoction of cedar sprouts or seneca snakeroot were valued as uterine stimulants to produce an abortion. It is very likely that Indian women knew of plants in their area that would stimulate menstruation or even act as an abortifacient. For instance, the ancients found juniper and artemisia (*Artemisia vulgaris*, mugwort), plants that are readily available on the plains, valuable for this purpose.[85]

The Arrival of "Civilization"

One thing that repeatedly stands out in evaluations of Native American medicine is that the Indian doctor knew how to treat most of the diseases and injuries to which he was accustomed prior to the arrival of Europeans. Gastrointestinal complaints, chronic skin disorders, rheumatism, some upper-respiratory infections, and various benign fevers responded well to Indian therapy. Native tribes lived in balance with their environment and its pathogens until foreign bacteria and viruses disturbed the balance.

Before the arrival of Europeans, though Native Americans may not have enjoyed an untroubled, romantic existence, life was mostly good. There were very few germs in their secluded environment. By contrast, Eurasian societies had been troubled with infectious diseases for thousands of years. Crowd maladies, often in the form of epidemics, spread through populated areas in Europe. Diseases had evolved out of the Eurasians' close association with herds of domesticated animals, a font of infectious disease that persists to the present. Because of their continuous exposure, generations of Europeans had developed a degree of immunity to such lethal afflictions as smallpox, measles, influenza, plague, tuberculosis, typhoid, cholera, and others.[86] But this was not true of the natives of America.

As the first European explorers arrived in the New World, they, and the animals that came with them, unknowingly brought viruses and bacteria that would decimate the indigenous population. By the time the *Mayflower* arrived in the New World in 1620, Europeans had been visiting New England for more than a hundred years. Probably smallpox came to this continent around 1525, influenza in 1558, diphtheria in 1614, and measles in 1618.[87]

When the first pilgrims arrived, between 1616 and 1622, a virulent pandemic spread through Massachusetts, New Hampshire, and Maine that wiped out nearly one hundred percent of the natives. A good case has been made by archaeologists that this scourge was viral hepatitis.[88] According to the leaders of the Plymouth Colony, who disembarked in 1620, the Indians "died on heapes." By robbing the decimated tribes' caches of corn, the pilgrims were able to survive. "And sure it was God's good providence that we found this corn," they said.[89] It is estimated that in the first one or two centuries after Columbus arrived in the Americas, the indigenous population of the New World declined by ninety-five percent.[90] With no genetic resistance or immunity, millions of Indians died. Population estimates of natives in North America in the fifteenth century vary. There may have been as many as twenty million. By the end of the nineteenth century there were only half a million.[91]

There was one condition that the natives traded to the whites, however—syphilis, a venereal disease. While Columbus and his men brought many infectious agents, it is accepted by most contemporary scientists that *Treponema pallidum*, the spirochete that causes syphilis, probably wasn't one of them. There are differences of opinion, but there is good evidence that syphilis was on this continent well before Columbus arrived, and it spread readily to the early explorers who lusted after the Indian women. (*Neisseria gonorrhoeae*, however, the bacterium that causes gonorrhea, was brought over the sea in Portuguese explorers' urethras.)

When Columbus's ships returned to Europe, syphilis spread furiously throughout the continent, and then into Africa and Asia. In the Native American population, the disease was characterized by genital sores and a slowly developing illness, but in Europe, the infection resulted in syphilitic pustules so extensive they covered the victim's body. Death from secondary infection was the usual result.[92] The explosive behavior of this illness in the European population—never before exposed to it and without any immunity—was similar to the American aborigines' reaction to the infections Europeans brought to them.[93]

In the West, the first whites to arrive were Spanish explorers, who were looking not only for gold but also for medicines. During the sixteenth century, people in Europe, whose medicine had been based on Greek and Islamic practices, began looking for new cures. Expeditions were sent from Spain to collect cinchona bark, cacao, ipecac, jalap, and sarsaparilla. This search into what is now Mexico and the American Southwest was dangerous. Scarce food and angry natives skilled with bows and arrows were among the problems of these early explorers, and the qualifications of the Spanish physicians on the trips were questionable. Wounds were cauterized with boiling oil, and injured men were purged and bled.

During the latter part of the eighteenth century, Spain introduced three dubious contributions to the New World: guns, horses, and epidemic disease. The infusion of guns and horses disrupted native life in many ways. Guns gave the Indian a power he had not had before and increased his aggressiveness. Tribes with firearms had an advantage, and that advantage was swiftly sought. The horse, too, increased violent encounters as warriors gained the mobility to make war over a greater area. "The progression was simple, but the changes were breathtaking: First had come the gun, next had come the horse, and then had come the smallpox."[94]

At first, isolated Indian tribes of the West were not exposed to the white man's sicknesses. But increased traffic from boats and horses in the mid-1700s brought the previously isolated groups into contact with European disease. Disease from sea traders on the Pacific Coast spread up the Columbia River, and travelers going from east to west transmitted contagion to the tribes on the upper Missouri in the late eighteenth and early nineteenth centuries. Soon, fur traders, gold-rush fortune seekers, and settlers followed. The native population was physically and physiologically unprepared for this onslaught.

Illnesses that were severe but relatively benign in the Old World were deadly to the Indians. Childhood diseases such as whooping cough, measles, and chicken pox were common in white people, and their mortality rate was not high. Not so for the Indian. For example, the Cayuse were struck hard with measles brought by early migrations of white people. The terrible fever inflamed their minds as well as their bodies, and the famous missionaries Marcus and Narcissa Whitman were blamed for the plague and killed. Other tribes were affected as well. James Willard Schultz reported that during the winter of 1859-60, hundreds of Blackfeet died of measles.[95]

Another viral outbreak for which the Native American was not prepared was influenza, a respiratory illness that spread rapidly. Influenza struck Crows in 1850, killing 150 people. Some of the Indians believed that trader Edwin Thompson Denig had inflicted the disease on them because they had stolen horses from him. To prevent further deaths, the Indians brought back nine of the horses.[96]

There was no specific treatment for any of these conditions that afflicted the natives, nor did the white population have any cure. Traditional white physicians could offer little except narcotics. Native healers believed that the demons that caused the illness had to be driven out of the body, so they resorted to harsh methods that occasionally hastened the death of a sick person. For instance, the debilitated and feverish patient was sometimes placed in a sweat lodge where moist heat could penetrate the body, then after an interval the victim was plunged into cold water. For common colds and arthritis, this kind of treatment was modestly effective, but for the desperately ill who were often near death, the shock frequently proved fatal.

Not all the illnesses that killed Indians were acute infections. Tuberculosis, for instance, was more insidious. There is evidence that some forms of that disease antedated Columbus's arrival. Skeletal remains in Peru and in southern Ontario have been found with tubercular lesions.[97] Some scientists feel that pre-Columbian tuberculosis was caused by an atypical mycobacterium that produced little cross-immunization. The Native Americans' lack of immunity doesn't explain the entire picture, however. Worsening social factors such as shoddy living conditions, crowding, poor nutrition, and alcoholism also played a large part. Whatever the explanation, tuberculosis, sometimes called consumption, in several different pulmonary and extrapulmonary forms, killed many Indians during the 1800s and well into the twentieth century.[98]

As one Indian survivor, Chilum Balum, said about the coming of the white man: "There was then no sickness; they had no aching bones; they had then no burning chest; they had then no abdominal pain; they had then no consumption; they had then no headache. At that time the course of humanity was orderly. The foreigners made it otherwise when they arrived here."[99]

"Many Scabs": Smallpox

Among the diseases Europeans transmitted to the native population, smallpox was the most devastating. This ugly contagion, sometimes called variola, spread like wildfire through the eastern tribes. Reverend Cotton Mather's cold, un-Christian observation illustrates the colonial attitude toward this tragedy: "The Indians in These Parts had newly, even about a Year or Two before, been visited with such a prodigious Pestilence as carried away not a Tenth, but Nine Parts of Ten (yea, 'tis said Nineteen of Twenty) among them: so that the Woods were almost cleared of those pernicious Creatures, to make Room for a better Growth."[100]

The smallpox virus was transported in all directions by traders and Native Americans. For a hundred years the fur trade brought Canadian merchants in contact with the Ojibwas, Crees, and Assiniboines. But

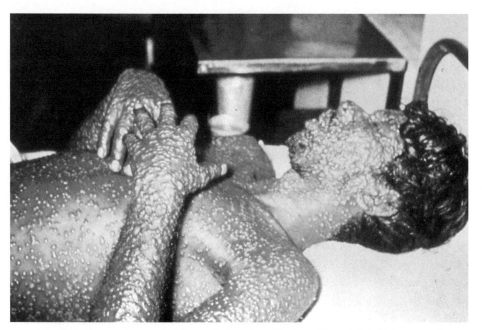

For three thousand years, smallpox shadowed civilization. This viral infection spread along trade routes, reaching the Americas in the sixteenth century. The disease tended to smolder in densely populated areas, sporatically erupting into a full-blown epidemic.
—Courtesy Immunization Action Coalition

according to Elizabeth Fenn in her book *Pox Americana*, this lucrative business was almost totally destroyed in 1781-82 by smallpox, the first epidemic that far north. The sickness and death caused such a severe cultural disruption that all trade ceased during the epidemic. In 1780 the disease was rampant in Mexico and Texas, and east to New Orleans. By this time the Comanches had horses, as did the Shoshones, and it is very plausible that horse travel helped spread the disease more rapidly. With wandering Plains tribes doing business and raiding over long distances, their contact with one another and with less mobile tribes probably conducted the disease from one location to another. [101] This may have been the first epidemic to strike the Plains Indians, but it was by no means the last.

Smallpox is characterized by a two-week incubation period of fever and malaise followed by a pustular eruption all over the body, an unremitting fever, and insufferable itching of the skin. The skin blisters, or bullae, fill with fluid, then burst and crust over; thus Native Americans called the disease "many scabs." Smallpox was highly contagious, easily transmitted by nasopharyngeal secretions or even dust in the air. Scales from the skin of an infected person were highly infective and retained the smallpox virus for weeks. Worst of all, the disease had no effective treatment.

In addition to the harm of the disease itself, it was almost impossible for the afflicted person not to scratch the itching lesions and open up raw surfaces to secondary infection, which was often fatal. Among other complications that led to death were hemorrhage and pneumonia. Those who survived were often left terribly scarred for life.

A few Indian tribes suspected that they had been infected with "many scabs" deliberately. Stories circulated that immigrants were giving the Indians blankets from sickbeds. Furthermore, in some instances, whites capitalized on the Indians' fear of the disease to manipulate them. In *Astoria*, Washington Irving tells of a Mr. M'Dougall, an early settler on the Pacific coast, who found himself in a confrontation with a large group of Indians. He called the chiefs together and said, "The White men among you are few in number . . . but they are mighty . . . I hold the small pox safely (and he drew out a small bottle and held it up) . . . I have but to draw the cork and let loose the pestilence, to sweep man, woman and child from the face of the earth." The chiefs were horrified. Thereafter M'Dougall was called the "the Great Small Pox Chief."[102]

Certain years were particularly bad for smallpox. In 1833 a party of Crows met a caravan of sick emigrants who unsuccessfully attempted to warn them off. After some of the Crows became infected, fear scattered the people over the countryside. This panicked escape may have prevented a few susceptible Indians from catching the illness, but many died. It was estimated that only about one in six or seven of those infected recovered. Denig reported that "More than a thousand fingers are said to have been cut off by the relatives of the dead."[103] Amputation of fingers as a memorial to the loss of a loved one was a common act of grief among Native Americans.

In June 1837 a boat arrived at Fort Union on the Missouri River with passengers sick from smallpox. By this time, travel up the Missouri was common, and steamboats regularly brought supplies, traders, and travelers of all kinds, as well as disease. Despite warnings, the Assiniboines, anxious to trade, insisted on coming into the fort. A smallpox epidemic of gigantic proportion followed, though Assiniboines from Canada had been inoculated for smallpox by the Hudson's Bay Company during a previous epidemic and were not affected. Denig, himself a survivor of the epidemic, gives us a vivid description of this terrible episode:

> 1000 souls contracted the disease at the same time . . . reducing them to 30 lodges. . . . Other bands coming in . . . caught the infection. . . . The dead were daily thrown into the river by cart loads. A singular characteristic of this disease was that two-thirds or more died before any eruption appeared. This event was always accompanied by hemorrhages from the mouth and ears. . . . The fever rose to a pitch of frenzy. . . . An Indian near the fort, named Little Dog, after losing his favorite child, proposed to his wife to kill the whole family before they were so much disfigured as to present a disgusting appearance in the future world. She agreed with the stipulation that he should kill her before the children.[104]

Denig says that some of the sick Indians were treated in the fort with purging and bleeding, but they all died.[105] There is a similarity between the hemorrhage that occurred in these people with little resistance to smallpox and fatal viral conditions now seen sporadically in African countries, Lassa fever and Ebola fever. These diseases are so rare and so fatal that no immunity has developed in the populations, and victims often terminate with massive and generalized hemorrhage.

Despite the compassionless attitude many whites expressed toward the Indians' plight, most white people were concerned about the sick Indians and tried to help. When the Gros Ventres on the Milk River were infected with smallpox in 1869, the government provided a hospital with blankets, supplies, and medicines. Nevertheless, 741 Gros Ventres died. The Indian agent, A. S. Reed, advised the Indians to scatter their lodges, which may have helped. Twenty-five miles away, Dr. Ash of General Sheridan's staff, in an attempt to stop the epidemic, vaccinated and moved the River Crow tribe across the Missouri River. Only thirty-five of them died.[106] (For more on smallpox, see chapter 14.)

"Water that takes away one's wits"

Infectious disease wasn't the only curse the white man brought to the Indian—he also brought whiskey. Colonial Americans used alcohol for medicine, as a tonic, and as part of their everyday life. During the nineteenth century in America, drinking was as much a part of life as food. It is estimated that by the time of the Civil War the consumption of alcohol in the States had reached an all-time high: over three gallons per capita per year.[107]

Liquor was traded to the Indians since the first white people set foot on the continent. The Teton Sioux first tasted whiskey during the seventeenth century and thought it was "sacred water."[108] Simply stated, trading alcohol was financially expedient for the whites. Aupaumut, a Mohican, said in 1722, "for as long as the Christians will sell Rum, our People will drink it."[109]

As white men came west, they found room in their packs for "spirits," for their own use as well as for trade. Lewis and Clark carried some with them as they traveled up the Missouri River, mostly to drink themselves, but sometimes they offered it to the Indians in trade. Imagine their astonishment when the Arikaras not only refused whiskey, but they shamed the whites by remarking that "they were surprised that their father (the United States Government) should present to them a liquor which would make them act like fools."[110]

In 1842 a man named Garrett, one of the first fur traders to introduce alcohol to the Plains Indians, traded whiskey for skins. Because the natives didn't like the taste at first, he added sugar to it. Five years later, the tribe was described as "a nation of drunkards."[111] Many Indians were completely powerless before its temptation. Some traded everything they had of value for the cheap rotgut provided by unscrupulous traders. E. C. ("Teddy Blue") Abbott left us a recipe for one of the concoctions traders sold to the Indians:

> You take one barrel of Missouri River water, and two gallons of alcohol. Then you add two ounces of strychnine—because strychnine is the greatest stimulant in the world—and three plugs of tobacco to make them sick—an Indian wouldn't figure it was whiskey unless it made him sick—and five bars of soap to give it a head, and half a pound of red pepper, and then you put in some sagebrush and boil it until it's brown. Strain into a barrel, and you've got your Indian whiskey; that one bottle calls for one buffalo robe and when the Indian got drunk it was two robes.[112]

By the time James Kipp, an American Fur Company trader, built Fort Piegan in Blackfeet territory in 1831, he knew how to get trade goods with what he called "a grand stroke of generosity." He sponsored a three-day drunk during which the Blackfeet were given gallons of "Indian" whiskey free of charge. The trader's "generosity" endeared him to the tribe, and in a few days he procured 6,450 pounds of beaver skins worth $46,000 in exchange for one barrel of whiskey, which made two hundred gallons of rotgut.[113]

Whites used "firewater" to cajole Indians to do their bidding not only in trade but in all negotiations. White traders and politicians capitalized on the Indian's alcohol-weakened body and spirit to manipulate him to the will of the white majority. Even such outstanding colonial leaders as Benjamin Franklin endorsed what remained the prevailing sentiment among white Americans up to the end of the nineteenth century: "If it be the design of Providence to extirpate these savages in order to make room for the cultivators of the earth, it seems not improbable that rum may be the appointed means."[114] The Christian culture that saw sin in the dress, religion, and mores of the natives didn't hesitate to use the evil of intoxicants to disrupt Native American culture. Alcohol's deleterious effect on people with no previous exposure to fermented grains begat the stereotype of the obnoxious drunken Indian and reinforced the notion that they were culturally and racially inferior to whites, i.e., savages.[115]

Of course, whites were at least as susceptible to the ugliness of drinking as Indians. For instance, trapper Beaver Tom, described in *Tough Trip Through Paradise* by Andrew Garcia, became "a half-mad, drunken maniac with the snakes, who was tied down in his saddle." Later Tom was "crawling around like a dog. . . . Every once in a while he picked up an imaginary snake." When he sobered up, Tom "swore by all the gods . . . that he had taken his last drink and that it was good-bye to whiskey forever." A short time later, however, he surreptitiously tapped the keg again.[116]

It could be argued that the Indian had more reason to turn to alcohol than did most white men, with his home and way of life undergoing destruction and his people sick with the white man's diseases. In time, the "water that takes away one's wits" would be a key factor in the devastation of the indigenous population.[117]

A Culture Degraded

Most Indian groups were proud and lived in a manner that had served them well for hundreds of years. They had great love for their country and appreciated its great rivers, forests, and wildlife. As the great Crow chief Arapooish said of his country along the Yellowstone, Powder, and Wind Rivers of Montana and Wyoming, "The Crow country is good country. The Great Spirit has put it exactly in the right place. Everything good is to be found there."[118]

As Europeans pushed native tribes off their lands, they disrupted entire societies, weakening them and making it progressively easier to push them farther. The Indians were soon at the mercy of newcomers with an entirely different agenda, who disapproved of their ways and looked on them as ignorant savages. Many tried to fight, but they were eventually overwhelmed.

Most Native Americans exposed to the pressures of "civilization" were affected similarly: their land was confiscated, disease depraved their friends and family, they starved as the buffalo disappeared, their men succumbed to alcohol, and their children were taken away to the "white man's school." Edwin Thompson Denig's descriptions of the state of health and living conditions of the tribes he knew in the early 1800s are graphic. Of the Arikaras, or Rees, of the Missouri River he wrote, "Both young and old of either sex are . . . tainted with the venereal disease. . . . The spaces between the huts are seldom if ever cleaned, animal and vegetable substances in . . . putrefaction are scattered about, and . . . fluxes, dysenteries, scurvy and other diseases prevail."[119] With these repugnant depictions, Denig is describing a once mighty tribe that was decimated by disease and loss of tradition. The Arikara comprised about thirty thousand persons in 1776, but several waves of smallpox wiped out thousands. By the time Lewis and Clark passed by, they had been reduced to only a few small villages.[120]

The mobility of the nomadic Plains tribes gave them a degree of protection from the intruders and their disease for a while. But eventually the white insurgency overtook them, too, and the simple expediency of staying alive took precedence over cultural heritage. Certainly in this state of devastation, there could have been little effort to preserve the past. With the hastened death of Indian elders and leaders, the reservoir of ethnic recollection was almost totally lost. With it a fund of valuable medical experience disappeared, at a great loss to mankind.

The Native American's life on the various reservations was not a good one. According to one witness, the nineteenth-century reservations were "shrinking islands dirty with lies and greed."[121] By 1882 the bison were gone from the plains, and periods of starvation and epidemics of disease further reduced these wards of the government to a pitiable circumstance.

The government's solution to the "Indian problem," European-style education, Christianity, and agriculture, failed miserably. By 1912, after a couple of decades of paternalism by the U.S. Department of the Interior, the reservation Indian's death rate was three times that of the white population. According to historian Diane D. Edwards, in one

Montana Blackfeet group of 1,200, examined just before World War I, ninety percent had trachoma and seventy-five percent had tuberculosis. (Trachoma, caused by the bacterium *Chlamydia trachomatis*, is a chronic eye infection that can cause blindness.) Edwards, writing in 1997, quoted an early student of Indian health who said, "While white Americans by the thousands enjoy the romance and color of the Indians, and love to sentimentalize about them, they do not give a whoop in hell whether they live well, die in misery, or just drag along in weary, broken despair."[122]

The health and welfare of today's Native Americans, most of whom are existing on reservations, is another story and one that is partly told every day by the increasing incidence of diabetes, alcoholism, fetal alcohol syndrome, cirrhosis, accidental death, suicide, and other preventable or partly preventable health threats.

Lewis and Clark

Keelboat Physicians

A turning point in American history.

—Bernard DeVoto[128]

THOUGH THEY HAD NO DEGREES, Meriwether Lewis and William Clark were the first healers from the so-called civilized part of the United States to come to the western frontier. Their previous army experience and later performance throughout the grand adventure qualified them as physicians at that time in history. The ability of Lewis and Clark to care for their entourage, and the medical services they were able to trade for help from the Indians along the way, made a major contribution to the final success of the venture now known as the Lewis and Clark Expedition, or the Voyage of Discovery.

While President Jefferson's paramount motive in organizing the expedition was to strengthen the nation and acquire wealth, he also valued science and wanted to learn about the fauna, flora, and people of this measureless unknown region. To lead the huge undertaking he envisioned, Jefferson chose his secretary, Captain Meriwether Lewis. In an unprecedented move, Lewis invited his friend Captain William Clark to participate as co-leader in "it's fatigues, it's dangers and it's honors."[124] The two had served together in the army, and now they formed a partnership that left indelible imprints on the history of the United States.

When the expedition left St. Charles, Missouri, the party probably totaled about fifty men, including a number of engagés and Clark's slave, York. On the way up the Missouri River, one man deserted and Sergeant Charles Floyd died. The engagés and several soldiers—two of whom had been dismissed for misconduct—left after the party's arrival at the Mandan villages, where interpreter Toussaint Charbonneau was hired, along with his Indian wife, Sacagawea, bringing the new total to thirty-two; the couple's infant son, Jean Baptiste, whom the men called "Pompey," made thirty-three.[125]

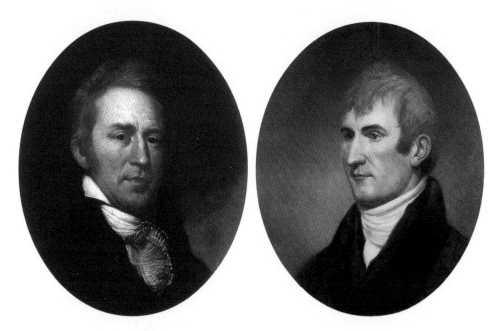

Portraits of William Clark and Meriwether Lewis by Charles Willson Peale.
—Courtesy Independence National Historical Park

In addition to Lewis and Clark's directive to explore the uncharted West, the president instructed the two captains to give the best medical care possible to the men in their charge, and to the natives along the way. Jefferson held the health and lives of the men of the expedition above all other considerations. It was under Jefferson's tutelage that Lewis strengthened his medical preparation for the momentous journey. Along with his other passions, Jefferson had a strong interest in medicine. He had written about medical subjects, corresponded with leading doctors of the era, and read extensively on the subject. His spacious library contained more than one hundred books on medical subjects, including surgery and anatomy. Jefferson was skeptical of some of the medical practices of his day. In one letter, he said of the ideal medical student, "His mind must be strong indeed, if it can maintain a wise infidelity against the authority of his instructors, and the bewitching delusions of their theories."[126]

Elliott Coues, a nineteenth-century physician and historian, later questioned why Jefferson did not send a professionally trained physician along with the expedition instead of relying on two army captains.[127] Others have also lamented this great "failure." There isn't any obvious explanation for the decision, except that Jefferson and many others of the time were skeptical of the value of physicians, and perhaps rightly so. The standard of medical practice was poorly established, and Jefferson probably recognized that there wasn't much difference between a physician and a well-trained layman. At one point, while traveling down the Ohio River, Lewis met Dr. William Ewing Patterson, who seemed eager to go, but he did not show up at the appointed time. According to Stephen Ambrose, "It was undoubtedly just as well; his [Patterson's] reputation was one of constant drunkenness, which may well have been the cause of his being late."[128] Another medical historian of the Lewis and Clark expedition, Dr. E. G. Chuinard, said the two captains gave their men better personal attention than was rendered by Revolutionary War doctors.[129]

Medical Training of Lewis and Clark

Both Lewis and Clark had gained practical medical experience as army officers. In colonial times, officers were responsible for the health of their men. Commissioned officers learned to use the lancet for phlebotomy and to vaccinate for smallpox, and they were familiar with minor injuries, jaundice, intermittent fever (malaria), diarrhea, venereal diseases, and other conditions that affected soldiers. Some, like Lewis, also had a working knowledge of herbal treatment.

Lewis's first medical instructor was his mother, Lucy Meriwether Lewis Marks. She was an herbalist of some renown, a "yarb" doctor (a term used then for herbalists) who grew her own medicines and was able to identify and use wild plants as well. Lucy taught her son this craft as she prepared and ministered to the illnesses of her family, neighbors, and slaves. "Even as an old lady, 'Grandma Marks' was seen riding about . . . on horseback to attend the sick," Ambrose noted.[130]

Later, in preparation for the expedition, President Jefferson arranged and paid for Meriwether Lewis to spend time in Philadelphia studying botany, zoology, and medicine. In the latter discipline, the young captain was tutored by Dr. Benjamin Rush. Rush had a reputation as a medical reformer, and during the Revolutionary War he served as a military surgeon and later criticized the deplorable care Continental soldiers were given in army hospitals. As a military physician he was ahead of his contemporaries in many ways. He was a proponent of vaccination for

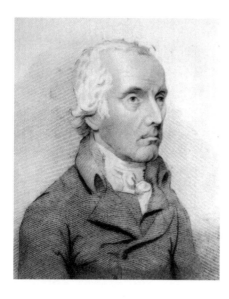

Dr. Benjamin Rush
—Courtesy National
Library of Medicine,
History of Medicine

smallpox, a diet rich in vegetables to prevent scurvy, abstinence from alcohol, and scrupulous cleanliness in the army camps.

Rush was a doctor of superior ethics and courage. During the 1793 yellow fever epidemic in Philadelphia, Rush and many of his fellow physicians stuck to their posts while, sad to say, some doctors left with their families for healthier places. Though Rush was as knowledgeable as any other physician of his time, he is, rather regrettably, best remembered for his strong belief in purging and bleeding. Of course, Rush wasn't the only proponent of these egregious methods, but he was the period's most vocal advocate, and his theories dominated the medical profession for many years.[131]

Dr. Rush had no medical peer in his day and was probably the best choice Jefferson could make to advise the expedition on how to protect against illness and what drugs and instruments to take into the wilds. Though Rush's recommendations showed an incomplete appreciation of the dangers and arduous circumstances of the wilderness, they also reflected the best understanding of the day, and some of them were of value. The good doctor suggested that if the explorers were fatigued or otherwise indisposed, they should rest and take fluids. If this and "a gentle sweat obtained by warm drinks" didn't cause improvement, an "opening of the bowels by means of one, two, or more purging pills" was indicated.[132] Following Rush's advice, the expedition carried fifty dozen of the doctor's bilious pills, a strong purgative containing calomel and jalap, which, according to Rush, would "gently open the bowels"—the understatement of the century.[133] This combination of drugs produced an explosive intestinal passage and became known by all who used them as "thunderclappers."

Rush's potent pills found their way into the armamentarium of medical kits after the yellow fever epidemic in Philadelphia, when the strong purge resulted in the passage of copious amounts of bile-colored material. This release of bodily waste supposedly diminished the jaundice of yellow fever sufferers. In reality, however, it was not beneficial; indeed, it was harmful. Nevertheless, for a long time doctors used these potent pills as a panacea. Once, when Clark himself was ill, he took five "thunderclappers" at once, but he didn't report any side effects from this excessive dose.

In addition to recommending purgatives, Dr. Rush preached that bleeding was beneficial for most ailments, even hemorrhage. In defense of bloodletting, he said, "Hemorrhages seldom occur, where bleeding has been sufficiently copious."[134] This implies that he and his contemporaries bled people who were already hemorrhaging. In some cases, the bleeding stopped when the blood volume and pressure became low; in other words, when the treatment resulted in shock. In spite of Rush's promotion of the value of bleeding, Lewis and Clark used the procedure sparingly.

While in Philadelphia, Lewis may also have gained much knowledge from Dr. Benjamin Smith Barton, an associate of Benjamin Rush and a professor at the medical school. Barton was known as the father of American "materia medica." Lewis bought his *Elements of Botany*, at a cost of six dollars, and carried it with him all the way to the Pacific and back.[135]

Clark's education had been much less formal than Lewis's, but he knew a great deal about the West and was an exceptional leader, a scientist, and a humanist. Of his early military experience he wrote, "I hate the recollection of the Sufferings of our Wounded. . . . No set of men in the like disabled situation ever experienced much more want of conveniancies &c."[136] During his military service, the notes he kept on his medical cases revealed him to be a careful observer and a pragmatic physician. His understanding of human nature and "hands-on" approach to health care made him a popular healer, especially with the Indians.

In St. Louis, while at Camp Dubois, Lewis and Clark were probably also given medical advice by Dr. Antoine Francois Saugrain, a colorful, four-foot six-inch Parisian doctor who was a friend of Benjamin Franklin.

Not only a physician, Saugrain was also a commercial manufacturer, an entrepreneur, and an inventor of barometers, thermometers, and matches. Saugrain made thermometers using mercury salvaged from the backs of mirrors. Although there is no record of a purchase of a thermometer, the Corps used one on the journey until it was broken.[137] These were not clinical thermometers, which had not yet been invented.

Drugs and Treatments

In Lewis and Clark's time, medical methods of the trained physician, the army medic, the home-remedy practitioner, the Indian healer, and others all melted together into a potpourri of health care practice. By the time the expedition started up the Missouri River, the two captains were prepared to treat many common medical conditions of the frontier such as "tumers" (inflammation with swelling), "biles" (boils), "pox" (syphilis), "charlick" (colic), and "biliousness."[138] Among the equipment the expedition carried were lancets, "pocket" surgical instruments, dental instruments, clyster (enema) and penis syringes, tourniquets, and "lint" for dressing wounds.

The Corps of Discovery's medical supplies included a number of useful drugs in common usage. The bark of the cinchona, also called quinine bark or Peruvian bark, from which quinine is derived, was of great value as an antifebrile agent. Quinine was known to be effective against "ague," or malaria.[139] Although there was no evidence of malaria infection during most of the long trip across the continent, the mosquito-infested Ohio and lower Missouri Rivers were a potential source, and some cases of malaria may have been prevented by the use of "barks" in the treatment of nonspecific fevers.[140]

Lewis was concerned about malaria along the Ohio River, where disease was endemic. In September 1803 he wrote, "The fever and ague and bilious fevers here commence their banefull oppression and continue through the whole course of the river with increasing violence as you approach it's mouth."[141] The expedition's medicine chest was ready for "ague" with plenty of Peruvian bark. Though the men never contracted malaria, the bark wasn't wasted. It was used against fever the way we use aspirin, and also as an ingredient of a poultice.

Glauber salts and saltpeter had limited use as wet packs to injured parts, and sometimes in dilute solution as an eyewash. The expedition also carried preparations for digestive problems and salves for treating wounds. Laudanum (tincture of opium) was valuable in the relief of severe

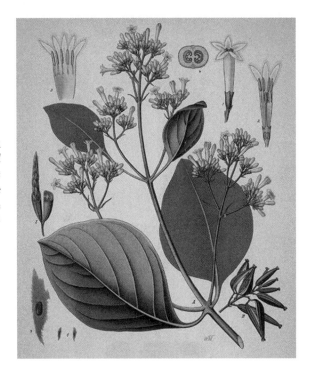

Cinchona (Cinchona succirubra), *whose wood is known medicinally as Peruvian bark or quinine bark* —From *A Modern Herbal* by Maud Grieve, 1931

pain. The captains brought nutmeg, cloves, and cinnamon to flavor oral medicines, and, of course, liquor, on its own or to enhance remedial concoctions. In addition to the drugs they brought, they employed various wild plants they found at hand in composing remedies.

Liquor was used not only as a medicine but also as a stimulant for flagging spirits and an antidote against the cold and wet. The last of the expedition's several kegs of "spirits" was finished off to celebrate both Independence Day 1805 and the successful end to the grueling portage around the Great Falls of the Missouri River. Alcohol may have been utilized as an anesthetic as well, since it was widely used in that era for this purpose.

The expedition also carried a variety of purgatives. The thrust of the medical philosophy of the time was to rid the body of toxins, and any treatment that caused an evacuation from the upper or lower intestinal tract was considered good therapy. Tartar emetic, a drug used to induce vomiting, was thought indispensable. Other salts and powders were also brought on the trip to use as laxatives and diuretics. Calomel (mercurous chloride), the cure-all of its day, was a strong purgative, and when incorporated into an ointment it was of great use in treating the skin manifestations of syphilis, a common venereal disease among the expedition's entourage. Lewis's tutor Benjamin Rush attributed almost magical powers to calomel, and it was a key ingredient in his infamous "thunderclappers."

In addition to the use of purgatives, doctors of the day recommended therapeutic bleeding for many ailments. Both captains knew how to bleed patients, but neither used the procedure as often as prevailing medical opinion dictated. For instance, Dr. Rush recommended bleeding to weaken and relax patients with a dislocated shoulder, but the captains did not bleed Sergeant Nathaniel Pryor when he dislocated his shoulder, which he did three times during the trip.[142] Clark wrote, "Sergeant Pryor in takeing down the mast put his Shoulder out of Place," and said that it took four trials before they were able to get the shoulder reduced.[143] We don't know the method of reduction they used, but the most popular routine at the time was traction on the affected limb, countered against the surgeon's foot in the armpit. It may sound crude, but this technique was used well into the twentieth century. Clark doesn't say if alcohol or narcotics were used as an anesthetic, but they probably were. Relaxation of the muscles of the shoulder and the arm is necessary to treat a dislocation properly.

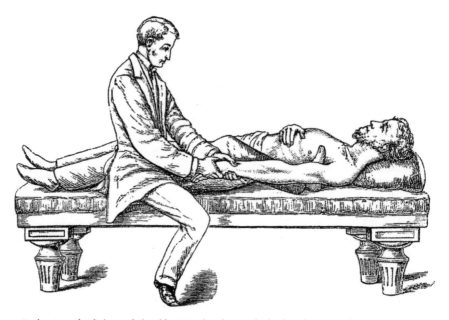

Reduction of a dislocated shoulder joint by placing the heel in the patient's armpit —From *The Science and Art of Surgery: A Treatise on Surgical Injuries, Diseases, and Operations* by John Eric Erichsen, 1884

The captains did employ the technique of bloodletting in some cases. They bled Sergeant Floyd during his fatal illness, and also Sacagawea, in an attempt to bring her fever down when she was suffering from a gynecological infection. Of course, this form of treatment did lower the temperature, but not in a beneficial way. Clark also treated pleurisy by bleeding. He recorded on January 31, 1805, "George Drewyer taken with Ploursey last evening. Bled and Gave him Some Sage tea, this morning he is much better."[144]

The captains were at times innovative in the techniques of venesection. Once during the portage around the Great Falls of the Missouri, Lewis did not have a lancet, so he bled one man who was "heated and fortigued" using his penknife, which he claimed "answered very well."[145] Apparently these healthy, young, vigorous, and superbly strong men suffered little from the "therapeutic" loss of blood.

Health Problems on the Journey

Skin inflamations, referred to as "tumers" or "biles," became a common ailment that troubled the troop throughout the journey. Poor personal hygiene, malnutrition, exposure to injury, and bacteria (probably a staphy-lococcus), all could have played a part in this painful and debilitating affliction. "Whitlows" (infection of the finger or toe that often lies under the nail and may extend to the underlying bone) were particularly troubling. Lewis commented that these abscesses, which cause severe throbbing pain, were "a complaint which has been very common among the men." The surgical skills of both Lewis and Clark were required in the treatment of some of these problems. Once, Clark wrote, he opened an abscess in a man's left breast that contained "half a point [pint?]" of pus.[146]

Other common problems, naturally, were fractures, joint dislocations, and lacerations. Foot injuries were particularly frequent, especially on the plains, where prickly pears grew in abundance, and along the rivers, where rocks were often as sharp as knives. There were also several injuries from unruly horses, but none was serious. Frostbite was another concern among the men and the natives as well. While at the Mandan encampment, Clark "sawed off" the gangrenous toes of a Mandan child.[147] Also at Fort Mandan, Clark wrote of his own men's frostbite in his journal, including, "my Servents feet also frosted and his P---s a little."[148]

Lewis and Clark themselves became sick on several occasions. The illness for which Clark dosed himself with five of Rush's special pills occurred at the Three Forks of the Missouri River in late July 1805. Lewis described Clark as "very sick with a high fever on him and much fatiegued and exhausted." He also reported that Clark suffered from frequent chills and constant muscle aches. According to Dr. Ronald V. Loge in an article for *We Proceeded On*, "A person . . . with these symptoms during the summer season in Southwestern Montana would usually be suffering from Colorado tick fever." Colorado tick fever, a viral disease transmitted by wood ticks, is endemic in this area of Montana. Further, Loge says, "The 1805 journal account of Clark's illness may be the first clinical description of Colorado tick fever, written by two good clinical observers."[149]

On one occasion, Lewis became ill when he was away from camp. Having no thunderclappers or other medicines to "clean out his system," he improvised with a liquid concoction made from chokecherry twigs. After drinking a large volume of this, his fever and gastrointestinal symptoms abated. The young captain must have recovered dramatically because the next day he walked twenty-seven miles.

Throughout the trip, diarrhea cursed everyone. On June 14, 1804, Clark noted, "The party is much aflicted with Boils and Several have the Decissentary which I contribute to the water."[150] In this observation Clark was probably right. There are many bacteria that may have caused the dysentery the men suffered, as well as a large selection of parasites carried by food and water that we now know can make humans sick.[151] The men were encouraged to dip their cups deep into the muddy Missouri to avoid the foul surface water, a procedure with little more than aesthetic effect, reflecting the era's lack of understanding of water contamination.

When we look at the kinds of food the explorers ate—much of which their bodies were not used to—the intestinal complaints are not surprising. There was a great variety of meat, sometimes poorly preserved, including elk, deer, horse, beaver, and dog. When labor was intense, each man might eat as much as ten pounds of meat a day, and beaver was the favorite variety.[152] If the hunting was poor, they were forced to eat wolf, hawk, and, at Fort Clatsop, whale blubber. Once, Lewis ate the small intestine of a buffalo, uncleaned and cooked in the coals of a fire. He didn't find it too displeasing at the time, but there isn't any record of the aftermath. Furthermore, some of the food obtained from the Indians, such as dried meat and fish, was probably contaminated with bacteria.

To provide sustenance during lean times, the Corps transported a large quantity of "portable soup," a dehydrated source of calories and vitamin C. The soup was stored in lead canisters, which Lewis planned on using to make bullets when they were empty. Because foodstuffs are impregnated with lead on prolonged exposure, it was fortunate that the explorers used the mixture only sporadically, or they might have developed lead poisoning. During the return trip, when the food supply was exhausted, the barely palatable soup, grudgingly lugged thousands of miles, supplied enough energy to allow the men to survive. It also probably helped to prevent clinical scurvy.[153] In addition, the expedition undoubtedly ate a variety of roots and bulbs they learned about from the Indians: camas (*Camassia quamash*), wapato (*Sagittaria latifolia*), and others, probably including Indian potato, cattails, and the bitterroot (*Lewisia rediviva*). Usually the plants were dried and pounded into flour to make into a bread.[154]

There was a lot of luck involved in the travelers' survival. For example, grizzly bear encounters were frequent, especially after they entered what is now Montana, but not one man was injured by a bear. One day, near the Great Falls, Lewis was chased into the Missouri River by a grizzly bear, charged by three bull buffaloes, and he awoke the next morning with a rattlesnake coiled ten feet away.[155] All along the Missouri River and especially above the Great Falls to Oregon, the Corps saw numerous rattlesnakes, but only one snakebite was recorded. Joseph Field was bitten on the ankle on July 4, 1804. Although he suffered local swelling and pain, Field responded to a poultice of bark and gunpowder.[156] Most likely only partial envenomation occurred, and he was spared the more severe and generalized toxic symptoms that can lead to death in some cases.

The expedition experienced a few near misses, but fortune seemed to be on their side in almost every case. Furthermore, none of the expedition members contracted any of the killer diseases of the era such as smallpox, yellow fever, malaria, cholera, or typhoid. The expedition's only death was that of Sergeant Charles Floyd on August 20, 1804. That the group suffered only one fatality is miraculous considering the difficulties and dangers of the long trek.

Floyd's death occurred early in the trip. He became sick on the way up the Missouri to the Mandan villages, where the Corps would spend their first winter. Early in Floyd's illness, Lewis bled the man, the usual procedure. In his journal on July 31, Floyd wrote, "I am verry sick and has ben for Somtime but have Recovered my helth again."[157] The recovery was an illusion, however. By August 19 his situation had become serious. The next day, Clark said that Floyd was "as bad as he can be ... no pulse." He died and was buried near the present site of Sioux City, Iowa. From what we know about Floyd's illness, his death was almost certainly due to appendicitis with rupture and subsequent peritonitis. The relief he felt on July 31 was not inconsistent with this conclusion: after rupture, a short period of improvement is not unusual. In that era, this ailment was referred to as "colic" or "locked bowels." It was common and almost always fatal. Even if the sergeant had been in a metropolis rather than the wilderness, he undoubtedly would have died, as appendectomy was an unknown surgical procedure at the time.

"Their favorite physician": The Corps among the Indians

The Corps arrived at the Mandan villages, on the Missouri River in what is now North Dakota, in October 1804. There the men constructed a small circular fort of timber covered with sod and twigs. It was a remarkably dry and warm enclosure in which the expedition passed a comfortable winter. A latrine was built about a hundred yards from the sleeping huts and the main building.[158] Little was known about sanitation then; the outhouse was more for comfort than for hygiene. Nevertheless, building a good latrine and placing it away from the living quarters was a wise move.

In February 1805, while at the Mandan villages, Lewis was present at the delivery of the teenage Sacagawea's baby boy. When her labor appeared prolonged, she was given a "dose" of crushed rattles from a snake—a folk medicine supposed to enhance labor. Although this charm was administered just before the child was born, Lewis didn't believe the material had any effect.[159]

The captains treated some of the Mandans' ailments at the expedition's winter camp, and later they doctored Chinooks, Klickitats, Nez Perces, and other natives along their route. Among the Indians' complaints were fevers, "Rhumitism," eye infections, and other ailments. Clark even splinted broken limbs using "broad sticks" and lint bandages. One morning, Clark saw four men, eight women, and a child for various complaints ranging from sore joints to hysteria. The hysterical woman was given thirty drops of laudanum, and liniment was dispensed for the painful joints.

Treatments as simple as an eyewash composed of white vitriol (zinc sulphate), lead acetate, sugar, salt, and rainwater was a popular item with many natives suffering from "soar" eyes. Most of the tribes along the Columbia suffered from eye disorders, ranging from simple conjunctivitis to blindness. Probably a myriad of diseases such as gonorrhea, syphilis, trachoma, and other infections were to blame for some of the more severe cases. Less serious problems were likely associated with gnats, mosquitoes, wind, blowing sand and grit, and sun glare. The captains' eyewashes, the only treatment available at the time, were apparently successful in many instances.[160]

The deplorable living conditions of many of the tribes along the route, particularly on the Columbia River, were lamented by both Lewis and Clark in their chronicles. The Samaritan contribution the captains made in the West was not exceeded by those who came later. Although Lewis was the expedition's physician-in-chief, it was Clark who developed a reputation as a healer among the natives. Of the Walla Wallas in May 1805, Lewis wrote in his journal, "My friend Capt. C. is their favorite physician."[161] In a demonstration of ethical responsibility, he added, "We take care to give them no article which can possibly injure them."[162]

Eventually the captains realized that the humanitarian aid they provided could benefit themselves as well. It was on the return trip up the Columbia River, in need of food and supplies but with their trade baubles long since bartered, they recognized that their medical expertise was a commodity and could be traded. While the expedition camped with the Nez Perces, waiting for the snows to melt before crossing the Bitterroot Mountains, historian Stephen Ambrose tells us, "Lewis did most of the smoking and talking with the chiefs, while Clark practiced medicine."[163] Every morning during their stay with the Nez Perces, Clark's patients were lined up and waiting. Clark's medical know-how paid for over sixty desperately needed horses.[164]

The captains also learned some medical lore from the natives. Both of them were impressed with the Indians' use of "sweat baths" in the treatment of certain ailments, especially rheumatism. On the way back, on the Columbia River, one of the soldiers suffered a severe, almost totally debilitating back disorder that was relieved with this therapy.[165]

The Indians also taught the explorers how to make pemmican, a staple food of the natives. This lightweight, nutritious, high-caloric preparation of dried meat and berries was a boon to the expedition. In addition, the natives showed them how to find edible plants and how to prepare skins for clothing. Another very practical skill the men learned from the Indians was how to castrate a horse properly. Stud horses were unruly and often dangerous, but some of the horses the soldiers castrated became infected; a few of them bled, and at least one died. A Nez Perce

Indian demonstrated how to avoid these complications. Lewis wrote, "He cut them without tying the string to the stone . . . he takes care to scrape the string clean from all adhering veigns before he cuts it."[166] Later, Lewis declared the Indian method of castration far superior to his, and some veterinarians still use this crude but safe procedure.

In regard to the Indians, President Jefferson, in his final instructions to Lewis prior to the expedition, included the specific instruction to "carry with you some matter of the kine-pox; inform those of them [the Indians] with whom you may be of its efficacy as a preservative from the small pox: & instruct & encourage them in the use of it."[167] Unfortunately, this presidential order was not accomplished. On his trip down the Ohio River, Lewis found that his supply of vaccine had "lost its virtue." He wrote to Jefferson for more, but a fresh supply never reached the captains.[168]

"Amorous contact": Venereal Disease

During the Corps's stay at Fort Mandan, the relatively lenient sexual mores of the Indians combined with the lustful appetites of the young soldiers guaranteed the spread of venereal disease. The Mandans on the Missouri River, and later the Shoshones, Nez Perces, and Chinooks along the Columbia, were a constant reservoir of infection, and at least eight men in the Corps of Discovery were infected with gonorrhea or syphilis during the trip. As E. G. Chuinard put it, the men of the expedition paid for "indulgences with Indian maidens with blue beads and venereal disease."[169] The Shoshones had only limited previous contact with whites, and Lewis was "anxious to learn whether these people had the venerial." Finding its definite presence in the tribe brought him to a conclusion that is only partly correct: "Gonaroehah and Louis venerae (syphilis) are native disorders of America."[170]

On January 14, 1805, at Fort Mandan, Lewis recorded "several" men "with the Venereal cought from the Mandan Women."[171] Clark wrote, "Generally helthy except Venerials Complaints which is very common amongst the natives and the men Catch it from them."[172] At this time in history, some medical men believed that syphilis and gonorrhea were simply manifestations of the same condition. Lewis and Clark correctly viewed them as two different afflictions, though it would be many years before the causes of gonorrhea and syphilis were discovered.

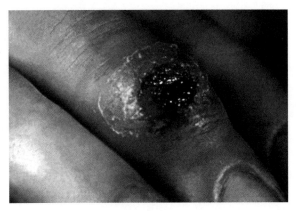

Extragenital syphilitic chancre. Syphilis has plagued mankind for thousands of years. The chancre usually develops on the external genitalia and is the first evidence of an infection. Until the discovery of penicillin, doctors relied on mercury compounds such as calomel for treatment.
—Courtesy Centers for Disease Control and Prevention

Syphilis (sometimes called Lues or French Disease) and gonorrhea were both endemic and epidemic in the native population. These conditions were certainly familiar to army officers, and their development among the men of the Corps was no surprise. The leaders' medicine chest was prepared with penis syringes, mercury salve, and calomel (mercurous chloride). To treat gonorrheal urethritis, penile syringes were used to inject a solution called saccharum (lead acetate) into the urethra. Gonococcal bacteria, transmitted through sexual intercourse, cause inflammation and a purulent discharge from the urethra. It is not nearly as serious as syphilis, and repeated treatments were usually effective.

Since the Renaissance, the accepted treatment for syphilis, and the one used by Lewis and Clark, was mercury. This heavy metal was administered in two ways. Mercurial ointments were rubbed directly into the skin, and calomel was given orally. When the patient's gums became sore from the toxic side effect of calomel, and the exterior symptoms, such as the skin rash or sores, disappeared, the drug was discontinued. We know now that the disappearance of symptoms doesn't mean that the disease is cured, though sometimes it must have been.

On January 27, 1806, Lewis wrote, "Goodrich has recovered from the Louis veneri [syphilis] which he contracted from an amorous contact with a chinnook damsel. I cured him as I did Gibson last winter by uce of murcury."[173] Six months later, however, both of these men exhibited the rash of the secondary stage of syphilis. Following the rash, there is a latent interval that can last many years before the terrible onset of tertiary syphilis, with its complications such as neurosyphilis, aortic aneurysm,

Charcot joints, and other terminal conditions. Both men died young, and it is possible that their shortened lives were attributable to uncured syphilis.

Some scientists now think that Meriwether Lewis himself acquired syphilis, and that his psychotic and bizarre behavior, culminating in his suicide in 1809, are consistent with symptoms of paresis due to tertiary syphilis. If so, he is only one of a long list of famous people who died as a result of this infection's progression to the central nervous system. A third of people with untreated syphilis progress to the tertiary stage. The debate over the cause of Lewis's death, whether it was suicide or murder, will probably never be settled. If it was suicide, syphilis may or may not have been a factor. Depression or alcoholism or both, and perhaps other unknown factors, are more likely causes. But Lewis may have been exposed to syphilis in August 1805, on his thirty-first birthday. Following a Shoshone tribal celebration, several of the men caught syphilis, and, although not recorded by either leader, it was reported that after this visit Lewis suffered for longer than a month from some mysterious illness. He made no notes in his journal for three months.[174]

Near Catastrophes

The Corps experienced a few—surprisingly few—incidents where members' lives were in peril. Lewis and a companion were nearly killed when they slipped off a cliff, but they managed to pull themselves back up. Others came close to drowning when boats capsized—many of the voyagers could not swim.

One of the most serious episodes was Sacagawea's illness in June 1805, at the confluence of the Marias and Missouri Rivers. Clark said on June 15, 1805, "Our Indian woman Sick & low spirited I gave her the bark & apply it exteranaly to her region which revived her much."[175] The next day, Lewis made comprehensive notes about the sixteen-year-old Sacagawea's condition. She was, he wrote, "extreemly ill. . . . This gave me some concern, with a young child in her arms, as from the consideration of her being our only dependence for a friendly negotiation with the Snake Indians on whom we depend for horses to assist us in our portage from the Missouri to the columbia river."[176]

Lewis bled her once and gave her opium, "barks," and mineral water.[177] He obtained the water from a highly sulphurous mineral spring located on a bench of land near the mouth of Belt (Portage) Creek.[178] Later, with obvious relief, he noted, "She feels herself much freer from pain. She complains principally of the lower region of the abdomen, I therefore continued the cataplasms of barks and laudnum which had been previously used by my friend Capt Clark. I believe her disorder originated principally from an obstruction of the mensis in consequence of taking could."[179] Her symptoms of pelvic pain, fever, and irregular menses are consistent with a diagnosis of pelvic inflammatory disease, an infection of the internal genitalia. The condition may have been the result of her recent pregnancy or gonorrhea or chlamydia, or a combination of the three.

The spring water probably supplied her with much-needed minerals and fluid lost during the prolonged sickness, and she recovered.[180] On June 17 Lewis reported, "The Indian woman much better today. I have still continued the same course of medecine; she is free from pain clear of fever, her pulse regular, and eats as heartily as I am willing to permit her of broiled buffaloe well seasoned with pepper and salt and rich soope of the same meat; I think therefore that there is every rational hope of her recovery."[181] Medical historian Dr. E. G. Chuinard writes that Captain Lewis's notes "are impressive because they are made by a non-medical man. His recording of the patient's complaints, his physical examination of her, the medication employed, and his genuine concern about her probably would not be exceeded by any physician of his time."[182]

Toward the end of May on the return journey, little Pompey became very ill with fever and swelling in his neck. Lewis accurately diagnosed his symptoms as related to teething (probably a secondary infection of the tonsils or throat with regional glandular inflammation) and considered his condition dangerous. The child was treated at first, in the standard of the times, with purges, including at least one enema. In addition, very hot poultices of boiled onions were applied to the swelling for several days, offering little relief except that the fever began to abate. On May 27, about five days after the onset of the illness, Lewis wrote, "Charbono's son is much better today."[183]

On the final leg of the trip, during a hunting expedition, Lewis was accidentally shot in the buttock by the partially blind boatman Peter Cruzatte. As Lewis describes the accident, "A ball struck my left thye about an inch below my hip joint, missing the bone it passed through. . . . The stroke was very severe. . . . I took off my clothes and dressed my wounds . . . introducing tents of patent lint into the ball holes. . . . I slept on board. . . . The pain I experienced excited a high fever."[184]

Fortunately, the wound was entirely within the soft tissue, and no bone or vital structures was injured. The lint apparently kept the wound open, to avoid a closed space that could harbor bacteria. As he recuperated, Lewis retained dedication to science. In severe pain and with a fever, he made a meticulous description in his journal of a type of cherry he had discovered along the bank of the river.[185] He measured and described the plant in scientific detail while lying prone in his pirogue, with a very painful posterior. Twenty-five days after the event, Clark wrote, "My worthy friend Cap Lewis has entirely recovered."[186]

True Physicians: "Humanity shown at all times"

By the time the Corps of Discovery returned to St. Louis in 1806, both Meriwether Lewis and William Clark were experienced physicians. They had successfully assisted in the delivery of Sacagawea's infant, and they had treated both mother and child for serious infections during the trip. They had also amputated gangrenous toes; sutured lacerations; treated many upper respiratory diseases and fevers; relieved diverse skin disorders and eye irritations; "cured" syphilis and gonorrhea; adequately immobilized minor fractures and reduced shoulder dislocations; and incised and drained abscesses, including whitlows.

Most of all, Lewis and Clark were kind, compassionate, humanitarian, and professional in their dealings with the natives and with their own men. One cannot read the journals without coming to this conclusion. As testimony to the accomplishments of Meriwether Lewis and William Clark, a member of the Corps, Private Joseph Whitehouse, expressed in his account of the great journey "my utmost gratitude . . . for the humanity shown at all times by them [the captains]."[187] The simple fact of their surviving the eight-thousand-mile trek—overcoming hardships, illnesses, physical discomfort, and almost daily brushes with death—is impressive. But more than that, the expedition carried forward a humanitarian medical duty, and Captains Clark and Lewis abundantly fulfilled that obligation. They were physicians in the true sense of the word.

THREE

Mountain Men
Hunting-Knife Surgeons

. . . and there wasn't any sound
Except a bridle made it. Then it came—
That funny sort of feeling, just the same
I had out there a little while ago—
A feel of something you could never know,
But it was something big and still and dim
That wouldn't tell. It seemed to come from him
Just looking down the Sandy towards the Green
That had been waiting yonder to be seen
A million winters and a million springs
And summers! 'Twas the other side of things—
Another world.

—From *The Song of Jed Smith*[188]

IMMEDIATELY AFTER THE Lewis and Clark expedition was completed in 1806, unprecedented numbers of trappers and fur traders began to come to the distant plains and mountains in what is now Idaho, Montana, Utah, Wyoming, and elsewhere. The creeks that drained into the Madison, the Jefferson, and the Gallatin Rivers had a "wealth of furs not surpassed by the mines of Peru."[189] With beaver hats in style in the metropolitan centers of the world, great profits were expected for trappers and traders. In 1830 beaver pelts were selling for $6 per pound in St. Louis, and each adult pelt weighed about two pounds. In a good season, two partners might trap as many as a thousand beavers and, by the standard of the times, become rich men.

63

In addition to its promise of wealth, the West was the setting of colorful legends of noble adventure. Men such as John Colter, Manuel Lisa, Jim Bridger, Hugh Glass, Jed Smith, and William Sublette were folk heroes, and tavern yarns of their exciting exploits were spun against a backdrop of snowcapped mountains, emerald forests, broad verdant valleys, crystal streams, and an abundance of nature's marvels. Such stories were powerful invitations to come west. To the few who would brave it, the exhilaration of risk and the sensuality of discovery were felt deep down in the vitals.

It is doubtful that anyone gave much thought to the health or welfare of these adventurers—neither the men themselves nor the entrepreneurs who planned and financed the expeditions. Each person chose his own trail and could not foresee how his passage would proceed. Survival depended on the weather, the natives, and other unpredictable factors. Every man was expected to travel light, live off the land, and look out for himself. The trapper's "possibles," or "fixins," were bare essentials, with no room for medical supplies. The typical outfit included a powder horn; a sack of musket balls; a flintlock pistol; a fifty-caliber gun; a knife with an eight- or ten-inch blade, sharpened to the hilt; and a leather "possible" sack containing an awl, extra flints, some extra powder, and perhaps some tobacco, sugar, and coffee. The trapper supplemented his provisions at the annual rendezvous, where liquor was the most popular item for sale.

Alcohol was the trapper's panacea for medical problems. It was the only anesthetic available, and most illnesses responded to alcohol, too. Whiskey was used in conjunction with sweat baths, herbal remedies, and many other treatments. In addition, coal oil was highly prized as a liniment, and bear grease was liberally applied to wounds of all kinds and used internally for sluggish bowels. Many mountain man remedies were copied from Indian culture.

Most trappers camped alone or in isolated small groups. Except during the most bitter winter months, they were nomadic, so they were seldom exposed to infectious diseases. The rivers and streams were clean, not yet contaminated with cholera or typhoid. But the risk of injury or death from exposure, violence, and accidents was high. At least a hundred men died while working for the American Fur Company. One early trapper, James Ohio Pattie, said that only 16 men out of 116 survived their first year's trapping experience in the Southwest.[190] There were exceptions, of course—Jim Bridger (Ol' Gabe) lived to be seventy-seven.

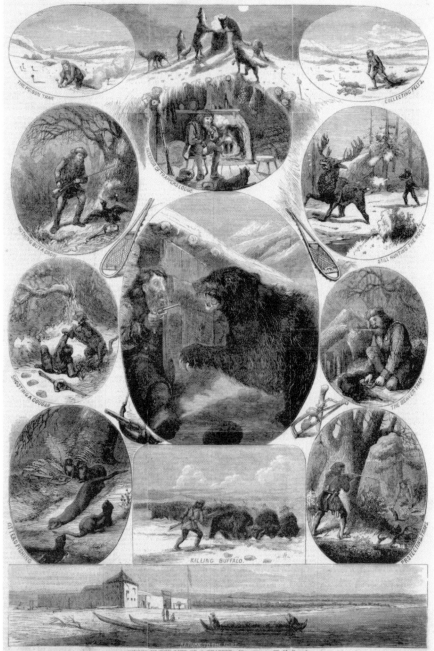

SCENES IN THE LIFE OF A TRAPPER. —[SKETCHED BY W. M. CADY.]

A mountain man's life was not an easy one. This drawing by William de la Montagne depicts some of the scenes of a trapper's life. —Courtesy Denver Public Library

Friends and Enemies

As Indian tribes grew angry with the seemingly endless line of strangers arriving in their midst, numerous unwary or unlucky trappers lost their lives. Trapper and outfitter Daniel T. Potts, after a particularly bad winter in 1827–28, wrote, "The Indians on one part and the hard winter on the other has been my sad ruin and have lost not less than one thousand dollars. The horses which the winter did not destroy, the early visits of the Black feet swept away with from twelve to fifteen scalps of our hunters."[191] Yet it is interesting how often the natives helped white people. Potts, while in the Wind River Valley, became separated from his companions and froze his feet. Unable to travel, he was rescued by friendly Indians.

Indians often knew better how to survive the rigors of the western climate. In 1835 three Canadian men were caught in the open by a furious blizzard. Their Indian guide urged them to huddle with him beneath some bedding for survival, but they refused. He saved himself by digging a tunnel into the snow, where he lay for twelve hours, then went for help. A search party from Fort Union uncovered the three men two days later. One man died, and another had his legs "sawed off with a wood saw" at the fort. The third man lost his feet, ears, and some fingers. The Sioux guide suffered only the loss of a portion of his ears and nose.[192]

Grizzly Tales

Along with other dangers, frontiersmen encountered a lot of ferocious bears. One early trapper, George C. Yount, said he sometimes killed five or six bears a day and had sighted as many as sixty in twenty-four hours.[193] In Jedediah Smith's most famous grizzly story, after being badly mutilated, he talked a young companion through the procedure of sewing up his extensive scalp lacerations and replacing one of his ears—undoubtedly the first recorded plastic surgery procedure in the West. Afterward, Smith mounted his horse and rode to camp.

Another legendary story was of Hugh Glass, who was mauled by a grizzly but managed to kill it with only his hunting knife. One of Glass's companions, Jim Bridger, found him and later described his face as "all scraped off." A day or two later, sure that he would die, his fellows took his "fixins" and abandoned him. How he survived in the wilderness, without a gun or knife, is a profile of endurance and courage. He eventually confronted those who left him for dead, but rather than wreak vengeance, he forgave them.[194]

Armed and Dangerous

While exposure to extreme weather, bear attacks, and other dangers regularly threatened trappers, the most serious injuries they suffered were usually gunshot and arrow wounds. "I once met a trapper," wrote Francis Parkman, "whose breast was marked with the scars of six bullets and arrows, one of his arms broken by a shot and one of his knees shattered; yet still, with the mettle of New England, whence he had come, he continued to follow his perilous calling."[195]

One old-timer described with startling nonchalance how his partner, Dick Somes, survived an attack by Pawnees. "Dick was as full of arrows as a porky-pine: one was stickin' right through his cheek, one in his meatbag, and two more 'bout his hump ribs. I tuk 'em all out slick, and away we goes to camp."[196]

Not all wounds were inflicted by hostile Indians. Trappers were a rough bunch ready to fight among themselves. The often-told tale of frontiersman Mike Fink and his friend Carpenter (first name unknown) illustrates this point. Fink and Carpenter often demonstrated their courage, marksmanship, and trust by shooting tin cups full of whiskey off each other's head. When during this dangerous game Fink shot Carpenter between the eyes, he claimed it was an accident, but the two had recently battled brutally over the affections of a half-Indian woman, and Fink had lost the contest. Another friend of Carpenter's, named Talbot, accused Fink of murder on the spot and shot him dead.[197]

In addition to intentional violence, accidents involving firearms occurred frequently. Andrew Broadus's forearm was shattered when the gun he was pulling from his wagon discharged. At first he refused amputation, the only treatment to prevent gangrene. As the mangled flesh putrified, the stubborn, suffering man finally relented. Luckily for Broadus, Kit Carson, the youngest person in the group but competent beyond his years, volunteered to do the surgery. He whetted his skinning knife, found a saw, prepared a hot fire to heat a searing tool for the stump, and removed the mutilated arm. Within days the stump was healed.[198]

Mountain Medics

As the previous stories show, when trappers needed medical care, it was often self-administered or administered by untrained companions. After he was struck by an Indian's bullet, "Peg Leg" Smith, a frontiersman in Missouri, amputated his own leg using a bullet mold as a hemostat, his razor-sharp hunting knife, and a tomahawk to chop the bone. Smith's only anesthesia was a few cups of a liquor known as Taos lightning, a mixture of Mexican aguardiente and raw corn whiskey.[199]

In 1838 Osborne Russell—an early frontier trapper and later a judge, cattleman, and merchant—also doctored his own wounds. He was camped with a few friends near Yellowstone Lake when the party was attacked by Blackfeet. Russell was hit with two arrows, which he immediately pulled out, then he managed to escape. He wrote, "my leg was very much swelled and painful but I managed to get along slowly on crutches." Later, he bathed the wounds in salt water and made a salve of castoreum and beaver oil. He says this eased the pain and "drawn out the swelling."[200] Russell survived his years as a trapper and lived a long life.

As self-reliant as the mountain men were, their survival often depended on one another. In a biography of Jed Smith, *The Splendid Wayfaring*, John Neihardt tells of an episode in which Smith's fellow trappers saved his life twice. A grizzly had mangled his thigh and would have killed him if his companions hadn't come to his rescue. But as he lay helplessly by the fire in camp, his two friends were killed and scalped by Indians. Hearing the shooting, Smith dragged himself painfully into the brush and watched as the Indians confiscated everything from the camp: food, blankets, pelts, saddles, livestock, and clothing. He was now alone in the wilderness, but he would survive yet again. Other trappers found him and brought him back to the main encampment on a litter. Within days, he was planning more adventures.[201]

There were no trained doctors in the wilderness, but a few mountain men passed as doctors. Richard Dunlop suggests that Kit Carson was one of the best hunting-knife surgeons in the West. During the Fremont expedition, Carson taught others how to extract an arrow. Sometimes it was necessary to push it through and cut off the head. If this couldn't be done, only the shaft was removed and the arrowhead was left in to be cut out later.[202] Other frontiersmen also became adept at removing arrows or bullets from their companions—"butchered out" was the term.

Most of the time, the mountain men used good judgment in knowing which arrows to extract and which to leave in place. Many of them knew something that physicians later learned the hard way: except in very superficial wounds, it is far better to leave the foreign body where it lodged than to destroy normal tissue, produce additional hemorrhage, and introduce infection. The trapper-surgeon also understood, as did the Native American, that opening and draining penetrating wounds were required to prevent infection from developing within the enclosed space.

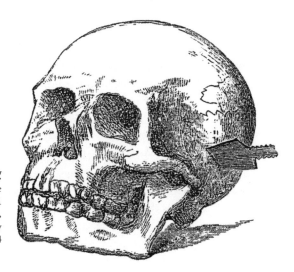

Indian arrow penetrating temporal bone —From *The Science and Art of Surgery: A Treatise on Surgical Injuries, Diseases, and Operations* by John Eric Erichsen, 1884

In addition to his surgical skills, Kit Carson had remedies for other maladies. For lice infestations, which were common, Carson tossed his clothes onto an ant hill, and while the ants feasted on the lice, he washed the miserable bugs off his body in a stream.[203] Paul C. Phillips tells about another trader reputed to be a skillful physician, William T. Hamilton. Though he had no medical training, Hamilton had a reputation of mythical proportions. Mountain men sought him out whenever they could, and some Indians preferred him over their own medicine men.[204]

One of the earliest fur traders to explore the West was Englishman David Thompson. As early as 1798, working for the Hudson's Bay Company, Thompson traveled to the Mandan villages on the Missouri River, and he had already crossed the Continental Divide and was working in the Peace River country when Lewis and Clark started up the Missouri in 1804. He later recorded his adventures in a memoir entitled *Narrative of Travels in Western North America, 1784-1812.*

Thompson was not only a businessman, explorer, surveyor, map maker, and student of native peoples and languages, but he was also a skilled healer. Amazingly, he was also a family man who brought his wife, Charlotte, and children with him on the trail much of the time, along with an entourage of trappers, their families, and helpers. The presence of women and children reassured the Indians they encountered that the party was peaceful, allowing them to mingle with the tribes in a friendly and personal way. This kind of frontier excursion was totally different from those of the American fur traders, who traveled alone or in small groups without their families.

Relying on natural intelligence, common sense, and some knowledge of medicine, Thompson rendered medical care to his family, his associates, and the natives. Once, while in the Flathead and Kootenai region, he treated many sick natives who suffered possibly from some form of measles, which he described as, "a violent Cold which generally ends in a Rash breaking thro' the Skin." Thompson prescribed a "Purge of Salts with a little Paregoric Elixer," which he claimed "soon eases them entirely." On another occasion, Thompson treated Kootenais stricken with a "violent Distemper" that he diagnosed as "Hooping Cough," of which several children died. For this illness Thompson administered doses of turlington (an elixir of balsamic resin).[205]

A few weeks after this episode, two of Thompson's daughters became ill with roundworms, a common intestinal disease transmitted from animals to humans. Twelve-year-old Fanny recovered, but seven-year-old Emma grew worse. Tirelessly, Thompson nursed his daughter and treated her with calomel, Carolina pinkroot, and castor oil, but she died. Over the years he lost several of his children to various afflictions, but he himself lived to age eighty-seven.

Backcountry Surgery

The first recorded surgical procedure in the West was a sagittectomy, the removal of an arrow. After Spanish explorer Alvar Nunez Cabeza de Vaca survived a shipwreck off the Texas coast in 1528, he and some companions were taken prisoner by the aborigines. His journal records the operation as follows: "Here they brought a man to me and said that a long time ago he had been wounded with an arrow through the right shoulder, and the arrowhead was lodged over the heart." According to the journal, the arrowhead traversed the cartilage of the chest. "I opened his chest. . . . I continued to cut . . . and with great difficulty I finally extracted it. . . . He bled profusely all over me." With strands of animal hair, Cabeza de Vaca "staunched" the flow of blood. Later the explorer-turned-surgeon removed the stitches and said proudly, "The wound I had made was no more apparent than a crease in the palm of the hand."[206]

Another famous tale of frontier surgery involved Jim Bridger. Ol' Gabe was whacked with two Blackfeet arrows in his back in 1832. His friend Tom Fitzpatrick was able to pull one of them free, but the other was too deeply imbedded. The sinews holding the shaft to the arrowhead were softened by Bridger's blood, thus the shaft separated and the projectile stayed in. Bridger's wounds healed, and the foreign object stayed in place until the Trappers' Rendezvous on the Green River in 1835. It so happened that Dr. Marcus Whitman, physician and missionary, was visiting the rendezvous encampment at the time. With difficulty and without anesthesia of any kind, Whitman removed the arrowhead from Bridger's back. According to Whitman, the three-inch-long arrowhead was bent and hooked at the point, and it was surrounded by "cartilege." The successful operation established Dr. Whitman's reputation, and he was kept busy throughout the rest of the rendezvous extracting arrowheads and bullets from other trappers and Indians. Years later, when Ol' Gabe was asked how he could have carried an arrowhead in his body so long, he answered, "In the mountains meat never spoils."[207]

Some mountain men's survival bordered on the miraculous. According to the stories, many injuries were extensive and contaminated. Of course we don't know how many of the injured died of infection, but at that time these hardy souls undoubtedly had considerable resistance or immunity to a multitude of potentially dangerous bacteria.

Dubious Legacy

As colorful as its history was, the fur trade changed the great western plains and Rocky Mountains forever, and not for the better. According to Malone, Roeder, and Lang in *Montana: A History of Two Centuries*, the fur trade began what would lead to "Montana's long and sad history of pillaging the environment, stripping the surface wealth, and returning little of the proceeds."[208]

The damage wasn't all ecological. Along with supplies and trading goods, the American Fur Company steamboats brought, in the nasal passages and lungs of the passengers, the diseases that killed thousands of Indians. Also on board were numerous casks of whiskey and the devastation it wrought. Civilization had arrived, only twenty years after the Corps of Discovery opened the way.

FOUR

Health on the Western Trails

Hope and Suffering

We left a dead man by the name of Middleton on the levee at St. Louis, and thought that we had left all the cholera with him. We were grievously disappointed, however. At noon . . . a boy, was taken and died the next day.

—Israel Shipman Pelton Lord, May 6, 1849[209]

IN 1849 DR. ISRAEL SHIPMAN PELTON LORD was restless in Illinois, tired of the failing economy and excited by the news of gold strikes in California. As a physician, he knew he could be useful—doctors would be needed on the trip and in the mining camps. Young, healthy, and adventurous, he and a few friends took off, choosing to travel overland. (The alternative was to go by ship via Panama.) A few years later, Lord returned to the States disillusioned by what he had seen. He wrote in a letter in 1851, "I think ninety-nine out of every hundred who shall hereafter go to California, are either madmen, fools—or radically unprincipled, and of course, dishonest."[210]

By the time of the gold rush that Dr. Lord joined, Americans had already been gazing hopefully west for many years. As early as 1824, long caravans of traders and emigrants began to follow the Santa Fe Trail through the Southwest. Along the way, they traversed a gauntlet of danger and disease, risking everything from wagon accidents to scurvy. A few of the early emigrant trains had doctors, but according to historian Louis J. Moorman, they "were commonly so incapable that travelers usually preferred amateur treatment by experienced traders and mountain men."[211]

As more trails opened up, religious groups also turned their attention toward the western expanse of America. In 1834 Pope Gregory XVI sent the Society of Jesus, also known as the Jesuits, to tend to the spiritual care of the Native Americans. Around the same time, American Protestants went west with a similar mission to convert the "benighted heathens." By the 1840s, many more had joined the migration, but with different objectives. Among these travelers were settlers in search of fruitful farmland; a disenfranchised religious group known as the Mormons, looking for refuge; and fortune seekers rushing to unearth the West's mineral treasures. While the dreams they pursued on the frontier varied, the path they followed to get there was invariably fraught with hardship and tragedy.

Missionaries

In the 1830s and 1840s, many young American Protestants were caught up in the nineteenth-century revival known as the Second Great Awakening. These believers were strongly committed to bringing "light" to the Indian tribes of the West. The first movement began in April 1835, when Reverend Samuel Parker and Dr. Marcus Whitman struggled up the Missouri by boat, then joined a fur caravan for the long overland journey to the Oregon Territory.

Parker and Whitman were quiet men from the East, in contrast to their escorts, who had been toughened by life in the wilderness and lived by their own rules. On the first Sunday of the trek, the preachers refused to travel on the Sabbath and, even more confounding to their hosts, refused the trappers' offer of alcohol. The mountain men took this as an insult of such magnitude that some even plotted to kill the missionaries. As luck would have it, however, an epidemic of cholera struck the party that day. As many of the trappers became sick, Whitman administered medical care and Parker served as a nurse. Although the men were bewildered by the missionaries' behavior, they were no longer resentful. During the rest of the trek, with every contact with natives on the trail, Parker and Whitman plied their religious effort.[212]

In 1838 Whitman returned to the Northwest with his new wife, several associates, including fellow Presbyterian minister Henry H. Spalding, and their wives to establish the first permanent settlement in the Walla Walla Valley, at a place called Waiilatpu. Whitman had earned a degree in medicine in 1832 at the College of Physicians and Surgeons of New York, and he was as well-educated as any doctor at the time. He and the other missionaries had brought a large supply of medicines, including smallpox "matter," but judging from their letters and diaries, the goal of the mission was primarily evangelistic rather than medical.

Among the followers to the Whitman's Oregon Mission were newly-weds Asa and Sarah Smith. "My desire is to go to that field where I can be of the most service to the cause of Christ," Asa wrote in requesting a missionary assignment.[213] Neither they nor the people who sent them appreciated the cultural differences they would face. On September 4, 1838, Sarah wrote in her diary, "Soon I hope to engage in the duties of a missionary life, instructing the ignorant, relieving the distressed & leading to virtue the degraded host."[214] When she penned this, Sarah had just completed a side-saddle horseback ride of nineteen hundred miles. During the trip Sarah suffered "almost a constant pain in my side & pressure upon my lungs." Her husband Asa, who had some medical training but not a complete course, treated her. "Have been bled and blister applied to my side."[215]

By the time the Oregon missionaries arrived, the local Cayuse were already distrustful of the whites who were coming into their country, and the missionaries were all but oblivious to the Indians' perspective. Furthermore, as we discover from their diaries, the evangelists' rigid, sanctimonious, and eccentric personalities clashed with one another. As one wife in Whitman's group wrote, "We have a strange company of Missionaries. Scarcely one who is not intolerable on some account."[216] They squabbled among themselves, which must have hurt their cause, both internally and in the eyes of the Indians.

With their energies splintered and their humanism channeled into proselytizing, the missionaries totally squandered their opportunity to bring some comfort and health to the natives and gain a degree of respect between the races. In late November 1847, the tensions came to a head. Whatever medical knowledge and supplies the Whitman missionaries brought to Oregon were overwhelmed by a deadly epidemic of measles among the Cayuse. Apparently blaming the missionaries for the devastation, the Indians killed Dr. and Mrs. Whitman and twelve others, tragically ending the story of the Oregon Mission of the American Board.

Meanwhile, the Pope's mission to begin the conversion of Native Americans was assigned to Father Pierre-Jean DeSmet. By 1841 this stouthearted priest, accompanied by Fathers Gregory Mengarini and Nicholas Point, had established St. Mary's Mission near present-day Stevensville, Montana. St. Mary's, the first Euro-American school, was a cultural center in the wilderness. During his extensive travels, DeSmet seemed to be impervious to danger. In a letter dated November 13, 1851, he wrote, "I escaped from a dangerous illness, from the attacks of wild beasts and enemies, from the smallpox and cholera. I passed through a camp where people were dying and rotting, alive, unhurt and untouched. I slept among the dying and dead for over a month, handling and attending on the cholera patients, and returned safe and sound. I had the happiness to place the holy waters of baptism on the foreheads of 1,586 children and adults, of whom many have since fallen victims of the two mentioned diseases, and are now forever happy."[217]

Following in DeSmet's footsteps was Father Anthony Ravalli, a well-trained and talented physician. A Jesuit who had studied medicine in Rome, Ravalli was skillful and innovative in his practice, and soon stories of his healing powers spread. In 1857 at the Colville Mission, an Indian woman who had hanged herself appeared to be dead, but Ravalli applied mouth-to-mouth rescucitation, and after forty-five minutes she breathed on her own. Needless to say, this enhanced the priest's reputation among the natives.[218]

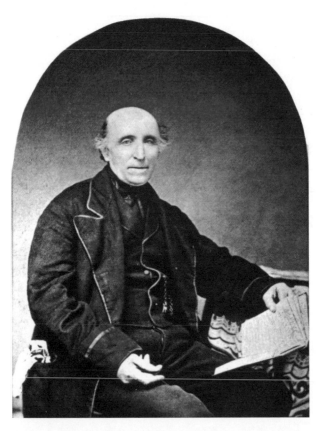

Father Anthony Ravalli followed in the footsteps of the legendary Father DeSmet. —Courtesy Montana Historical Society, Helena

As Dr. Wilfred P. Schoenberg, a well-known Portland, Oregon, Jesuit scholar noted, "At this time priests were not allowed to practice medicine without special permission from Rome. Some missionaries practiced a nonprofessional kind of medical help."[219] With or without permission from Rome, Ravalli brought medical knowledge that was truly a godsend for the Flathead Indians and for the white people of the Bitterroot Valley. He prepared his own medicines, and his treatments for frostbite and fractures were ahead of their time. Even after he became partially paralyzed by a stroke, he continued to serve the sick and dying for four more years. His death in October 1884 was mourned by the entire territory of Montana.[220] Unquestionably, his contributions and those of other Jesuits to the practice of medicine in the West, especially in western Montana, were significant.

"Every man his own physician": The Mormons

Unlike Protestant and Catholic missionaries, the Mormons came to the Rocky Mountains not to "save" the Indians, but to escape persecution. After Mormon leader Joseph Smith was murdered by a mob in Illinois in 1844, the members of the Church of Jesus Christ of Latter-Day Saints, led by Brigham Young, began a long and perilous journey west in search of a new home. It is estimated that twenty-five hundred wagons left on the initial trip, which started at the Mormons' winter quarters in Council Bluffs, Iowa, followed the North Platte River through Nebraska and Wyoming, and ended near the Great Salt Lake in Utah. Some pulled carts, some rode in wagons or on horseback, some walked leading livestock. They faced storms, rough terrain, and disease, but they made it to Salt Lake in July 1847. Over the next two decades, more than seventy thousand Mormons made the same pilgrimage.[221]

Like those of other overland pioneers before and after them, the Mormon emigrants' journey was filled not only with choking dust, treacherous mud, maddening insects, and difficult weather, but also with bad water, scarce food, sickness, and, all too often, death. Death, especially from cholera, was such a frequent occurrence on the trail that bodies were buried quickly and the trains moved on.

Among the many Mormon practices that significantly influenced the West was the church's form of medical care. The Mormons applied a system of herbal medicine called Thomsonianism, which Joseph Smith, the founder of the church, had chosen for his followers. Smith despised

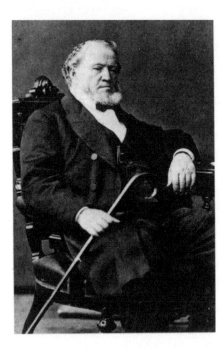

Mormon Church leader
Brigham Young —Courtesy
Utah State Historical Society

physicians. Early in his life his brother died after calomel treatment by an allopathic doctor. Smith's followers embraced his attitude toward medical matters as firmly as they did his religious beliefs.

The Thomsonian motto was "Every man his own physician." The system's originator, Samuel Thomson, born in 1769, was a self-taught practitioner who through trial and error found herbs that caused physical responses in sick people. Among his teachings were that heat was a manifestation of life and cold was the cause of all disease. Relying on plants such as *Lobelia inflata* (Indian tobacco) to cause puking, cayenne pepper to heat up the body, enemas, and vapor baths, Thomsonian medical practices worked as well as any other of the period and, since they did not use harsh treatments, probably better. By 1852 laws had been passed in Salt Lake that made Thomsonians the only legal medical practitioners.[222]

Mormons in the Great Basin used urine in many treatments. It was used for chapped skin, sore eyes, and earache, and it was given internally to babies with the croup. Baby urine was valued by some Mormons as a cosmetic to improve the complexion.[223] Perhaps these therapies were in direct response to the proverb, "Drink waters out of thine own cistern." Urotherapy is an ancient practice used in many ethnic cultures. The chemical urea is known to benefit external inflammation, and we know that hormones such as estrogen, melatonin, urokinase, and others can be extracted from urine and used for specific medical problems.[224]

During the Mexican War, the U.S. government recruited five hundred Mormon men to create a wagon trail across the Southwest to San Diego. Although the "Mormon Battalion" did not face any enemy guns, they did suffer injuries when a group of wild bulls attacked them. The army doctors' standard treatment for wounds consisted of bleeding and blistering. Mormon leaders had instructed the soldiers to rely on their own herbal medicines. The expedition had two deaths, which the Mormon soldiers believed were due to the army doctors' treatments with mercury.[225]

The movement of religious groups into the West had a substantial impact on the region's development. By the end of the nineteenth century, nearly every faith was represented in the Great Plains: Protestant, Catholic, Mormon, and many others. Whether or not the groups themselves brought specific medical know-how, the presence of the pious encouraged more families to settle on the frontier, eventually creating better schools, hospitals, and public health in the formerly wild West.

"Sickness and death attended us"

Once the primary westbound trails had been blazed and tested, mass migration began. Between 1840 and 1870, more than half a million emigrants headed west, bound for Oregon, Utah's Mormon colonies, the California goldfields, or far-flung mining camps. The major migration began after January 24, 1848, when the cry of "Gold!" echoed across North America from Sutter's Mill in California. Within ten years, more discoveries in the Rocky Mountains, in the Black Hills, and in Wyoming caught the attention of thousands more restless fortune seekers. With this migration, as Elliott West put it, "the republic changed in size, purpose, and values. The two gold rushes helped knit its parts into a newly imagined union—sure in its blessings, imperial in vision, blindly arrogant, naively confident of a future of untarnishable luster."[226]

But the luster did become tarnished. About the same time gold was discovered, ships from Europe arrived in New York and New Orleans with passengers sick with cholera. Asiatic cholera, with its severe diarrhea, was so devastating that it could wipe out whole wagon trains. Its cause was unknown at that time, and there were many erroneous theories. A few suspected the true culprit: infected drinking water. Some

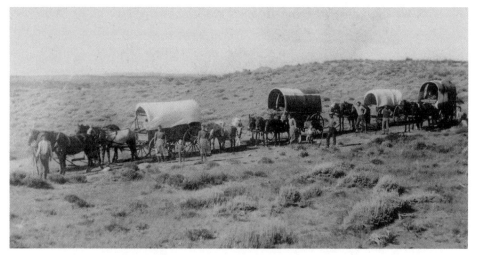

Thousands came west by wagon. Disease and injury plagued these hardy pioneers.
—Courtesy Denver Public Library

doctors, like Dr. George Davis in 1850, warned his party not to drink "Slew water" and encouraged them to drink only from running water.[227] Immigrant George Gibbs in 1849 said, "A man died today of cholera. . . . He was seen drinking copiously of swale water. . . . Two hours after he was attacked with the disease and at night was buried."[228]

Against the killer cholera, the best medicine a doctor had to prescribe was opium, called by some "the soothing monarch of medical powers." It relieved pain and slowed down the increased bowel action and cramps. Still, many doctors of the era believed that strong purges like calomel were indicated. Of course this made the already dreadful flux even worse. Doctors did not understand dehydration, fluid balance, or the need for electrolytes. Today during epidemics of cholera, many victims are saved by the simple replacement of fluids, volume for volume. In those days, survivors of this illness depended on strong constitutions, luck, and good nursing care. (For more on cholera, see chapter 14.)

In addition to cholera, diseases such as malaria, typhoid, measles, diphtheria, scarlet fever, and smallpox all took their toll. One diarist mentions that a man died of "iricipilus"; erysipelas is a serious and highly contagious form of streptococcal infection. The emigrants were undoubtedly troubled by undiagnosed conditions as well, not to mention accidents, which were frequently fatal. Kenneth L. Holmes, in *Covered Wagon Women*, says that a conservative estimate of the number of deaths from disease on the trails west between 1842 and 1859 is twenty thousand, an average of ten graves per mile.[229]

Lucia Loraine Williams wrote to her mother in September 1851 of her overland trip. "We have been living in Oregon about 2 weeks, all of us except little John, and him we left 12 miles this side of Green River. He was killed instantly by falling from a wagon and the wheels running over his head." Of her three-year-old daughter, she wrote, "Helen has been sick nearly all of the way and at the time that John died she was getting a little better. . . . She was continually sick. We think that she had scarlet fever. . . . She came out with a fine rash accompanied by a high fever. . . . Her throat was sore and she vomited blood several times."[230]

Anna Maria King, writing to relatives from Oregon in 1846, described the journey: "We had plenty of flour and bacon to last us through. . . . All this sickness and death attended us the rest of the way."[231] King's party suffered epidemics of measles, whooping cough, and "fever." On one leg of the trip, there were fifty deaths, and later a family drowned crossing the Columbia River.

Mormon newlywed Lucena Parsons saw more death during a few weeks in 1850 than most people do in a lifetime. On June 23 she wrote, "The boy that was sick died about noon. . . . These are hard times for us but it is harder for the sick. Nothing for their relief it seems." The next day, "Last evening there was 3 more died out of the same family. One was a young lady & there was a child." Fellow Mormon Sophia Lois Goodridge's diary contains a similar battery of sad events: "June 25. Crossed the creek this morning. Passed 5 graves." "June 26. One man sick with cholera. Died and was buried in the forenoon." "June 27. Sister Green died of cholera this morning. Brother Blazerd taken sick."[232]

Recalling his childhood emigration many years later, Elisha Brooks wrote, "A picture lingers in my memory of us children all lying in a row on the ground in our tent, somewhere in Iowa, stricken with the measles, while six inches of snow covered all the ground and the trees were brilliant with icicles. A delay of a week to enjoy the measles put us on our feet again and we drove on."[233]

As Brooks's semifacetious comment about "enjoying" the measles suggests, any rest period was welcome, even if it was spent suffering. The schedule of a wagon train was rigid. Most emigrants began their trip in May and had only about five months to travel before winter set in. The urgency forced families to continue regardless of health. In many cases nothing, not even death, slowed the caravans. One father whose child was ill wrote, "The trubel was, they wood not stop to docter thar sick. They wood kep a roling on."[234]

A wagon train on Ute Pass in Colorado in 1885. The trip west was arduous and dangerous.
—Courtesy Denver Public Library, Colorado Historical Society, and Denver Art Museum

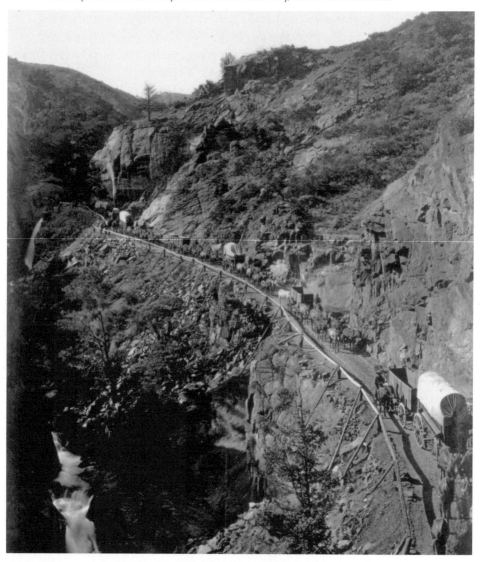

Scurvy: "As common as damaged flour"

Besides cholera and other deadly diseases, emigrants slogging across the country faced an often fatal condition known through the ages as scurvy. Whereas cholera occurred in epidemics and spread furiously, scurvy was slow in onset but just as deadly in time. Scurvy is simply a vitamin C deficiency, and although it had been recognized for hundreds of years, the cause and cure was not completely understood or even believed by many. Dr. I. S. P. Lord was as knowledgeable as any other physician of his time, but he demonstrated a lack of appreciation of the cause of scurvy in 1850 when he wrote, "scurvy as common as damaged flour. . . . And yet we seem to have pure air, soft crystal water, wholesome food, cooked well and regularly, and comforable sleep."[235]

After months on the trail—as well as in gold camps and military barracks—eating a diet of beans, salt pork, boiled beef, pancakes, and other staples of the time, people on the frontier developed scurvy. In the early stages, the victim might develop a few blemishes due to hemorrhage under the skin, swelled joints, or loose teeth. Days or weeks later the person would be totally debilitated and coughing blood. An observer described one terminal patient: "Darling with some cough, diarrhea & bloated all over, with one leg swelled full. He had applied to a doct. & got salivated [treated with calomel]. He called it Scurvy."[236]

Scurvy resulted in death unless the sufferer ingested a rich source of vitamin C, such as certain fresh vegetables, fruits, and wild plants. By trial and error, some caregivers discovered herbal vegetables that prevented scurvy—for example, pigweed (*Chenopodium album*). Watercress, high in vitamin C, readily grew along many western streams, but sadly most immigrants and even doctors did not realize its power as an antiscorbutic.[237]

Apparently, white people did not take into account that Indians and mountain men seldom suffered from scurvy. An old-timer could have told the greenhorns about his diet, copied from the Indians, which prevented scurvy. "Red muscle meat will do you in the settlements, maybe so where you can get plenty of greens and vegetables. But on the prairie you will have the cow's insides for choice marrow, lights, heart and tongue, warm liver spiced with gall, and best of all guts–plain guts–and raw at that!"[238] This may have turned the stomach of most pioneers, and they likely wouldn't have believed it worked anyway. (For more on scurvy, see chapter 6.)

Indian Attacks

In addition to disease, pioneers faced the threat of violence from Indians. In the early days, the danger from hostile natives was considerably exaggerated by some travelers and embellished by many newspaper writers. It is documented that more deaths occurred from gun accidents (most overlanders carried firearms they were ill-equipped to handle) than from Indian attacks. But in the 1860s, after the Bozeman Trail was established through Sioux country, the Indian wars became bloody. With the building of this ill-fated trail, the Cheyennes, Arapahoes, and Sioux, furious at the expanding settlement and destruction of game, launched a concerted campaign against stagecoaches, emigrant trains, mail stations, and ranches along the Platte and Missouri Rivers.

One of many hair-raising stories of the "Bloody Bozeman" involved thirteen miners with $25,000 in gold dust, who in July 1863 decided against advice to float home down the Missouri from Fort Benton. A group of Sioux soon attacked them. The miners had a cannon on their makeshift boat and fired it at the Indians, but the recoil shattered the boat and it sank. The Sioux killed all the miners, whose bodies were never found. The warriors, seeing no value in the yellow stuff the miners were carrying, dumped it in the river but kept the buckskin bags.[239]

The Sea Route

In addition to the famous (and infamous) overland trails west, there was an alternative route to California: traveling by ship. The sea journey entailed sailing to Panama, crossing the Isthmus overland, then taking another boat north to San Francisco. A much lengthier trip involved sailing all the way around South America.

For travelers headed to California, going by sea was thought to be safer than going overland. While it may have been safer from angry Indians, the "Argonauts" who chose the fifteen-thousand-mile ocean voyage found it was certainly not safer from illness. The cabins were small and airless, the ships overcrowded, and the sanitary conditions primitive. Temperatures aboard the ship could be scalding, seasickness was common, and when the traveler debarked to cross the Isthmus of Panama, the trip across was miserable. Heat, mosquitoes, fevers, combined with, as one doctor remembered, "bad coffee, the barking of dogs, squealing of pigs . . . torrential rains [and] flea-bitten nights."[240]

Food and water onboard were often of doubtful quality. Doctors placed quicklime and other chemicals in the water to make it more potable, but this did not prevent illness. One ship, the *Golden Gate*, sailing from Panama to San Francisco in August 1852, had 84 deaths from cholera within days after leaving port. The *Uncle Sam* lost 104 out of 750 passengers from the same illness. There was also yellow fever. One passenger, Frank Marryat, boarded a steamer out of Panama that was overrun with this disease, now known to be a virus transmitted by mosquitoes. Marryat wrote, "We could hear the splash of bodies as they were tossed overboard."[241]

Pioneer Caregivers

Almost all emigrant parties in wagons and on ships had among them a few physicians, or at least someone who was addressed as "doctor." Often the doctors gave their services willingly and without thought of reward. But their numbers were few, so the bulk of treatment and nursing care fell to the women. Facing everything from toothache to "locked bowels,"

A pioneer family, Henry Smith with wife and children, heading west to Colorado in 1893 —Courtesy Denver Public Library, Colorado Historical Society, and Denver Art Museum

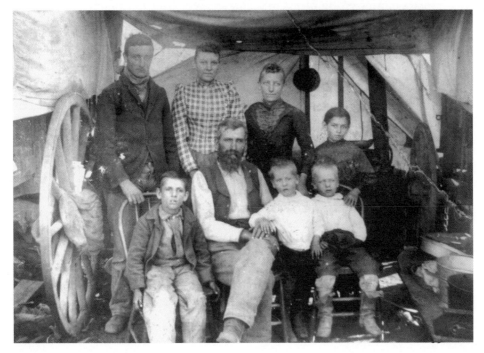

frontier wives, sisters, mothers, and grandmothers rose to the occasion. (For more on women caregivers and home remedies, see chapter 7.)

In many instances, the best the women could do was to make sick and dying loved ones as comfortable as possible. When Mary Matilda Surfus's daughter developed diphtheria on August 14, 1883, the worried mother wrote, "Ina is bad. . . . It took all my time and attention to care for Ina." When the girl became much sicker a few days later, Mary wrote, "We fixed a swing bed in the wagon and she lay on it and the jolts did not hurt her." Ina became delirious, could "scarcely breath," and hemorrhaged from her throat. She died on August 20, just six days after becoming sick.[242]

Some pioneer women practiced preventive medicine. Margaret A. Frink, while preparing to travel to the goldfields in 1850, took measures to prevent scurvy. Among the provisions for the long trip, she included "one peck of potatoes and a bushel of cucumbers and a supply of vinegar."[243] No one in her family developed scurvy during the journey.

When the emigrants reached their destinations, some of the great suffering they experienced on the trail was relieved. In many parts of the West, the United States Army had stationed units and built forts outfitted with military surgeons and even hospitals. The medical officers and military hospitals were always willing to treat civilians, giving travelers and newcomers better medical care than they might otherwise have received. (For more on military medicine, see chapter 6.) In addition, a motley group of doctors and amateur healers came west along with the rest of the pioneers and set up practices in mining camps and other settlements. Some of these places, however, had health problems of their own.

FIVE

Gold Camp Sawbones
Life and Death in the Western Mining Districts

*I little thought that the first digging I would
do in California would be digging a grave.*
—Quoted in Anthony J. Lorenz, "Scurvy in the Gold Rush"[244]

FROM THE EARLY 1850s until the early 1900s, gold and silver were magnets that pulled folks west. Thousands of fortune seekers were buried along the trail or at sea, but of those who arrived at their destination, the death rate continued to be high. New arrivals met with as much disease and danger at the goldfields as they had on the trip to get there, if not more. During the first two years of the California gold rush, ninety thousand immigrants had arrived, and "of this number, it was roughly estimated that one-fifth had found graves within the first six months after their arrival."[245] Dr. Israel Shipman Pelton Lord, upon his arrival in California, wrote in his journal on December 23, 1849, "People die here, I reckon, for 28 were buried day before yesterday."[246]

The Asiatic cholera, scurvy, and infectious diseases that stalked the trails settled in and around the mining camps, where the crude and unsanitary living conditions were an ideal environment for illness. Ships, wagons, and mule trains poured into California and, later, other areas of the West, bringing supplies, livestock, passengers—and disease. Towns became congested with people and animals, but no one understood sanitation or public health as we know it today, and health regulations were unheard of. Creeks and other water sources near the sprawling masses were contaminated with human waste and garbage. People coughed and sneezed openly and spit at random. Respiratory diseases such as influenza spread easily among people congregated in dank, poorly ventilated spaces. This firsthand description of a mining camp on the Sacramento River in 1850 offers a glimpse: "This whole concern is surrounded with filth. Bones, rags, chips, sticks, horns, skulls, hair, skin, entrails, blood, etc., etc., etc."[247]

Impure water and poorly preserved food caused various forms of dysentery, and inadequate diets resulted in nutritional deficiencies, especially scurvy. Historian Anthony J. Lorenz claims "one can conservatively estimate that 10,000 men died of scurvy, or its sequelae, in the California Gold Rush, half of them in the winters of 1848 and 1849. . . . Its victims outnumbered those of cholera."[248] One group of miners who seldom suffered from scurvy were the Chinese. They had learned to coax vitamin-rich vegetables out of the soil no matter where they were forced to live. White people were amazed that the Chinese ate green gourds, green pumpkins, and green squash, but eventually they realized that this "strange" diet prevented scurvy.[249] (For more on scurvy, see chapter 6.)

Throughout the West, mining camps rose and fell according to the mineral supply, so they tended to be jerry-built, ephemeral, and hectic places. Because the miners never knew how long they would stay, they usually lived in tents, shanties, makeshift shacks, or worse. Those who failed to find—or found and lost—their fortune in the diggings slept wherever they could, on the floors of drafty buildings or the cold ground.

The silver-mining town of Jimtown, Colorado, 1883. Sanitation was not a prime consideration in the mining camps, so infectious diseases spread easily. —Courtesy Denver Public Library, Colorado Historical Society, and Denver Art Museum

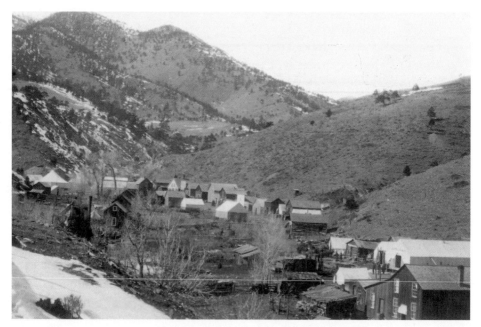

Some miners were called the "sawdust gang" because they slept on the sawdust floors of the bars. In these primitive and unclean conditions, infections spread rapidly. Clearly, survivors of illness in the gold camps had great resistance as well as luck.

Besides the prevalence of disease in the mining camps, the violent culture, dangerous working conditions, excessive drinking, and depressing environment meant further deaths from murder, accidents, and suicide. One doctor's wife in California wrote, "In the space of 24 days, we have had several murders, fearful accidents, bloody deaths, whippings, a hanging and an attempt at suicide and a fatal duel."[250] The camps had an atmosphere of desperation, and lawlessness reigned. According to one estimate, during the first five years of the gold rush, there were 4,200 murders and 1,400 suicides.[251] Accidents were also common and added significantly to the death toll.

Most of the accidents were related to the work itself. In the mine shafts were the dangers of cave-ins, falling rock, dynamite explosions, scalding water, and fires. In winter, further injuries came from exposure to bitter cold that froze poorly protected feet, hands, and other body parts. Other accidents happened in camp, where the unrestrained consumption of alcohol led to all manner of mishaps.

The rich silver deposits of the Comstock mines in Nevada came with a price in life and limb. The mines were built on top of a hydrothermal region, so the miners, in addition to all the other hazards of their profession, were exposed to superheated water. The heat and steam caused scaldings, and the poorly ventilated work spaces led to upper respiratory diseases. The dangers were remedied gradually, but not soon enough to save the many who died or were permanently disabled. To make life worse at Comstock, the miners had no toilet facilities and literally worked in a cesspool. Human excretions mixed with all the other detritus in the mines, producing an obvious source of infection.[252]

As more mineral wealth was discovered, mining communities sprang up in nearly every state in the West, and in virtually every one of these often evanescent settlements, health hazards were similar—dangerous and filthy working conditions, alcoholism, violence, malnutrition, and a multitude of contagions. Colorado miners suffered from all these problems, but in addition, with the high altitudes, they experienced a range of symptoms including headache, fatigue, lightheadedness, and pulmonary problems, now lumped under the term "altitude sickness." In this rarefied atmosphere, pneumonia became a major killer—even the healthiest miners succumbed to it.[253]

There was also a lot of tuberculosis in high-elevation mining camps. Many tuberculosis sufferers came west hoping that the dry, cold mountain air would help their "consumption." Thus were others exposed to the disease, a chronic, debilitating, and untreatable pulmonary illness. Dr. L. Rodney Pococke, the first physician to establish himself in Helena, Montana, came west from St. Louis in 1863 for the benefit of his consumption. He died two years later, earning the dubious distinction of being the first person to be buried in Helena. That winter was particularly bad, and Dr. Pococke lived in a cabin "poorly chinked" and "covered with a layer of loose, thin dirt."[254] His weak lungs could not tolerate such an environment. (For more on tuberculosis, see chapter 14.)

Though women and children were few in early mining towns, in time families began to settle in and around the more permanent camps. As they did, living conditions improved, but childhood diseases crept in. Diphtheria, whooping cough, measles, scarlet fever, and others were often epidemic in western communities, bringing sickness and death to children and sometimes adults as well.

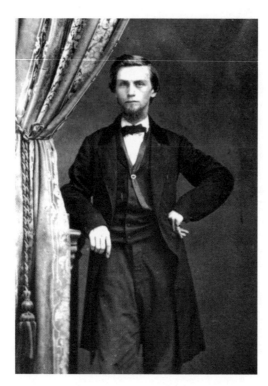

Dr. L. Rodney Pococke,
the first person to die and
be buried in Helena
—Courtesy Montana
Historical Society, Helena

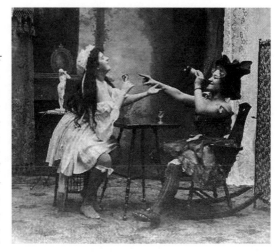

Soiled doves. The spread of venereal diseases due to prostitution was a problem in the mining camps. Tragedy stalked these "ladies of the night" in many ways—some suffered violence, many became addicted to alcohol or narcotics, and a number succumbed to infections such as tuberculosis. —Courtesy Timothy Gordon Collection, Missoula, Montana

Eventually, the settlers began to demand better medical treatment, and some mining towns built hospitals. These hospitals were among the first nonmilitary medical facilities on the frontier. (For more on mining-town hospitals, see chapter 11.)

"Hurdy-Gurdy Girls" and Sexually Transmitted Diseases

In the early years, before the influx of families to the West, most mining-town residents were single men, and the majority of the women were prostitutes. Using Helena, Montana, as an example, between 1865 and 1886, prostitution provided the largest source of paid employment for women.[255] Prostitutes were often called "hurdy-gurdy girls," among many other names; the term is derived from the hurdy-gurdy organs commonly played in dancehalls.

Miles City, the quintessential cowboy town of log buildings along the Yellowstone River, had, according to the November 1881 issue of the *Yellowstone Journal*, "32 saloons in our town and they all do good business." As if to neutralize this statement, the article continued, "We will have a church soon." Prostitution, too, was thriving in Miles City, with at least six whorehouses: Annie Turner's Coon Row, Mag Burns's 44, Connie Hoffman's, Frankie Blair's, Cowboy Annie's, and Fanny French's Negro house.[256] The prostitute, in the minds of some men, filled a special niche, and a kind of chivalry existed. One miner said, "Many's the miner who'd never wash his face or comb his hair if it wasn't for thinkin' of the sportin' girls he might meet in the saloons."[257]

Prostitution was accepted as a necessary evil wherever men outnumbered women on the frontier. In fact, society tacitly condoned the practice, on the principle that giving men a place to satisfy their primitive urges made "decent" women safer on the streets. Enterprises such as saloons and dancehalls perpetuated this belief in their own interest. Thus brothel districts, often called "tenderloins," could be found in most towns, and hardly any cluster of people, even in the most obscure outposts, was without a local "house of ill repute."

The hurdy-gurdy girls presented special health problems, the most obvious one being venereal disease. Gonorrhea, a urethritis caused by the organism *Neisseria gonorrhoeae*, was the most common. In males, it is quite obvious when an infection occurs, but females may be symptomless, and a prostitute could infect many men. For this reason, any discussion of venereal disease, and gonorrhea especially, has to include an understanding of prostitution and its place in the frontier communities.

Treatments for gonorrhea and syphilis had not changed since colonial times. Gonorrhea was suppressed by urethral injections and irrigations. The old standbys, calomel and mercurial ointments, overpowered the external evidence of syphilis. Although these treatments may have prevented some transmission of disease, the infected patient was still at risk for delayed complications. Later in the nineteenth century and in the early twentieth century, patients with syphilis were treated with heavy metals, arsenic and bismuth, injected intravenously or intramuscularly. This had a beneficial effect and probably cured some cases, but not all. These treatments did serve to eradicate the chancre and rash, and probably minimized transmission. But until the invention of penicillin in the 1940s, untreated and undertreated syphilis killed thousands of people and placed many more in mental hospitals. (For more on venereal disease, see chapter 14.)

Being exposed daily to dirty and sometimes diseased men, at a time when hygiene wasn't high on the personal agenda of most people, a prostitute might acquire any number of infectious illnesses. In addition to venereal disease, many of these women developed tuberculosis, which was, as previously mentioned, a common disease in mining camps. Alcoholism and drug addiction were other occupational hazards, as was violence. Most of the men these women dealt with drank heavily and were often brutal. It was not unusual for prostitutes to be beaten or even murdered.

"Fallen doves" also faced the constant danger of unwanted pregnancy. Few birth control methods were available during this period, and those that existed were primitive and unreliable. The most common contraceptive used in this area was some form of barrier to stop the spermatozoa from reaching the uterine canal. For this purpose some women used homemade pessaries of beeswax or other gummy substances. Affluent urban women had access to more sophisticated devises such as condoms and vaginal "tents" made of eelskin. Some homemade preparations, taken orally or used as a douche, were thought to act as a contraceptive, abortifacient, or spermicide, and the ladies of the demimonde probably tried some of these folk remedies. Among the preparations used in douches were "alum, pearlash, sulphate of zinc, or infusions of white oak bark, red rose leaves, nutgalls, or plain water."[258]

Many prostitutes discovered that the regular use of opiates caused disruption or total cessation of menses, and it is possible that they used these drugs as a form of birth control. Whatever precautions, if any, these women used, certainly they sometimes failed. Abortion was usually an option in such cases, but it was one that carried the inherent danger of infection and possible death. A few frontier doctors performed this procedure, and it's conceivable that among the working girls themselves someone might have "specialized" in this service. In unskilled or careless hands, abortion was particularly risky. Of prostitutes who gave birth, most gave the baby away for adoption or to an orphanage.

Most prostitutes were unfortunate women who had been abused or abandoned. Only a few got married and attempted to live a socially acceptable life. The vast majority led dehumanizing existences and were treated with contempt. Their living conditions were usually abysmal, and their lives were filled with despair, physical and verbal abuse, unwanted pregnancy and abortion, alcohol, opium, and disease. Suicide, perhaps unsurprisingly, was common. Among prostitutes in Helena, Montana, in the late 1800s, author Paula Petrik noted, "Blanche Mitchell shot herself; Kitty Williams committed suicide by taking an overdose of morphine . . . and Nellie Summers . . . ended her life with whiskey laced with arnica."[259] Petrik concluded, "For every one of Matt Dillon's Miss Kittys or Bob Dylan's Lilys, there were hundreds . . . who lived and died in poverty. . . . Evidence from the Comstock suggests that comparatively few prostitutes left the criminal community before they died."[260]

Doctors who attended the "ladies of the night," for whatever reason, had to use discretion, lest they tarnish their reputation among the more persnickety citizens, especially the "upright" ladies of the community. Yet these "bad" women often contributed to the community—for example, by nursing the sick during epidemics. One pioneer of Philipsburg, Montana, said of prostitute Nellie Talbott, "In later years I learned from old miners she was a good woman and did many charitable acts, and always took care of the sick and helpless."[261] Talbott was said to be beautiful and cultured, but she developed a severe cough, probably tuberculosis. When she was no longer able to "entertain," her gambler husband deserted her and took her savings. After this she worked as a scrubwoman until she died.

By 1880 Helena, Montana, the mining town that called itself the "Queen of the Rockies," developed pangs of remorse about its outrageous past and attempted to restrict prostitution. Community leaders, probably at the behest of their wives, wanted the red lights out of sight. It doesn't appear that the elite cared much about what happened to the women themselves, nor were they too concerned about the public health aspects of the business. One person who did care was R. H. Howey, an educator, minister, publisher, social reformer, and newly elected alderman. In *Strange Bedfellows*, a study of prostitution in Helena, Paula Petrik writes that Howey differed from his peers in his revolutionary idea that men were partly responsible for the existence of prostitution. In one speech, he said, "All sin and fault is laid at the doors of the women; no charity is expressed for them. . . . Some mercy should be shown them. . . . It is an evil arising from the vile passions of men that made them what they are."[262]

Doctors in Gold Country

Seeking their fortune along with everybody else, some doctors found after arriving in the gold camps that they could make more money attending the sick than prospecting. An ounce of gold, which might take all day or longer to dig, was worth sixteen dollars, and that was what many doctors charged for a house call. As one discouraged forty-niner complained, "Dierea, piles, gravel, chills, fever and scurvy begin to make their appearance and I ain't well myself. . . . There has been three doctors or things they call doctors working at me for some time. . . . Have now paid out all my gold to the doctors and they leave me worse in health." Another miner wrote, "The doctors charge pretty well. They charge for pills as if they were diamonds, and bleed a man of an ounce of gold and an ounce of blood at the same time."[263]

Doctors, like other fortune seekers, were always ready to move on to the latest hot spot. Many mining-town transients, including doctors, lawyers, merchants, gamblers, and prostitutes, came to "mine the miners" out of their hard-earned gold dust. But the hustle sometimes worked both ways. One doctor newly arrived at Deadwood, Dakota Territory, treated a miner's badly shot-up arm and was paid with a sack of gold dust. Later he found out that it was not real gold. After that he always carried a bottle of testing acid with him.[264]

Mining-camp doctors were often justifiably leery of their professional colleagues. Not only was there a great deal of suspicion among the different medical sects at the time, there was also rivalry and territoriality. Practicing in Placerville, California, previously known as Hangtown, a Dr. Hullings, described as a large, belligerent, swaggering man, had frightened off all other doctors who tried to hang their shingles in the community. Then Dr. Edward Willis came to these diggings and hung his diploma on the wall of the tent that served as his office. It wasn't long before Hullings stalked into the tent, tore up the diploma, and spat tobacco juice in Willis's face. This was a mistake. Willis challenged Hullings to a duel, which ended in the newcomer's favor. The good Dr. Willis then settled into a quiet medical practice.[265]

Especially in the far-flung mining towns, anyone calling himself a doctor was usually accepted at face value. During the boom in Bannack, Montana, in the 1860s, at least twelve men who called themselves doctors drifted into town. Even legitimate doctors didn't come to these hardscrabble places for humanitarian reasons, but to dig for gold. Some of the physician-miners, failing to make their "pile," returned to their profession. Some had offices, often in a tent, but they practiced mostly out of saddlebags. The doctor's paraphernalia were carried either on horseback or in a buggy, and he treated his patients at their home or wherever they happened to be.

Many of the mining "gulches" were so isolated they had no resident doctor. A few doctors rode the circuit and made regular visits, sometimes accompanying a clergyman. Men of the cloth often rode circuits in rural areas, including those in the West. The progress of these traveling physicians and preachers on their missions to heal body and soul was often slowed by poor trails, bad weather, and stream crossings.

In their saddlebags, pocket cases, or leather handbags, doctors carried their tools of the trade, often referred to as pocket instruments: scissors, scalpels, probes, a bistoury (a special knife for enlarging bullet and arrow

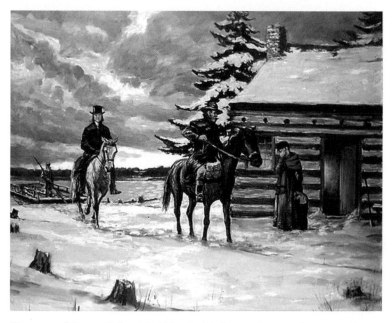

"Doctor and Circuit Rider, 1820" by Carl Rakeman. Some early western doctors made rounds with circuit-riding clergymen. While the physician tended the sick, the circuit rider offered spiritual solace to the families. —Courtesy Federal Highway Administration

tracks), needles, tweezers, sutures, and clamps. Some carried amputation saws and knives as well.[266] Muslin was valuable as a bandage, and at that time lint was used to staunch bleeding and to keep wounds open and draining.

Frontier doctors often used whiskey as anesthesia, even when ether and chloroform were available. They knew whiskey well and trusted it. Liquor was used as a general medicinal for a variety of ailments—if nothing else, an ounce or two worked as a great mood elevator. And if a doctor used any antiseptic at all, it was drinking whiskey sloshed into the wound.

Doctors in the farther reaches of the frontier were usually the last to hear of, not to mention accept, new medical ideas. In the mid- to late 1800s, a time of considerable medical progress, dissemination of medical advancement was almost entirely by word of mouth. Growth of medical knowledge is layered like the growth rings of trees, and different places show different patterns of accomplishment. Many western practitioners, due to ignorance, by preference, or sometimes out of necessity, used the naked ear rather than the stethoscope to listen to the chest and never learned to use the ophthalmoscope or even the thermometer. Some continued to prescribe calomel as a purge and still blistered the skin as therapy. There also remained a persistent belief in "laudable" (i.e., valuable) pus as essential to healing.

In the light of the enormous advances made by medical science during the twentieth century, it is hard for us to envision how those physicians practiced as they did. Knowing little or nothing about germs, they did not completely understand the transmission of infectious diseases, and they diagnosed ailments without modern tools. The frontier practitioner relied primarily on common sense and experience.

Surgical instruments, late 1800s. Left to right: Nelaton's probe; bullet screw; forceps; bullet extractor; bullet forceps; hook splinter forceps
—From *The Science and Art of Surgery: A Treatise on Surgical Injuries, Diseases, and Operations* by John Eric Erichsen, 1884

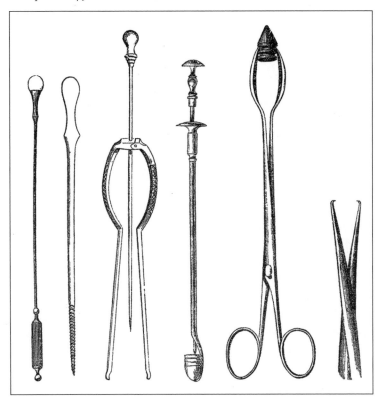

Barroom Surgeons

Although helpless in healing infectious disease, many frontier doctors were skilled trauma surgeons. In the tempestuous environment of the gold camp, guns were used all too often to settle disputes. Thus mining-town doctors gained a good deal of experience with gunshot wounds and other injuries. Because of the high risk of infection, the sometimes crude tools, and the often inadequate anesthesia, surgeons had to have great confidence, be adept with a knife, know anatomy well, and operate with speed.

During most of the frontier era, there was little or no appreciation of microbes, and operations were performed with unsterilized instruments, perhaps washed only in creek water prior to use. The patient was immobilized on a makeshift table, stuporous from whiskey and laudanum. Operations then were restricted to the external surface of the body; doctors knew that to open the abdomen or other body cavity invariably led to fatal infections. With bare, unwashed hands and in meager light, the surgeon did his work, tying off gushing blood vessels, probing wounds for bullets, suturing lacerations, and amputating limbs. Dressed in regular clothing contaminated from daily wear and contact with other patients, the surgeon might let his cigar ashes fall into the open wound as insects buzzed around the room.

A patient's survival depended largely on luck, the surgeon's skill, and his own vigor. One Montana man fell on a circular saw, cutting through several ribs and lacerating his lung. Dr. John B. Buker put the ribs in place, stopped the flow of blood, and patched the lung. The man recovered.[267] The frontier surgeon performed procedures that today require special instruments, advanced anesthesia, and a team of professional assistants. Yet many patients came out of it without so much as a fever.

It was in his surgical skill that a doctor gained his reputation. Any operation he performed was a matter of public interest. When Dr. Charles Fox Gardiner elected to remove a huge tumor from a woman's scalp, a self-appointed commentator shoved his way into the office to report on the operation to the crowd waiting outside. Through an open window, he announced each step of the procedure. At the end, he said, "She's doing fine, folks. . . . It's all over but the shouting." The crowd cheered and fired off a couple of shots in jubilation, then escorted the doctor to the saloon to celebrate.[268]

One of the most colorful pioneer doctors was Armistead H. Mitchell. From his headquarters in Deer Lodge, Montana, Dr. Mitchell traveled by

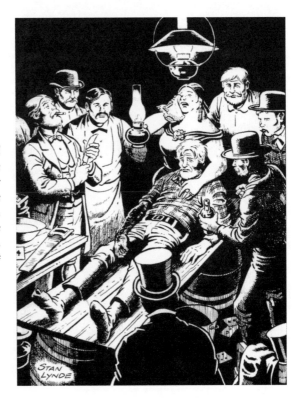

Operations performed in a barroom were typical of frontier medical care during the settlement of the West. This kind of practice evolved out of necessity.
—Courtesy Stan Lynde

horseback from place to place. It was said that he had drifted to Montana from the mining camps in California about 1865, and that he "was ready for any type of surgery with a good drink warming his veins and a butcher knife in his hands."[269]

One Saturday, in the mining camp of Bear Town on the Little Blackfoot River, Mitchell was called on to treat the badly burned arm of a miner named Shorty. The night before, in a drunken stupor, Shorty had fallen into his own fireplace and almost incinerated his arm. In the town's store/saloon, an operating table was prepared with planks and whiskey barrels. Of course, the anesthesia was whiskey, and Mitchell went to work amputating Shorty's arm while the owner of the establishment spread sawdust on the floor to soak up the blood. After the operation, Shorty hopped up and invited his friends to join him and the "doc" in a round of drinks.[270]

Mitchell became one of Montana's outstanding physicians, a founding member of the Montana Medical Association and one of the organizers

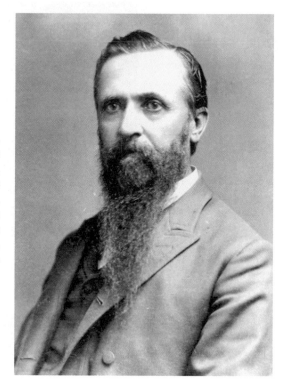

Armistead H. Mitchell. During the gold rush, a few doctors rode a circuit, making regular visits to isolated mining camps. Mitchell was one of the most interesting circuit riders. —Courtesy Montana Historical Society, Helena

of the mental hospital at Warm Springs. His reputation was so commendable that the *New Northwest* said of him, "If it is true that a good share of the benefits of medicine depend upon the degree of confidence that the patient has in the physician, Dr. Mitchell could go over this country and cure half the ailments with a pocketful of flour and a pint of *aqua pura*."[271]

Dr. Ira C. Smith, a frontier surgeon in Virginia City, was innovative, especially in orthopedics. He built supports for broken legs that he elevated with pulleys and strings. Once when a broken leg refused to stay in place, he nailed the bones together using carpenter's tools. The bones held, and the patient recovered the use of his leg.[272]

No study of gold camp doctors would be complete without mentioning Tombstone's amazing Dr. George E. Goodfellow.[273] An innovative surgeon, Goodfellow gained a national reputation for the development of some technical operative procedures. His first successful case was the first recorded laparotomy in Arizona, performed July 13, 1881, on a nine-day-old abdominal wound sustained from a .32-caliber bullet.

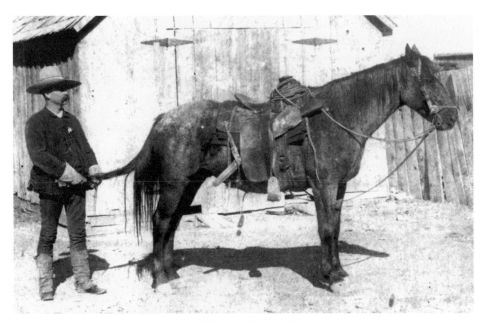

Dr. George E. Goodfellow, a famous Tombstone surgeon.
—Courtesy Arizona Historical Society

Tombstone, Arizona, was an angry place, and few civilian doctors, before or since, ever saw more lawlessness than did young Dr. Goodfellow. Fights with fist, knife, and gun as well as hangings were common. Not only treating most of the survivors, but also doing autopsies on some of the dead, Goodfellow developed an advanced understanding of trauma and ballistics. What's more, he shared his studies and observations with colleagues. Goodfellow's postmortem reports show a degree of meretricious humor. His examination of a gambler killed over a card game showed, "the body to be rich in lead but not too badly punctured to hold whiskey."[274]

Goodfellow followed Lister's method of surgical antisepsis completely and carbolized everything—the instruments, the sponges, the surgeon's hands, and the field of surgery. He even sprayed carbolic acid solution around the room. Word of Goodfellow's skill in saving men with heretofore fatal abdominal gunshot wounds spread throughout the Arizona Territory. There were few hospitals, so Goodfellow's operating suite was usually a dingy, drafty room or a smoky, dimly lit bar.

But not even Goodfellow could save everyone. When his colleague, Tombstone county physician Dr. George C. Willis, was shot in the groin, he died of hemorrhage so fast that there was no time for surgery. In September of 1891, Dr. Goodfellow was asked to operate on another colleague, Dr. John C. Handy. This prominent Tucson doctor was shot in the abdomen by his wife's divorce lawyer. Goodfellow arrived in Tucson ten hours after the incident. With the help of several other doctors, he sutured more than a dozen holes in Handy's intestines. Dr. Handy died just after the last stitch.

Goodfellow called Winchester rifles and carbines the "toys with which our festive or obstreperous citizens delight themselves."[275] People on the frontier preferred large-caliber weapons, and they used more powder behind the ball than was used back East. Thus gunshot wounds could cause death within an hour from hemorrhage. For this reason Goodfellow recommended immediate surgery in such cases, to repair the damage. While this is a questionable practice, Goodfellow did save a few lives. Eventually Dr. Goodfellow left Tombstone and set up practice in Tucson. Later he taught medicine and surgery.

Dr. John C. Handy, circa 1890, in front of his Tucson office with his horse and buggy. Handy, shot in the abdomen in 1891, died from his wounds in spite of heroic surgical efforts by his colleague George E. Goodfellow. —Courtesy Arizona Historical Society

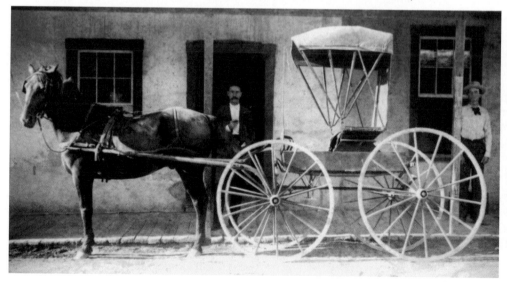

Doctors in the Line of Fire

In addition to keeping doctors busy, guns were also used to "motivate" them. When a cowboy brought his wounded brother to see Dr. B. F. Bancroft in Denver, he told the doctor that if his brother died, he would kill him. The man's arm was badly wounded, and the doctor performed an amputation. The patient survived. Later, Dr. Bancroft told friends that he wasn't too worried because he was also armed, and that if the patient showed signs of dying, he would have known it before the cowboy did.[276]

Another surgeon who had to deal with outlaws was Jerome S. Glick.[277] Dr. Glick was not a miner and came to the gold camp of Bannack, Montana, for the sole purpose of practicing medicine. He had good credentials. But on one occasion his surgical skill led him into a dangerous position with the notorious Plummer gang. In March 1863 Henry Plummer, the charismatic outlaw and ironically elected sheriff of Bannack, chose Dr. Glick as his physician after the sheriff of Virginia City, Henry Crawford, shot him in the "trigger arm."[278] According to Glick, Plummer's henchmen took him to a secret place where, under threat of death, he treated Plummer's bullet wound and its almost inevitable subsequent infection. The frightened doctor recommended amputation, but the gunslinger sheriff refused it. As Glick was preparing to work on the wound, one of the men said, "I just thought that I'd tell you that if you cut an artery, or Plummer dies . . . I'm going to shoot the top of your head off."[279] Rather than probe for the bullet and risk further damage, Glick performed a simple debridement and left the bullet track open to drain. The wound healed, saving Plummer's arm and presumably Glick's life.

As the gang continued their violent activities, Glick was required to make additional "house calls" on injured gang members, under a strict code of silence. Glick's servitude to the criminals ended in January 1864, when vigilantes hanged many of the members of the gang, including Plummer. The doctor's testimony had helped to seal their fate. Some claim Glick had an overactive imagination, and that when drinking, "he was apt to see things."[280]

There are many hair-raising tales about close calls doctors experienced in the routine pursuit of their profession. They were threatened at times by disgruntled patients, and because they had narcotics, desperate addicts intent on getting a fix were a constant threat. Sometimes when a person's life was at risk, a doctor's "no" was not accepted as an answer. In Montana in the 1880s, a man asked an elderly doctor named Wentworth to come and attend to his wife, who was having her first baby. When the doctor refused, the man pulled a gun and made the doctor ride ahead of him. According to the story, "It all turned out alright."[281]

In the violent climate of the frontier, many doctors learned to arm themselves. Around 1880, in Helena, Montana, Dr. Charles K. Cole was returning from a visit to a miner's sick wife when a thief, brandishing a gun, demanded his watch and money. The doctor refused, and the assailant shot him in the left wrist. Using his good arm, Dr. Cole pulled his own gun and shot his attacker. The injured man fled. Later, after he had dressed and treated his wrist wound, the doctor was summoned to a cabin in a remote part of town. There, to his surprise, was the bandit he had shot. Dr. Cole removed the bullet from the thief's abdomen. After the man recovered, he worked for Dr. Cole as a stableman to make amends and to pay for his treatment.[282]

Chinese Medicine on Gold Mountain

Most Chinese immigrants came to the West with the gold rush and during the westward expansion of the railroad, when they were sorely needed as laborers.[283] For cultural reasons and for safety against persecution, they clustered together, establishing their own communities within communities. Most of these "Chinatowns" were crowded slums. Essentially they were male societies, since most of the workers were men who left their families in China and sent their wages home. Of the few Chinese women, most were prostitutes. In 1880, half of the fifty-six prostitutes in Helena, Montana, were Chinese.[284]

The Chinese population in the western states and territories reached a peak of about eight percent in 1880. By the turn of the century, barely two percent remained.[285] The Chinese were simply not wanted. Although they came primarily as miners, a few found other employment, working in laundry houses, cleaning homes and businesses, peddling wares, cooking and serving in restaurants, or toiling at whatever menial tasks white intolerance allowed them to do. The editor of the *Avant Courier* of Bozeman, Montana, illustrated this bigotry when he wrote that the "celestials," as he called them, were "worthless pagans . . . a detriment to any country outside the Mongolian empire."[286]

The racism was so rampant that in 1873 the Elko County Hospital in Nevada refused admission to Chinese patients. In response, the Chinese community in Elko built their own hospital, directed by Dr. Ken Fung. A graduate of the School of Medicine and Surgery in Canton, Dr. Fung was as qualified as any American physician of the day.[287]

In general, the Chinese stayed healthier than other groups. For example, in 1870 and 1880, the mortality rate for white people was twice that of the Chinese in many parts of the West.[288] Some of this was due to their diet. They ate many vegetables containing vitamin C, which prevented scurvy. In addition, interestingly, the fact that they were ostracized kept them away from the mainstreams of society where contagion was spread.

Chinese doctors used primarily herbal treatments, but they also offered acupuncture and other services. Acupuncture, a time-honored technique, was sometimes associated with shamanism and magic. The Chinese also had an ancient tradition in surgery. As early as the second century in China, doctors were performing amputations.

In spite of the whites' oppression of the Chinese, Asian medicine was very important to the frontier West. Because there was often a shortage of American physicians, white patients seemed more than willing to consult Chinese doctors. A large proportion of the Chinese doctor's patients were women who felt that white doctors were unsympathetic

Office and apothecary of Dr. Huie Pock, Butte, Montana. In the West, especially in the mining and labor camps, Chinese medicine appealed to both white and Chinese cultures. —Courtesy Montana Historical Society, Helena

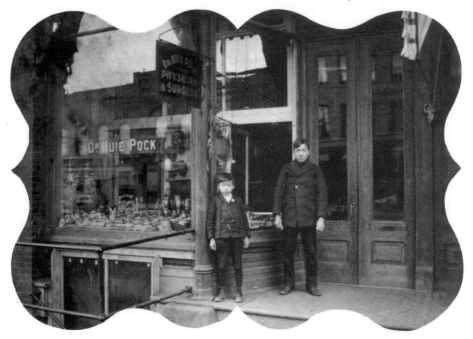

to their special complaints. Chinese physicians tended to be more compassionate toward women. One Chinese physician who became successful in both cultures was Dr. C. K. Ah Fong. Trained in China, Dr. Ah Fong arrived in California about 1869 with many other Chinese. By the 1880s he was practicing Chinese medicine in the mining communities of Idaho. When the gold played out, he moved to Boise, where, in spite of great opposition, he was licensed to practice medicine by the state of Idaho in 1899.[289] In Carson City, Nevada, Mrs. Chow Sing Huey served as a midwife for many women and was said to administer to the Paiute community as well.[290]

The Chinese immigrants who practiced medicine were usually a class of merchant-doctor-pharmacists. Chinese physicians offered cures for everything from hangovers to gonorrhea. One well-established liniment and sometime tonic was made by thrusting a live rattlesnake into a pan of alcohol; the resultant solution was used to treat arthritis. It was also said to cause contraction and tightening of flaccid tissue, offering a "painful but effective cure for impotency."[291] The elixirs Chinese healers prescribed for impotence were very popular. White men seemed perfectly willing to swallow "rattlesnake wine," tiger-bone liquor, and other unusual substances, including a tincture made of the ground penis and testis of a seal.

Even after the mining and labor camps closed, Chinese medical practitioners continued to treat the non-Chinese.[292] One of the reasons Chinese medicine appealed to white people was that the herbal medicines were often less harsh than Euro-American treatments. They also seemed more effective for female complaints, sexual disorders, and psychological symptoms. As Paul D. Buell points out, "The mountain West became a new Chinese frontier, a place where ancient traditions, including medical and pharmaceutical theories and practices, could flourish and continue to evolve."[293] Practitioners like "Doc Ing Hay" had hundreds of herbs and animal parts to choose from in the Kam Wah Chung Pharmacy in John Day, Oregon. He also provided an "opium den" in his home office.[294]

An unfortunate contribution the Chinese made to the frontier was opium use. Opium dens were common in the West, often run by Chinese proprietors. It was said that the Chinese laborer was paid one dollar a day and spent half of it on opium.[295] Desperately injured, sick, or miserable workers used the "black pill," an overdose of opium, to commit suicide. Among the white population, many gamblers, prostitutes, and others also succumbed to the temptation of opium. Until it was outlawed, the drug was readily available in pharmacies and from independent peddlers.

SIX

Unsung Heroes

Army Surgeons on the Frontier

The bravery, the skill and the foolishness of the Custers and the Renos, the Crooks and the Gibbons will be debated for many years, but the surgeons who accompanied these men on their campaigns will likely remain unremembered.

—Mary Gillett, "United States Army Surgeons and the Big Horn-Yellowstone Expedition of 1876"[296]

EMPHASIZING THE UNSUNG HEROES of the military's medical service, Mary C. Gillett, historian at the U.S. Army's Center of Military History in Washington, D.C., wrote, "The army surgeons of the 1870s practiced medicine that was up to the highest standard of the time, and they practiced it under circumstances that would intimidate modern physicians. Furthermore, while they cared for the sick, they were themselves in greater danger of contracting disease than anyone else was. And while caring for the wounded they were in greater danger from enemy attacks than anyone else was."[297]

Military doctors were burdened with many different responsibilities beyond the daily sick call. They had to see to it that the soldiers' living conditions were decent and that the water supply was safe. They had to inspect the kitchens, supervise the hospital, maintain a pharmacy, and perform as a military officer on various boards and courts-martial. Furthermore, the military doctor was expected to accompany field campaigns, and he had to be ready to take to the field whenever conflict erupted. Truly the army doctor was just as important to the military as the combatants.

A qualified army physician, especially one with war experience, understood the importance of isolation during epidemics, knew of sanitary precautions in building latrines and disposal of garbage, and recognized the preventive value of personal hygiene. He was skilled in the treatment of injuries, and he was aware of the complications of infection from compound fractures and from overzealous attempts to remove bullets and arrows from the chest or abdomen. He was prepared to work in hastily constructed field hospitals and trained to move his patients when necessary by whatever means were available.

In addition to their official duties caring for the soldiers, doctors at western army posts treated sick and injured civilians, including migrating settlers, passing travelers, and local Native Americans. At the end of the Mexican War in 1848, the government sent the army out to build posts on the frontier to protect migrating caravans of Americans moving to Oregon, California, and other points west. Although Congress never formally authorized the army to give the civilians medical treatment, the

Pocket surgical kit issued by the U.S. Army, used by Dr. Mary Walker during the Civil War —Courtesy National Museum of Health and Medicine, Armed Forces Institute of Pathology, Washington, D.C.

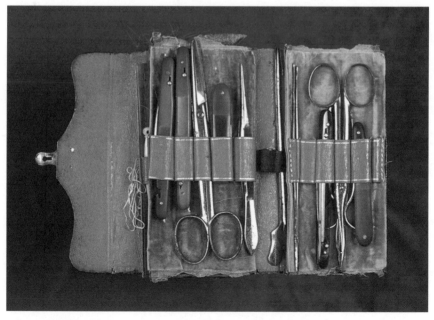

posts took in injured and sick overlanders whenever a military doctor or medical supplies were available.

Caring for so many people was not an easy task in the remote locations of military camps. There were often delays before doctors, equipment, and medicine reached newly established posts. But even with limited supplies and without formal authorization, the humanitarian effort expanded as more military presence was established. At Fort Laramie, Wyoming, in 1850, assistant surgeon S. P. Moore said, "I presume I saw and prescribed for every sick emigrant passing the fort, and many were necessarily left under my charge."[298]

Volunteer doctors at Fort Riley, Kansas, carried out a health care program for civilians, equipping their horses with saddlebags specially made for medicines and instruments, sometimes using a mule-drawn ambulance to assist them. During a diphtheria epidemic in the late 1880s in New Mexico, Dr. Henry Lippincott rode a wide circuit to render medical aid.[299] On occasion, both soldiers and civilians were vaccinated for smallpox.

In one famous case, Lieutenant Walter Reed, the post surgeon at Fort Robinson, Nebraska, during the late 1800s, treated Jules Sandoz ("Old Jules" as he was later memorialized by his daughter, Mari Sandoz) for a crushed ankle. The compound fracture, after eighteen days, had become infected and was draining bloody pus, the leg was swollen and discolored, and Jules was delirious and emaciated. He would have died already if he had not had such a strong constitution, and exceptional medical care was now called for. But the testy Sandoz refused an amputation, threatening the young lieutenant with, "You cut my foot off, doctor, and I shoot you so dead you stink before you hit the ground."[300]

Dr. Reed forwent the amputation and treated the infected wound. He probably debrided all the necrotic tissue; removed any foreign material such as bone fragments, clothing bits, or dirt; and closed suppurating spaces that could harbor infection. Against all odds, after two months of keeping the wound open to air, Old Jules not only survived but lived many productive years. The two men became lifelong friends.[301]

Riding on expeditions and riding out to treat civilians meant army doctors spent a lot of time in the saddle. Assistant acting surgeon Wallace Edgar Sabin, for example, lived and practiced for long periods in tents, exposed to the elements and Indian attacks. It was calculated that over a span of fifteen years, Dr. Sabin traveled 10,180 miles on horseback, a record unexcelled by any other officer of that period.[302]

When there was a civilian community near the post, army doctors often established a private practice as an additional source of income, riding back and forth between the fort and the town. In times of inactivity, some military doctors pursued other interests, studying botany, zoology, and even archaeology. The army encouraged such extracurricular activities. Edgar Mearns requested duty as an army surgeon at Fort Verde in central Arizona so he could pursue his interests in desert flora and fauna. For four years he accompanied the cavalry on scouts after Apaches, where he "removed arrows from trooper's backsides . . . and collected plants and animals when time allowed."[303] He wrote the first description of an unusual species of quail now known as Mearns's quail.

Medical Training in the Military

Positions as surgeon or assistant surgeon in the army were sought after because the pay was usually more than a doctor made in civilian practice. During and after the Civil War, to be accepted as a commissioned military surgeon, doctors had to have established credentials and pass a demanding examination. After finding, early in the Civil War, that many doctors were incompetent, the army learned to be careful in selecting its medical personnel, and it established rigorous examinations. The test given to those who aspired to be a military doctor covered many subjects, not just medicine. In addition to anatomy, pathology, physiology, general therapeutics and materia medica, forensics, toxicology, and surgery, the doctor was expected to have a broad knowledge of the world, including geography, mathematics, and foreign languages. The examination might last as long as a week, and many candidates failed. In 1877, only 21 of 185 doctors passed the exam.[304]

The test given to prospective military doctors in 1879 included questions that indicate the progressive state of the art of medicine at that time. Three of them were: 1) "Discuss the etiology of suppuration and the means of preventing it, or in case it exists, of relieving and curing it"; 2) "What are some of the best methods of treating the hands and field of operation before and during operative work?"; 3) "Describe briefly the subject of fracture of the cranium, diagnostics, effect and treatment."[305]

Any enlightened physician of this era, especially a recent graduate of a credible medical school, knew how to prevent infection with disinfectants and soap and water, and had been taught the importance of sterilized surgical instruments. He knew to drain an infected wound or abscess of purulent material. If he were especially well instructed, he might also know the different kinds of recently discovered bacteria that caused infection. Even neurological complications following head injury and the use of a trephine to elevate depressed fractures of the skull were appreciated by the well-educated. All this intelligence had developed in America since the Civil War.

During the Indian wars, the army became desperate for doctors and hired contract surgeons from civilian sources. These men were given no rank and wore no uniform. A number of these doctors had flunked the army's test, but during this period "the rules were bent."[306] One writer compared the contract surgeon's status with that of the mule: "The mule," he said, "without pride of ancestry or hope of posterity, neither horse nor ass, unloved and unlovely, the recipient of contumelious language, was the army's standby and salvation in the field in time of trouble."[307]

Some contract doctors unable to obtain a regular commission spent long careers in this secondary capacity. Others never intended to have a military career and accepted the lot of a contract physician as a paid trip to the West, where they hoped to seek their fortune. In the last few decades of the nineteenth century, many army physicians left the service and founded a practice in the burgeoning western communities, where they were sorely needed.[308]

Post Sanitation and Disease

During the Civil War, more soldiers died of disease than on the battlefield—bacteria were deadlier than bullets. In that conflict, there was essentially no sanitation as we view it today. One Civil War doctor later described his experience: "We operated in our blood-stained and often pus-stained coats. . . . We used undisinfected instruments from undisinfected plush cases, and still worse used marine sponges which had been used in prior pus cases and had been only washed in tap water. If a sponge or instrument fell on the floor it was washed and squeezed in a basin of tap water and used as if it were clean."[309]

Gradually there grew a better appreciation of the importance of sanitation. Medical care of soldiers has always improved from war to war. In the Civil War, the incidence of mortality from disease was fifty-three per thousand soldiers; during the Spanish-American War, the rate dropped to sixteen per thousand; and in World War I, only twelve men per thousand died from illness unrelated to battle.[310]

Nevertheless, at frontier posts during the Indian wars, very few commanding officers understood the value of prevention of illness, and many

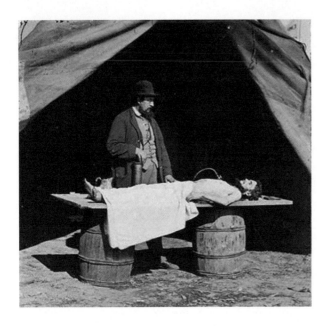

Civil War embalmer working on a soldier's body —Courtesy Library of Congress

were unwilling to support a doctor's efforts toward better sanitation and health.[311] Army doctors had very little authority, and much of the time the medical officer's hands were tied by military protocol. Why, one might ask, were unwholesome conditions allowed to persist? There probably isn't any one answer. Too often, officers in charge, out of ignorance and lack of respect for a medical officer's opinion, ignored their doctors' recommendations. Sometimes it was a matter of rank.

As late as 1898, during the war with Spain, the schism between the medical department and the officers of the line had tragic consequences. More than twenty thousand cases of typhoid occurred during the five months of this war, and more than fifteen hundred of those were fatal, compared to only 280 soldiers killed in action. A board of military physicians found that camp pollution was the greatest sin committed by the troops in 1898.[312] The bacillus that caused the disease and its mode of transmission were known by that time, and the epidemic could have been prevented simply with proper disposal of human excrement.

Disease was also a tremendous scourge during the Indian wars. Part of the problem was that army pay was so low, living conditions so dismal, and morale so poor that almost any volunteer was accepted. Post surgeons complained in their reports that advanced syphilis, scrofula (tuberculosis of cervical lymph nodes), epilepsy, and alcoholism were found in many of the new recruits.[313] As doctors had learned during the

112

Civil War, a myriad of streptococcal diseases attacked soldiers with poor personal hygiene crowded together in inadequately ventilated barracks. Erysipelas and scarlet fever, streptococcal infections with serious complications, could spread rapidly and decimate whole companies.

Furthermore, epidemics of cholera, typhoid, measles, smallpox, and other diseases were a constant threat to anyone living on the frontier. Naturally, army doctors watched for the beginning signs of an epidemic because isolation of the first case safeguarded other potential victims. But the onset of an outbreak of typhoid or cholera could be abrupt and unexpected, and within hours, many victims might be felled by disease, including the caregivers. History is replete with stories about the courageous attention to duty of medical people during epidemics until they collapsed themselves. During an 1867 epidemic of cholera at Fort Harker, Kansas, Dr. George Sternberg continued to treat patients even after his wife died of the disease. Later he, too, suffered this dreadful diarrhea, but he survived. At Fort Lyon, Colorado, during the same epidemic, the military surgeon there also lost his wife to cholera, but he kept to his duty until he succumbed himself.[314] (For more on epidemics, see chapter 14.)

Cholera was one of the worst examples of the many types of dysentery that bedeviled soldiers and civilians alike. It is characterized by the sudden onset of excruciating abdominal cramps and continuous diarrhea. The massive loss of intestinal fluids led to critical dehydration. Cholera was one of the most rapidly fatal conditions known; sometimes death occurred within a few hours. The need to replace lost fluids was not understood at that time, and the therapies of the day sometimes made the condition worse. Survival depended on the individual's general health and probably on the number of bacteria (*Vibrio cholerae*) he or she had swallowed.

Typhoid was another epidemic that struck military camps and other groups on the frontier. It was usually more insidious in the beginning than cholera, but victims died just as readily. Caused by the bacterium *Salmonella typhi*, typhoid is epidemiologically similar to cholera and usually comes from ingesting water contaminated with human feces. The main symptom was diarrhea, but the patients could be profoundly ill with fever and prostration. Relentless cases developed bloodstream infections and sometimes fatal peritonitis from perforation of ulcers in the small bowel.

In warmer, more humid climates infested with mosquitoes, malaria and "fevers" referred to as "effluvial" were endemic. The prevailing theory was that poisonous vapors from swampy, stagnant water and garbage dumps caused malaria (from *mala aria*, bad air), or "ague" as it was called. The malarial parasite was not yet recognized, and no one knew until the turn of the century that the mosquito was the vector. Malaria was a disease of the East and Midwest, but migrants sometimes brought the fever with them. Unlike cholera and typhoid, malaria had an effective treatment—quinine.

It was difficult to distinguish malaria from typhoid, hence the term typho-malaria was commonly used. Since many conditions were accompanied by fever and malaise, an exact diagnosis for any given illness was not always possible. For instance, the diarrhea seen with scurvy was often confused with several forms of gastrointestinal disease.

By the 1880s most caregivers appreciated the value of isolation, rest, and nursing care in the treatment of febrile illness. Doctors no longer purged and bled patients, at least not to the extent as before. But during the Civil War, the use of calomel as a purge was still nearly sacrosanct. One outstanding doctor, Surgeon General William Hammond, believed that purgative drugs caused more deaths than they prevented and tried to get calomel and the puking drug tartar emetic removed from the military pharmacies. But so strongly were these substances supported by his colleagues that he was eventually court-martialed and discharged from the army.[315]

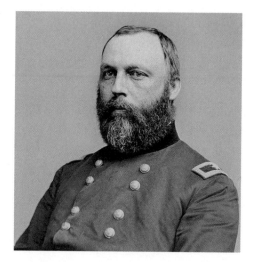

Brig. Gen. William A. Hammond, Federal Army Surgeon General. Early in the Civil War, Hammond unsuccessfully tried to stop the military's use of calomel and tartar emetic.
—Courtesy National Library of Medicine, History of Medicine

For many years even wounds were treated with these old methods. In 1847 Dr. John Strotter Griffin, traveling with the Army of the West to San Diego, treated soldiers with lance and bullet wounds with purging, bleeding, and blistering.[316] Because allopaths, or "regular" doctors, were more likely to use cathartics, it was a popular joke that the "patient of a homeopath might die of the disease, while a patient of a regular [doctor] might die of the cure."[317]

Scurvy and Poor Nutrition

At first it is surprising to learn that a simple vitamin C deficiency called scurvy rivaled cholera as the number-one killer on the frontier. But knowing the dietary habits of the first white people to come west, it is no wonder. A soldier's diet typically consisted of salt meat, bread, lard, coffee, and hardtack; miners and immigrants subsisted largely on cornmeal, beans, and salt meat.

For thousands of years, scurvy had been a leading cause of death in armies, on ships, in frontier towns, and anywhere that diet was inadequate. Some called it "the explorer's disease." Not until 1870 did the so-called civilized world understand that a diet deficient in fresh vegetables or fruit caused scurvy. This was another example of medical discoveries lost, rediscovered, and lost again. Intermittently for hundreds of years, the cause of scurvy was recognized and then forgotten. There were undoubtedly many other conditions related to inadequate diet that developed in army camps. It was not uncommon to see night blindness in scurvy patients, now attributed to a deficiency of vitamin A.[318]

The 1819-20 Long expedition, one of the earliest recorded expeditions into the Rocky Mountains, was devastated by scurvy. There were three hundred cases and one hundred deaths from the disease. It is sadly apparent that the company's physician, Dr. Edwin James, a well-known botanist, geologist, and surgeon, was not knowledgeable in the prevention and treatment of scurvy. The doctor observed that the hunters, who spent much of their time away from camp, did not develop the disease. Afterward it was learned that they had eaten green herbs and wild garlic in the woods. This discovery would later save the life of Maximilian, Prince of Wied, who became sick with scurvy while at Fort Clark in 1834. A cook who had been with the Long expedition remembered the bulbs and fed them to the prince, and he recovered.[319]

Army surgeon James A. Mullan, brother of Captain John Mullan, was sent in 1860 to watch over the health of the men under his brother's command. Twenty-five men developed scurvy, but Captain Mullan reported that all the cases "yielded under the care of my brother."[320] Dr. Mullan had prescribed fresh vegetables and vinegar. This simple and folksy remedy indicated an advanced understanding of the disease.

Once the cure for scurvy was discovered, army doctors needed to know how to diagnose it. It was important that physicians recognize the early stages of scurvy in order to treat it and prevent it from developing in others. Doctors learned to look for small hemorrhages around the hair follicles of the skin, an early symptom. Progression of the illness resulted in bleeding gums, loose teeth, and sometimes large areas of hemorrhage in the skin. Cavalry soldiers commonly developed hemorrhage in the "saddle area" of the buttocks and thighs. The course of the disorder was progressive, leading to inanition, lassitude, and death. Scurvy in children developed differently; it was recognized by tenderness on the surface of large bones where blood collected under the periosteum, the fibrous covering of bone. Children also characteristically developed knobby hemorrhages along the attachment of the ribs to the sternum, producing the so-called "scorbutic rosary."[321] Luckily, even in severe cases, the consumption of vitamin C-rich foods produced a dramatic recovery.

As the military expanded west, vegetable gardens, managed by the post surgeons, became the army's first line of defense against scurvy. In addition, the doctors scoured the countryside to find edible wild plants containing vitamin C. By 1878 the army's exam for physicians required knowledge of the cause, symptoms, course, and treatment of scorbutus.[322]

Venereal Disease: "A night with Venus, a lifetime with mercury"

Nearly every army camp listed venereal diseases as persistent problems, almost endemic in their frequency. Army doctors had a great deal of experience with venereal disease. During the Civil War, prostitution was rampant. *The Medical and Surgical History of the War of the Rebellion*, written in 1888, reported a rate of eighty-two cases of VD per one thousand men.[323] In the West it was even worse—incidences of syphilis and gonorrhea in New Mexico were three times higher than the national military average during the Civil War. Whorehouses sprang up near most army camps in the West, and some prostitutes traveled with soldiers as "wives" or worked as laundresses. Taverns and brothels were lucrative enterprises in frontier towns, attracting soldiers and civilians alike.

Camp doctors stayed busy treating the external manifestations of venereal disease, a urethral discharge in gonorrhea and the skin sores of syphilis. Their medications included calomel, mercurial salves, and irrigating solutions, though these did little for deep-seated, systemic pathology. A common joke at the time was "A night with Venus, a lifetime with mercury."[324] General Tasker H. Bliss said facetiously that post surgeons had little to do except "confine laundresses and treat the clap."[325] Clearly this was not true, but the comment does speak to the prevalence of the problem. (For more on venereal disease, see chapter 14.)

Wilderness Woes

Doctors working in remote areas had to be prepared for anything. At Fort Concho in 1878, screwworms from blowflies plagued the men. Tarantula bites were so common that *Harper's Magazine* featured an article on the subject. Wild animals also carried the threat of the greatly feared condition known as hydrophobia (rabies). Rabies is always fatal, and from the descriptions of eyewitnesses, no death was more agonizing or appalling to watch. The symptoms of encephalitic rabies include bizarre, sometimes aggressive behavior and spasms of agitation, disorientation, and fear of water (hence the name hydrophobia). Increased salivation and difficulty swallowing, described as "frothing at the mouth," also occurs. The victim finally collapses into a terminal coma and dies. (For more on rabies, see chapter 8.)

One incident of rabies took place on a pleasant August evening in 1868, when a mad, snarling wolf charged through the streets of Fort Larned, in western Kansas Territory. The raging animal snapped at everything—people, dogs, tents, even bed clothing. Stumbling into the post hospital, the wolf bit Corporal Mike McGuillicuddy as he lay in bed. From there, it attacked a group of soldiers, wounding two more men and a dog. Finally the animal was shot. The base surgeon treated the three men's bites with silver nitrate cautery. One month later, McGuillicuddy and the dog died of hydrophobia. The other two men did not develop the disease.[326]

In 1872 fifteen men died of rabies at Fort Dodge. This time the infection was carried by skunks. Rabid skunks were common on the Great

Plains, and some of them lost all fear of humans and even came into the tents. Other carriers included raccoons, coyotes, bats, and foxes.

Wounds and Infections (Hospital Gangrene)

History and experience taught doctors that most combat wounds involved soft tissue (skin and muscle), primarily on the arms and legs. It was fully appreciated, too, that the longer an injury was left unattended, the more likely infection was to develop, causing protracted disability or death. The rules for proper wound treatment in the nineteenth century were not appreciably different from those recommended by Napoleon's surgeons, nor from those of the sixteenth-century French surgeon Ambroise Paré, whose teachings on the treatment of gunshot and other war injuries were followed into modern times.[327]

Injuries contaminated in the field or in hospitals by a bacterium called streptococcus led to infection, which in turn led to gangrene. The experienced military surgeon knew that neglected wounds or those containing foreign bodies must be left open and not sutured closed, so as not to foster this condition. Limbs that developed gangrene required amputa-

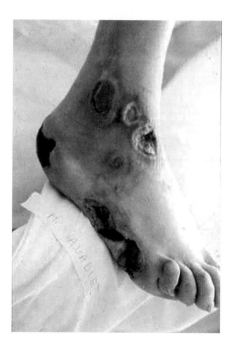

Gangrene of a foot. Any condition that compromises the circulation to an extremity can result in gangrene. Amputation to arrest gangrene was one of the most common surgical procedures during wartime.
—Courtesy Centers for Disease Control and Prevention

118

tion before the infection spread through the body and to vital organs, causing death.

An article in the *Marine Corps Gazette* offered this description of the dreaded condition: "The skin sloughed off.... The flesh around the injury changed color to 'reddish, greenish, purplish or black,' and the gray edges of the opening grew wide at the rate of half an inch an hour. Arteries and even bones were rapidly exposed and the stench of rotten meat filled the air. As his skin turned gray, the patient's breath became sickly sweet, his body alternated between chills and sweats, and his pulse grew even faster, even feebler."[328]

Is it any wonder that Civil War soldiers with arm and leg injuries begged for amputation, or that surgeons were willing to cut off limbs with only minor apparent damage to prevent such terrible consequences? In the case of "hospital gangrene," a few Civil War doctors stumbled onto a preventive. Well before there was an understanding of germs, some physicians were beginning to suspect that something spread from pus-filled wounds to clean ones. In 1862, while assigned to a large hospital at Portsmouth Grove, Rhode Island, Dr. George M. Sternberg, who later became one of the foremost bacteriologists in the United States, witnessed

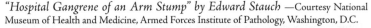

"Hospital Gangrene of an Arm Stump" by Edward Stauch —Courtesy National Museum of Health and Medicine, Armed Forces Institute of Pathology, Washington, D.C.

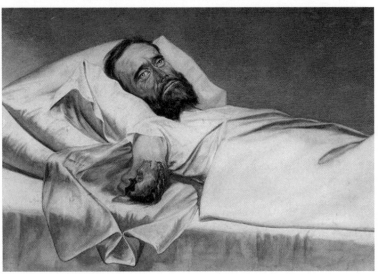

an epidemic of hospital gangrene. As small wounds became large ones and clean cases became dirty, it soon became apparent that the doctor in charge had used the same dressings over and over. Dr. Sternberg transferred all uninfected cases to other wards and treated the others by cleaning the wounds and applying clean dressings. The hospital was scoured and whitewashed, and the epidemic subsided. If these findings had been passed on to other military surgeons, thousands of lives could have been saved.[329]

Another infection that could develop in improperly debrided injuries was gas gangrene. The bacillus that causes gas gangrene, *Clostridium perfringes,* thrives in dead tissue. It is estimated that over one hundred thousand German soldiers died of this complication in World War I.[330] Tetanus (lockjaw) was another bacterial infection caused by contamination and from which many soldiers perished. The dirt on many battlegrounds was polluted from grazing animals that carried anaerobic organisms such as *Tetanus bacillus* and *Clostridium perfringes,* and all open wounds and perforations were exposed. American army doctors had thoroughly learned of the danger of contamination during the Civil War, and by the turn of the twentieth century, there were few competent practicing doctors, civilian or military, who didn't understand how to treat contaminated injuries correctly.

Even without modern medical treatment methods such as intravenous fluids, blood expanders, transfusions, antiseptics, and antibiotics, most injured personnel responded favorably to the medical care that was available. Narcotics eased pain, and the comfort afforded by nursing care, psychological support, and rest lessened shock and aided in recovery. The human body is very resilient. And resiliency was what was needed to survive on the frontier.

Arrow Wounds

The Native American's expert use of the bow and arrow in battle presented a new challenge to the frontier military physician. Few doctors had previous experience treating arrow wounds, so they were forced to learn about it through trial and error combined with common sense. Dr. Joseph H. Bill, assistant surgeon at Fort Craig, New Mexico Territory, developed the first instruments for treating arrow wounds and the technique that guided other military doctors faced with these kinds of perforating injuries.[331]

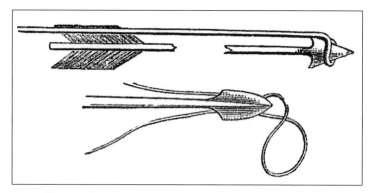

Bill's Snare for the extraction of arrowheads —From *The Science and Art of Surgery: A Treatise on Surgical Injuries, Diseases, and Operations* by John Eric Erichsen, 1884

A skilled Indian bowman could accurately shoot six arrows per minute. If a soldier was struck with one arrow, he was likely to soon be hit by another.[332] Purposefully Native American war arrowheads were loosely attached to the shaft, using animal material such as tendon or ligamentous tissue or an organic glue. When this material became wet from the victim's blood, the connection was weakened. With such an insecure bond, the arrowhead usually stayed in when the shaft was pulled out, becoming a source of potential infection. Furthermore, an attempt to remove an arrow by the injured soldier or helpful comrades could not only produce additional tissue damage, it also made the doctor's job more difficult. Without the shaft as a guide, it was often hard for a surgeon to find and remove the arrowhead. Soldiers were warned not to pull out arrows, but most did anyway.[333]

In spite of the difficulties, army doctors had a good record in treating superficial arrow wounds. Most of the fatalities were from cerebral, abdominal, and chest penetrations. Fortunately most arrow wounds involved the upper extremities because by reflex combatants used their arms as shields. The Surgeon General's report of August 17, 1871, listed forty cases of superficial arrow wounds without one fatality or serious complication.[334]

With experience, the military doctor developed special methods in the treatment of arrow wounds. First he explored the wound with his finger to determine the location and attitude of the foreign body and what anatomical structures it was near. Sometimes he used a bistoury—

a long, thin, probe-tipped knife fashioned to cut in two directions, from the inside out—to enlarge the track of the arrow. This allowed the projectile to be extracted more easily and enhanced drainage. Experienced surgeons fashioned various probes, forceps, and snares to help extract arrowheads. Some used a wire loop, blindly guided by a finger, to encircle the arrowhead at the base, then tightened the loop and—if the surgeon was lucky and strong enough—pulled the arrowhead out. This bloody, painful procedure was performed in the field hospital or even on the battlefield. When available, chloroform, morphine, or whiskey dulled some of the pain, but much of the time, no anesthesia was used.

Dr. Elliott Coues, a famous military doctor, ornithologist, and historian, became an expert on arrow wounds while stationed at Fort Whipple, Arizona Territory. He wrote, "A regular part of my business for two years was the extraction of Apache arrow-heads."[335] Dr. Coues once removed an arrow from a young man's chest while the patient sat on a barrel and he sat on a stump, "the heat and flies intolerable." The arrowhead was lying near the large subclavian artery, but the artery was "luckily quite uninjured," and the procedure was successful.[336]

War Stories

As a rule, military doctors, with their rigorous training and their mettle tested on the battlefield, were competent and conscientious physicians, and many became leaders in their profession. One outstanding example was George Miller Sternberg, who eventually served as U.S. Surgeon General. Dr. Sternberg was a veteran of the Civil War and had a long career with the army. His creative research in microbiology saved thousands of lives. Stationed at Fort Walla Walla, Washington Territory, in 1877, Sternberg had just arrived for duty when the Nez Perces began to attack. He was sent to render assistance at the Battle of White Bird Canyon, and soon after that he tended troops at the Battle of the Clearwater. Dr. Sternberg stalked the battlefield in the dark, only a few yards from the Indian lines, to reach some of the wounded and bring them in. One man, in serious condition and losing a great deal of blood, required immediate surgery in the field. His assistants held a blanket up to hide the light of a candle from the enemy while he operated. In spite of the precaution, Nez Perce sharpshooters fired at the light, so Dr. Sternberg had to finish in the dark. Miraculously, none of the medics was hit, the surgery was completed successfully, and the patient survived.

After several more confrontations between General O. O. Howard's command and Chief Joseph's warriors, Dr. Sternberg was ordered to take twenty-seven wounded soldiers back to safety. This was no small order, as he had an inadequate number of wagons in which to carry them. Emulating the Cheyennes he had fought against, the doctor ordered several travois built to transport the wounded. During the formidable trip to Fort Lapwai, which took almost a week on the trail, young Major Sternberg cared for the injured and even amputated one soldier's leg when massive bleeding developed.[337]

Another remarkable army doctor was Walter Reed. Dr. Reed, a first lieutenant in the Army Medical Corps, was part of the team that discovered the vector and transmission of yellow fever, and, like Sternberg, he later served as Surgeon General. In December 1880, after the massacre at Wounded Knee, Reed was sent to Fort Keogh, near Miles City, Montana. Arriving three weeks after the battle, he treated one officer, a Lieutenant Hawthorne, whose life was saved when a bullet struck his pocket watch. Dr. Reed meticulously removed the mainspring, ratchet wheels, glass, and watchcase from Hawthorne's abdominal wall. There is no record of whether the watch was repaired.[338]

Torturous Ride

Just eight days before General George Custer's appointment with destiny at the Little Big Horn, General George Crook's forces, camped near the Rosebud River, were attacked by an estimated fifteen hundred Lakota and Northern Cheyenne warriors under the command of Crazy Horse. The fight raged for hours, frequently in hand-to-hand combat. The battle cost the army at least nine soldiers killed and nineteen wounded. There were no arrow wounds because by then the Indians had guns, and they used cylindrical bullets that produced greater tissue damage than the standard ball.[339]

One of the officers, Brevet Colonel Guy Henry, was shot in the head, and his story alone demonstrates the courage and fortitude of these men. The bullet smashed both of Henry's cheekbones, his nose, and one eye. He nevertheless attempted to lead another charge, but overcome with shock he finally fell to the ground. His wounds were dressed at a small aid station in the nearby woods. After the battle, the army began the retreat south. To make the trip, Henry was placed on a litter suspended between two mules fore and aft. Army surgeons supposedly preferred mules to horses because they took smaller steps, giving the wounded

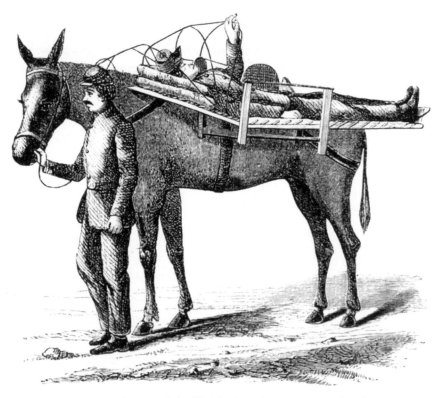

Transportation of a wounded soldier by horse litter. Horses and mules were often used to evacuate the injured during the Indian wars. —Courtesy National Library of Medicine, History of Medicine Division

soldier a smoother ride.[340] On several occasions doctors had requested that badly injured patients be transported on an Indian-style travois—parallel poles rigged as a litter and pulled behind a horse—but the army "brass" always refused the request. Some believed the refusal was based on a reluctance to copy anything from the "savages." Travois were used sometimes, however.

In their hurry to leave the battlefield, the troops forced the mules to trot much of the time—the stolid Henry admitted later that this was the worst part of his long odyssey. Because Henry was positioned feet first between the mules, the rear animal's thick skull repeatedly bumped the man's badly injured head until someone saw this and turned his body around. Unfortunately, this position put him in danger of the lead mule's kicking him, and he was in fact kicked in the face once. Henry suffered further when the litter struck a boulder—he was thrown to the ground and rolled down an incline. After surviving this, he was nearly washed away in the current while the mules were fording the Tongue River.

By the time he reached Fort Fetterman, having traveled three hundred miles on a litter, Colonel Henry was totally blind and severely anemic, but alive. Amazingly, he eventually returned to full duty. When asked later about the experience, Henry replied that it was "nothing remarkable."[341]

Doctor's Last Stand

Army surgeon James DeWolf did not survive the famous attack at the Little Bighorn River, nor did his associate, Dr. George Edwin Lord. Dr. Henry Renaldo Porter, however, did live to tell about the bloody battle: "We made this retreat on a dead run, the Sioux running right alongside of us shooting, and in some cases pulling our men off their horses and then killing them. Several were killed by my side, and the Indians were within ten yards on either side, firing all the time."[342]

As soon as he could, Dr. Porter improvised a "hospital" on the top of what would later be called Reno Hill. It was no more than a shallow depression in the earth with "sagebrush walls, an operating table made of sand, and the blue canopy of heaven for a roof."[343] Into this barely protected space, the Sioux chief Gall and his warriors lobbed arrows without showing themselves. Coming from above with high trajectory, the arrows struck the unprotected soldiers. "Many . . . died that way, and in death lay face down, an arrow rigid and upright in his back."[344] Dr. Porter worked throughout the first night, under attack, with over fifty wounded in his care. With only flickering candlelight and without anesthesia, the intrepid physician cleaned and dressed wounds, removed arrows, probed for bullets, and amputated limbs. Though fully occupied, at intervals the frustrated Dr. Porter grabbed a rifle and fired a few shots at the Indians.

Colonel John Gibbon's Seventh Infantry, with assistant surgeon Lieutenant Holmes O. Paulding, were among the first to discover the grisly scene on the Little Bighorn battlefield. The young physician was ordered to assist Dr. Porter. In a letter to his mother, Dr. Paulding wrote, "We found a horrible sight & did all we could for the wounded of whom only 50 got in, the rest being killed."[345] At first, hand litters were used to move the wounded, but this method proved an "utter" failure. Mule litters were then constructed from timber frames and thongs of rawhide cut from the horses' carcasses, topped with blankets and canvas. During the exhausting evacuation process, the weather changed to heavy rain. Eventually the soldiers reached the mouth of the Bighorn River with their suffering cargo, where the steamer *Far West* waited. "I was nearly dead with the fatigue of the past 3 days & nights. . . . You bet I didn't make much bones about going to sleep for 3 hours," Paulding said.[346]

"Horrible state of affairs"

The Battle of the Big Hole was one of the most intense conflicts in the annals of the Indian wars.[347] The Nez Perce War had begun the previous June, when tensions over the U.S. government's takeover of Nez Perce land erupted in violence and the Nez Perces, under the leadership of Chief Joseph, began an exodus to flee the country. On August 9, 1877, in the predawn hours, civilian volunteer troops under Colonel John Gibbon infiltrated and surrounded the Nez Perces' camp on the Big Hole River. After a premature first shot from an overeager soldier, Gibbon's men began firing at the tepees.[348]

In spite of Gibbon's superior arms, better-trained soldiers, and the element of surprise, after twenty-four hours of bloody combat, the Nez Perces, led by Chiefs Joseph, White Bird, Looking Glass, and others, had gained the upper hand, then escaped with their wounded. When the Indians left, Colonel Gibbon, who was wounded in the left thigh, and his troops huddled together behind pine trees and waited for assistance.[349] Gibbon counted his dead at twenty-nine and his wounded at forty. In his official report he classified twenty of the injured as serious or severe.[350] Without a surgeon or medical supplies, the injured men were left to their own devices, making bandages of shirttails, spitting tobacco juice into their wounds, and cauterizing raw gashes by sprinkling them with gunpowder and igniting it.[351]

General Howard had left the previous day from Idaho to relieve Gibbon's men. Accompanying him were two army doctors, surgeon Charles T. Alexander and assistant surgeon Jenkins A. Fitzgerald. The two doctors arrived with an advance escort in the early morning of August 11, and they immediately went to work. Dr. Fitzgerald later wrote his wife that the wounded were in a "horrible state of affairs . . . suffering intensely."[352]

The most seriously injured included Lieutenant William L. English, with an abdomen wound from which he died eleven days later, and Sergeant William W. Watson, with a shattered left hip that also proved fatal. Another seriously wounded man was Private Charles Alberts, who was shot in the chest. A companion on the field wrote that, "from the bubbles of air in the flowing blood," he knew the bullet had punctured the lung.[353] Apparently someone sealed the wound, or blood clots developed to plug the hole, preventing a fatal pneumothorax, and Private Alberts survived.

The rest of General Howard's relief column appeared on August 12. Howard described the scene: "So many wounded; nearly half lying cheerful, though not able to move, many white bandages about the head and face; some arms in slings; there were roughly constructed shelters from the heat."[354] It seems that in one day's time, the aid rendered by Drs. Alexander and Fitzgerald had alleviated much of the soldiers' suffering.

Meanwhile, more help was on its way. Civilian relief groups were organized in Butte, Deer Lodge, and Helena, then they joined forces and headed toward the Big Hole. In all were six surgeons, twenty-eight light wagons and ambulances, and two companies of volunteers.[355] From Helena, some Sisters of Charity of Providence came to offer their nursing skills. According to the August 14 *Butte Miner*, the supplies included "four gals. brandy, 2 gal. whiskey, 50 yds. bleached muslin for bandages and some lint, 2 cases of surgical instruments, $75 worth of medicine, 1 case each of strawberries, peaches, oysters and sardines."[356]

Army medical wagon, Civil War. This shows a demonstration of the use of anesthesia in amputations. —Courtesy National Museum of Health and Medicine, Otis Historical Archives, Washington D.C.

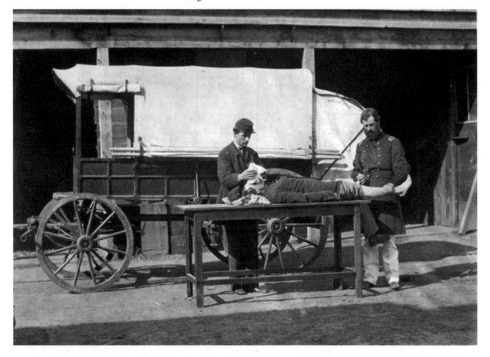

The relief party was requested to make camp about fourteen miles from the battleground and wait for the wounded. At the Big Hole, the approximately thirty injured soldiers were loaded onto army wagons, which, General Howard wrote, were "hard, shaky things . . . at best."[357] As soon as the wagons arrived at the relief camp, the civilian doctors and nurses went to work. The *Butte Miner* reported that "They did not stop to eat or rest until all the wounded had been aided."[358]

After dark, the doctors and nurses worked by the light of lanterns hung on the ambulance wagons. The scant supply of ether and chloroform was soon used up, and it was necessary to immobilize some of the wounded men by force during painful procedures. The volunteer doctors had had years of "on-the-job training" at frontier gold camps, where they had honed their skills treating injuries from mine accidents, ranch and farm mishaps, barroom knife- and gunfights, and Indian skirmishes, and they ably met the challenge. As soon as possible, the suffering soldiers were again loaded onto wagons, on which they were transported to the newly built St. Joseph's Hospital in Deer Lodge, approximately fifty miles away. Rattling over rough trails and through swamps and creeks, the patients arrived at the hospital around noon on August 16, six days after the battle.[359]

G. O. Shields, writing in 1889, recorded and charted the survivors' injuries from the Battle of the Big Hole.[360] Of the forty wounded survivors, twenty were listed as "serious," and only two died. Knowing the outcome of this group of patients gives us a yardstick with which to measure the quality of medical practice of the era. It is a commendable record. The two army physicians, Alexander and Fitzgerald, deserve a lot of the credit, but because they had to continue the mission with General Howard, they could not stay with their patients. The volunteer frontier doctors finished the job admirably.

The Battle of Wounded Knee

Perhaps it is fitting that such a terrible, bloody blunder as Wounded Knee marked the last battle of the Indian wars. The tragic showdown at Wounded Knee Creek has been examined by many credible historians from many different viewpoints. Although the exact number of Indian casualties is not known, the official figure has been set at 153 dead and 44 wounded.[361] On the army side, according to Mary Gillett, 29 soldiers and an Indian scout were killed and 30 were wounded.[362]

The morning of December 29, 1890, was warm and pleasant but charged with tension when Seventh Cavalry troops surrounded Big Foot's Miniconjou band camped on Wounded Knee Creek, fifteen miles from Pine Ridge, South Dakota. As the Indians were surrendering their weapons, someone from somewhere fired a shot, and the troopers opened fire. The echoes of the gunshots were clearly heard at Pine Ridge by Dr. Charles Eastman, the reservation physician, and his bride-to-be, Elaine Goodale.[363]

Charles A. Eastman was a Lakota Sioux, but he had never lived on a reservation and had no preconceived ideas about the plight of his kinsmen. After he graduated from medical school, he applied for a position as physician on one of the Sioux reservations.[364] Eventually he was assigned to the one at Pine Ridge. From his own description in *From the Deep Woods to Civilization*, he arrived in a November dust storm and saw the reservation as a stark and desolate place. Nevertheless, he was "alive with energy and enthusiasm."[365]

On that fateful day in December, by late afternoon the wounded had begun to pour in at Pine Ridge. The army casualties were sent to an army field hospital, but most of the forty-four wounded Indians were brought to Dr. Eastman. To hastily prepare a hospital in the Episcopal mission chapel, the pews were torn out, the Christmas tree and decorations pushed out of the way, and the floor was covered with straw and blankets on which to lay the victims.[366] "There we laid the poor creatures side by side," Dr. Eastman wrote. "Many were frightfully torn by pieces of shells and the suffering was terrible." Even though army physicians volunteered to help, Eastman found that "The tortured Indians [would] scarcely allow a man in uniform to touch them." He did have the help of several volunteer nurses, including Elaine Goodale. Nevertheless, "we lost the greater part of [the patients]."[367]

As if conditions were not bad enough, a raging blizzard struck. A few days later, as soon as travel was possible, Eastman led a group to the battle site to look for survivors. As his gloomy expedition struggled through the drifts of snow, they found frozen bodies scattered several miles from the scene, "as they had been relentlessly hunted down and slaughtered."[368] The Indians accompanying Eastman began to cry and sing death songs.

Each body was dug from the snow and chipped out of the ice to make sure no flame of life still flickered. Eastman searched in places he thought he himself might have hidden, and the strategy was successful.

He and his men found ten survivors. Sadly most of these partially frozen wounded did not live another day. Of the experience, Dr. Eastman wrote, "All this was a severe ordeal for one who had so lately put all his faith in the Christian love and lofty ideals of the white man."[369] There was one gratifying recovery, however. Hearing a muffled cry, the searchers discovered a baby girl, frostbitten but breathing, sheltered in a shallow hole beneath her mother's frozen and mutilated body. The baby girl, later known as Lost Bird, was adopted into a white family.[370]

The injured casualties at Wounded Knee were the first patients to come under the care of the army's new Hospital Corps. Until then, military surgeons had had to do everything themselves—treat the injured, nurse the recovering, arrange for transportation of the wounded, and generally oversee the entire operation, all under battlefield conditions. After the establishment of the Hospital Corps, field surgeons examined the wounded, then placed a tag on each patient describing his injuries, whereupon trained corpsmen handled their care accordingly and evacuated them to hospitals. With the new system, according to Mary Gillett, both wounded soldiers and wounded Indians were efficiently attended to in the field hospitals. The care of all wounded in this battle was far superior to that received in any previous military conflict. (For more on military hospitals, see chapter 11.)

SEVEN

"Granny Remedies"
Pioneer Women and Folk Medicine

I don't want a doctor. I want a woman!
—Pioneer Nannie T. Alderson, in *A Bride Goes West*[371]

FOLK MEDICINE DATES as far back as mankind. Found in a Neanderthal burial cave in Iraq was sixty-thousand-year-old pollen from species of plants that are still traditionally used to treat wounds, dysentery, asthma, inflammation, toothache, and other ailments.[372] Scores of remedies passed down through generations came west with the pioneers. Some were useless, but many of them worked. Who would have believed that igniting an herb called mugwort (*Artemesia vulgaris*) and letting it smolder against the little toe of a pregnant woman would have an effect on the fetus? Researchers tested this Chinese practice and found that of fetuses in a breech position, seventy-five percent rotated to the normal and safer headfirst position before delivery, where in the control group, only forty-eight percent rotated.[373]

In the latter part of the nineteenth century and into the twentieth, the profession of medicine was so anxious to escape its history of "purge, blister, and bleed" and accept science as its icon that it abandoned credible folk treatments handed down since antiquity. This is unfortunate. Recent clinical trials of some "alternative" therapies have shown intriguing results. In addition to the mugwort study previously mentioned, saw palmetto extracts were found to improve urologic symptoms in patients with benign prostatic hyperplasia, and one Chinese herbal formulation improved symptoms of irritable bowel syndrome.[374]

In spite of the medical profession's aversion to it, folk medicine, called "granny medicine" by some, was practiced in nearly every community in the West. Through trial and error a heritage of "cures" and nostrums developed. There were literally thousands of home remedies, and each family had its favorites. Though most of these methods were directed

131

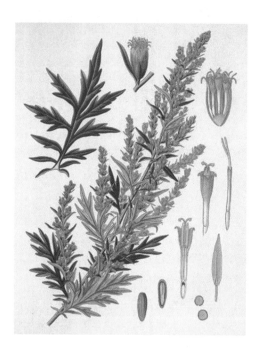

Mugwort (Artemesia vulgaris) —From *A Modern Herbal* by Maud Grieve, 1931

at symptoms and were not curative, few cures of any kind existed at this time in history.

Bernard De Voto, a famous historian of the West, wrote, "On the frontier ... the family doctor was the housewife, or grandma, or a neighbor who had a reputation in occult wisdom, or some beldame who was supposed to be gifted at magic. . . . We may safely assume that at one time or another everything which grew in the fields, forests, and swamps played a part in family medicine."[375] There was a "receipt" (recipe) for every illness that came along or needed to be prevented. Certainly many of these treatments relieved symptoms, especially if accompanied by rest and good nursing care.

"The true spirit of nursing": Frontier Women as Caregivers

Since the earliest of times, women have always played a major role in medical care, though their contributions were seldom officially recorded. From the beginning, the male-dominated profession of medicine refused to recognize the value of women in the healing arts. History does tell us, however, that since antiquity it was usually the women who gathered herbs and prepared medicine, bathed the infirm, nursed the sick, and delivered babies. In the American West, tale after tale describes women's roles as caregivers on the long trip from the so-called civilized world to the wild, untamed frontier. Many pioneers were nursed through sickness and injury by mothers, aunts, sisters, and grandmothers on the trail and in the pubescent towns of the western frontier.

Frontier women were caregivers in the true sense of the word, and they represented the first line of defense against disease. For a long period in American history, these pioneer women, whose only reward was the satisfaction of helping others, devoted themselves to the sick. Many of them learned about medicine from their mothers, and a few might have read books on health. Some knew a good deal about herbs. Mostly, however, they used common sense and relied on their own experience with illness and injury. More important than what they knew was the fact that they cared. It is doubtful that any of these humble people thought of themselves as exceptional or had ever heard of Florence Nightingale.

Most communities had midwives and women who specialized in tending the sick. A few scattered anecdotes about these selfless, unpaid, and underappreciated women survive, but the full story may never be told. An unnamed "negro" woman, said to be the slave of Dr. Benjamin C. Brooke, nursed many prominent citizens in Helena, Montana,

Caregivers on the frontier came from different walks of life. Taken in Gilt Edge, Montana, about 1897, this is a photograph of Martha Jane Canary, the notorious "Calamity Jane," who was a nurse. —Courtesy Montana Historical Society, Helena

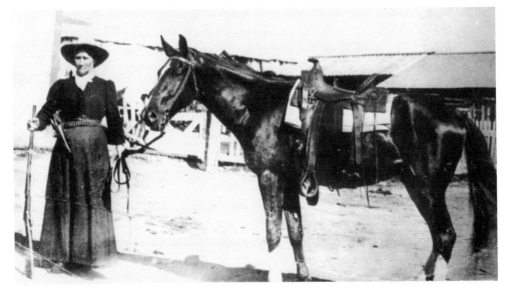

including the family of territorial governor Sidney Edgerton.[376] Martha Jane Canary, better known as "Calamity Jane," was a frontier nurse. Her vices were legendary, but few know that she served as a nurse in Billings, Montana, before there was a hospital, and her contemporaries described her as caring and competent.[377]

Occasionally Indian women gained reputations as healers. Not all white people trusted Native Americans, but some early settlers accepted their services, if only out of necessity. Most Indian women used herbal medicine and were experienced in treating wounds. One time at Fort Union, when the child of famous fur trader Alexander Culbertson and his Blackfeet wife, Natavista, was sick with croup, Natavista allowed the child to be treated with the white man's remedies, but they did no good. She persuaded her husband to call an old Blood "squaw" who had a reputation as a nurse. When this medicine woman arrived, she heated rocks, poured water on them, and immersed the child's room in steam. During this procedure, she chanted a song that was part of the cure. Father Nicholas Point heard the chants and rushed into the house. He chastised Culbertson, saying, "How do you suppose that I can win these people from their pagan practices if you allow them to bring them into your homes?" The pragmatic Culbertson nevertheless permitted the woman to continue her treatment, and the child got well.[378] This nameless Indian lady had a great deal of common sense—many forms of respiratory disease respond well to vapor. Native Americans had been using the sweat lodge for this purpose for a long time.

Most of the women who served as nurses in their communities also had their own broods to raise and worked with the men on the farms. Mrs. Rodney Simmons Barnes, who arrived at Fort Benton, Montana, from Canada in 1883, had sixteen children of her own. Nevertheless, she found time to care for others as a practical nurse and midwife.[379] Broadwater County, Montana, was fortunate to have Mrs. Mary Powell Jenkins, who nursed the sick and delivered babies in Toston, Townsend, and Radersburg from 1888 to 1912. According to her daughter, Mary had "no formal training in nursing, but she had the true spirit of nursing . . . service . . . when and where it was needed."[380]

Home on the Range

Most newcomers to the plains had been used to better circumstances. Having left their cozy homes back east, they now lived in sod houses, lean-tos, or tarpaper shacks with dirt floors, insulated only with newspaper. Fuel

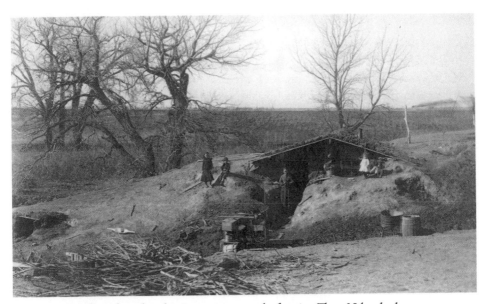

Families adapted to the circumstances on the frontier. These Nebraska home-steaders built their home using the sod and wood available. —Courtesy Nebraska State Historical Society

was usually scarce, and water was often hauled great distances from rivers or creeks of uncertain quality. Still, to a degree, the relative isolation of the homestead was more healthful than conditions in the East because there was less exposure to disease. Sometimes epidemics nevertheless found their way into even the most remote communities. Dr. Camilla Anderson said that, when she was a little girl, her house in tiny Sidney, Montana, was like Grand Central Station. On one occasion, some visiting immigrants from Denmark brought scarlet fever. She contracted the disease, and the illness swept through the community, causing the deaths of at least two people.[381]

When times were hard, most homesteaders were trapped, barely able to survive but too poor to leave, and for many there was no professional medical care available. Distances were great, and transportation was unpredictable, difficult, costly, and time-consuming. A few doctors settled in the burgeoning communities along the railroads, waterways, and trails, but even then, their services were expensive. Most pioneers' first response to sickness was to employ folk remedies and tender loving care.

Even though their "receipts" had limited therapeutic value, the ministrations of mothers and grandmothers provided symptomatic relief, gave warmth and comfort to enhance rest, and allowed the patient's natural defenses to mobilize. This was good nursing care by anyone's definition. Who among us, during an illness with fever, muscle aches, congestion, or a tormenting cough, has not felt better thanks to soothing vapor and aromatic ointments gently rubbed onto the chest? After a long period in bed, who hasn't appreciated a sponge bath, clean sheets, and cool, smooth hands massaging a sore back?

In *A Bride Goes West*, Nannie T. Alderson, who homesteaded with her husband in the 1880s, a hundred miles south of Miles City, wrote, "Taking the law of averages into account, we got off very easily during the years we lived so far from a doctor. We never had a serious illness. We had a few accidents." She said her husband had a "rough competence" at surgery and a natural sense of what to do when someone was hurt. All the ranchers kept sheets of surgeon's plaster to bind up a broken limb. "In all the years of our life on the ranch we never had a doctor for the children but twice," Alderson said. When she left Kansas for the frontier, a friend gave her a homeopathic kit with many bottles of "little white sugary pills," and directions for treating illnesses such as colds, fever, and stomach trouble.[382] This "drug" supply apparently worked for her family. Here is major support for the idea that faith plays a large part in the curative art.

Frontier women were often left alone for days—sometimes weeks or months—while their husbands worked elsewhere to supplement a measly farm income. One summer while her husband was away, Mrs. Alderson had a miscarriage. The hired men were terrified. When they suggested that they get the doctor, who was a hundred miles away, she scolded them, saying, "I don't want a doctor. I want a woman!" A woman who had just moved into the territory came and nursed Nannie back to health.[383]

Mrs. Alderson's attitude was not unusual. Frontier women did not turn to men for emotional support, but to "other women, companionable mothers, aunts, sisters, cousins, friends—allies of a lifetime."[384] Women almost never discussed their feelings, and certainly not their intimate health problems, outside this close-knit sorority. Men seldom used definite language to describe "woman troubles"; a man whose wife was pregnant might make some vague allusion to her "condition."

Many women had a baby every year, and children were often sick. Concern for the children was the greatest cause of anxiety to frontier families. The pioneers may reluctantly have accepted hazards such as potential household and barnyard accidents, poisonous snakes, and fire, but the deep fear of the unknown when a child developed a fever, rash, sore throat, or stomach pain hung like a pall over frontier homes. There were no magic cures, and all too often a family had to bury one or more of its little ones.

It was usually up to the mothers to doctor and nurse their offspring. If they were lucky, they might have a neighbor to help, perhaps a "yarb doctor" or someone with knowledge of "Indian" medicine. Where else could they turn? We are distracted today at the primitive methods and unscientific remedies that held the trust of those untrained homesteaders, but the diseases that killed the pioneers either no longer exist or are preventable or easily cured with the miracles of modern medicine. Seldom in modern society does this terrible fear clutch at the hearts of parents of small children.

It was not uncommon for families to be stricken with two or more epidemic diseases at once, such as smallpox with scarlet fever. One Christmas in Minnesota, Harriet Godfrey, whose husband had gone to

The Harvey Andrews family at the grave of their nineteen-month-old son, Willie. Death hovered close over the lives of the pioneers. —Courtesy Nebraska State Historical Society

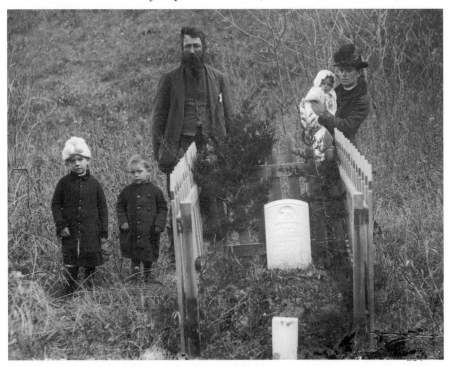

Montana, had to nurse her several children back to health after such a bombardment. An outbreak of measles was followed by an eruption of boils. Her eight-year-old daughter Kittie had a dozen boils on her face and scalp. Infections such as this sometimes led to "blood poisoning" (a bloodstream infection, or septicemia) or even to brain abscesses, but Mrs. Godfrey treated her child's condition successfully with "mustard." Then, just as this crisis subsided, all her children developed whooping cough. Both whooping cough and measles were serious maladies with many potential complications, but it seems the Godfrey family was blessed not only with a superb caregiver, but with some luck as well. During the weeks of illness, Mrs. Godfrey "got along without a physician," relying on the herbal medicines she had prepared herself.[385] Truly, the homestead mother was the key to health on the frontier. She has no equal in the annals of the pioneer West.

Home Remedies and Patent Medicines

Every frontier home had a variety of nostrums and remedies. Most family medicine chests contained a variety of dried herbs called "simples," such as feverfew, fleabane, boneset, rhubarb, oak of Jerusalem, thyme, marjoram, and many others. Obviously, some served two functions, as medicine and as food seasoning. Some were bitter (the more bitter the better), to ease dyspepsia; others were tasty, like sassafras, which was used to "cleanse" or to "thin" the blood. Sweet sarsaparilla was popular as a blood purifier and a tonic. Part of its appeal was the unsubstantiated belief that it could restore sexual vigor in men. Impotence was a very common fear, and sarsaparilla was one of many preparations that were in demand to counter it.

Although birth control was a nearly taboo subject in the 1800s, many frontier women kept some kind of substance, passed down from mother to daughter or friend to friend, that was trusted as a contraceptive or emmenagogue. Many people, especially men, influenced by religious and societal beliefs, felt that anything pertaining to sex should never be discussed and viewed the prevention of unwanted pregnancies as sinful. Nevertheless, unknown numbers of wives kept hidden some herb thought to be a contraceptive or an abortifacient. Pennyroyal (*Mentha pulegium*) and seeds of Queen Anne's lace (flowers of the wild carrot, *Daucus carota*) were among the most popular substances for this purpose. Women also taught each other to make and use pessaries, douches, and various spermicides. Much of the information was questionable, such as

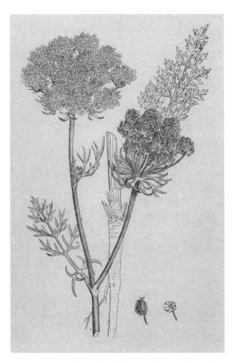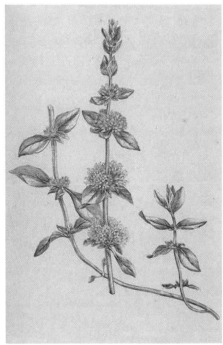

The seeds of Queen Anne's Lace (Daucus carota, wild carrot), *pennyroyal* (Mentha pulegium), *and other plants have been used as contraceptives for thousands of years.* —From *A Modern Herbal* by Maud Grieve, 1931

using coal oil as a douche. Pessaries were fashioned out of materials such as beeswax or citrus peel. Some of these methods worked, but they often led to infections.[386]

Many of the staples of the frontier medicine kit were store-bought. Some were intoxicants, kept under guard by the family caregiver. One of these was the opium tincture known as laudanum. A few drops would be given orally for severe pain. There were few laws regarding drugs until the early twentieth century, and drugstore owners—whether pharmacists, doctors, or laymen—could dispense whatever the public demanded, including narcotics.

Whiskey was another drug that homesteaders frequently used, taken straight or mixed in elaborate concoctions. Used both internally and externally for a vast number of common ailments, "medicinal" whiskey was deemed indispensable by many people, even teetotalers. Pioneer

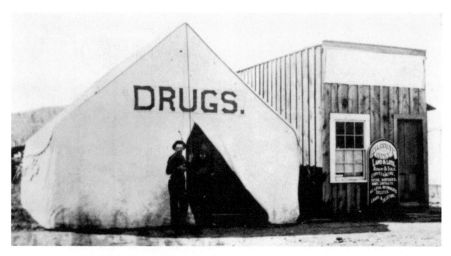

Shannon and Hall's Drug Store, Coulson, Montana, an early river town, 1882. Drugstores were not far behind the settlers in frontier communities. This one obviously appeared in a hurry. —Courtesy Montana Historical Society, Helena

housewives, including some who saw liquor as an instrument of the devil, were skilled at mixing various alcoholic remedies. For indigestion, a solution of rhubarb bitters or cayenne pepper mixed with whiskey was rubbed into the abdomen, often combined with whiskey and water taken internally.

Castor oil was the classic cure-all of the nineteenth and early twentieth centuries. A potent laxative made from the castor bean, it was used as the main medicine of choice in many families during that era, when purging the bowels was considered a panacea. Castor oil combined with calomel emptied the intestinal tract and left the patient weak and dehydrated. Nevertheless, it was one of the most respected medications of the day, frequently prescribed by physicians and mothers alike.

Snake oil, the ingredient that became synonymous with bogus medicines, was popular at one time as a liniment for sore muscles and other ailments. Well-known Montana cattleman Conrad Kohrs testified in his diary to the healing powers of snake oil. In the early 1860s, Kohrs was nearly totally disabled with rheumatism. Oil was rendered from sixty to seventy snakes and used to bathe the rancher's aching joints. According to the patient, the result was miraculous. Kohrs's business partner, Johnny Grant, used skunk oil for the same purpose. He said that "the smell is

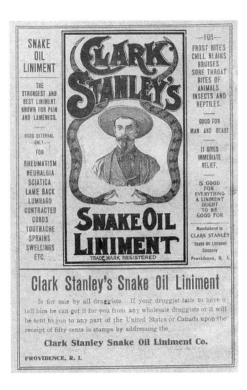

Clark Stanley liniment. Snake oil was respected as a cure-all by many frontiersmen. —Courtesy National Library of Medicine, History of Medicine Division

Castor oil, a powerful purgative, was a mainstay of home remedies.
—Courtesy National Library of Medicine, History of Medicine Division

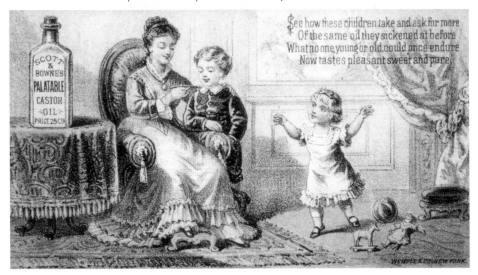

awful . . . but the relief one feels of getting rid of that annoying pain . . . is worth trying."[387]

In time, most family pharmacies included patent medicines. Perhaps there was a bottle of Kickapoo Indian Sagwa, which the pitchmen claimed was a cure for liver complaints, scrofula, chills and fever, or "whatever ails." A bottle of Warner's Safe Kidney Cure (most backaches were attributed to kidney disease) might also have been included on the shelf. Lydia Pinkham's vegetable tonic was accepted as a panacea for women's complaints, from minor menstrual cramps to cancer of the uterus. If nothing else, the high percentage of alcohol in most "patent" medicines contributed to a temporary feeling of well-being. Though the charlatans who sold this stuff were mostly quacks, the home caregiver believed in the curative powers of these concoctions, and a patient's faith often has a significant impact on his or her recovery.

Most folk medicines were used with adequate-to-good symptomatic results, even putting aside the placebo effect. Modern skeptics have to

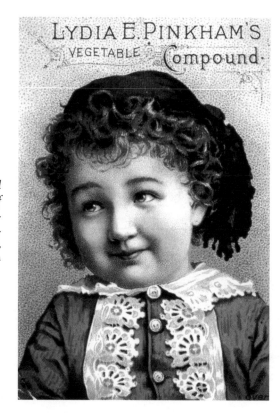

Lydia Pinkham was a real person. She made a lot of money with her tonics for female complaints. —Courtesy National Library of Medicine, History of Medicine Division

admit that many folk remedies were scientifically valid. It is hard to fault some of the frontier reliables. For instance, cold witch hazel applied with cotton balls to hemorrhoids after a hot "sitz" bath served as an astringent and vasoconstrictor, and variations of this treatment still give relief to hemorrhoid sufferers. Mashed strawberries used as a facial cleanser to alleviate acne was beneficial because of the fruit-acid. Even today, a few gastroenterologists, looking for mild laxatives, are recommending old favorites such as a mixture of rhubarb, fruit juice, and honey. And the classic home remedy of rich, hot, nutritious chicken soup for upper-respiratory illness has never gone out of style.

For injuries, family healers used poultices of slippery elm and cornmeal to relieve burns; wet tea leaves, which contain tannic acid, also benefited burned skin. Chronic sores were sometimes treated effectively with mold from bread or cheese—positive results may have been due to an antibiotic in the culture. A plaster of mustard or other irritating substances applied to the skin eased the ache of bruises, arthritis, and pleurisy. Sugar, seldom thought of as a drug, was used for hundreds of years to help heal wounds. Applying sugar to a fresh wound dried it out and inhibited bacteria growth.

Other commonly used remedies were more dubious. There is little support for poultices of fresh cow manure (a sometime favorite) applied to wounds, snakebites, and infections. It is highly doubtful that diphtheria responded to mashed snails and earthworms or that a tea made from chimney soot relieved rheumatism. And it would be hard to prove scientifically that a bag of asafetida hung around the neck prevented the common cold or whooping cough, or that an onion carried in a pocket could ward off smallpox, or that passing a horse collar over a child's head three times made him immune to a contagious illness.[388]

As these examples illustrate, frontier "cures" were often a combination of old lore, superstition, and everyday ignorance. A horseshoe placed under the bed allegedly relieved toothaches, and it was thought by some that touching the hand of a corpse benefited cancer. A firmly believed treatment for snakebite was to apply fresh animal flesh to the bite to prevent a toxic reaction to the venom. The animal most commonly sacrificed for this purpose was a chicken, easily obtained in most farmyards, but sometimes fresh deer liver was used. For diarrhea, or "looseness of the belly," it was recommended that one "take the yard or pizzle of a buck, reduce it to a powder, put a spoonful of the powder in a bottle with a pint of spirits; take this solution in small quantities, every hour, till relief is obtained."[389]

As people of different cultures crossed the oceans and prairies, they brought their own favorite medicines. The Basque influence can be seen in Nevada, where a foot soak of dried mustard and wood ashes in water was used to ward off colds; whiskey and lemon juice mixed with hot water was taken for sore throats; and tobacco smoke blown into the ear was thought to ease earache. Garlic and onions were also popular medicines among Basques. Garlic soup was drunk for upper respiratory illnesses, and garlic cloves were placed in wounds to enhance healing. Applying half a yellow onion to an infection was believed to bring it to a head. Basques also used superstition. To treat a wart, blood from a cock's comb was applied to the wart, then the comb buried along a road, where it was thought to transmit the wart to the next person who passed by.[390]

Chinese medicine, not really folk medicine but an ancient discipline markedly different from European practice, is described in some detail in chapter 5. Chinese doctors practicing in western communities offered a variety of herbal remedies as well as moxa cautery, acupuncture, and traditional bone setting. In spite of widespread prejudice against the Chinese, Asian treatments were very popular among whites.

Words of Advice

There were several manuals available to the frontier family to guide them in their home doctoring. Stillman Jones, of the small farming and railroad town of Harlowton, Montana, remembers that his mother relied on *The Cottage Physician*, a book for home use that listed methods of prevention and treatment for diseases, accidents, and household emergencies.[391] The publishers of *The Cottage Physician* stressed that it was intended to be an adjunct to proper medical attention, not a replacement. A perusal of its pages confirms that is was up-to-date for its time, and it undoubtedly served home caregivers well. Jones recalls the mustard plasters applied to painful chests and aching joints, and medicine flavored with lemonade and peppermint extract, which his mother prepared according to this book. A mixture of niter, sugar, and water "seemed to cure stomach problems," he said.[392]

Another health manual often found in the homesteader's house was called *The Doctor Book*. Some doctors found it difficult to endorse these books. One Idaho physician allowed that one chapter in *The Doctor Book*, entitled "What to Do Until the Doctor Comes," was invaluable. But he proclaimed the rest of the book "a damned nuisance."[393]

Indeed, the greatest problem with home treatment was that proper medical attention might be postponed in favor of nostrums. There are numerous examples of people with appendicitis, incarcerated hernias, bowel obstructions, gall bladder disease, pneumonia, severe injuries, and other ailments who arrived at the doctor's office too late. On the other hand, the harsh treatments of some frontier doctors were just as likely to cause harm.

Timeless Wisdom

As already noted, modern-day scientists are discovering that many of the "old-time" herbal medicines contained valuable chemicals. Robert and Michele Root-Bernstein, in their book *Honey, Mud, Maggots, and Other Medical Marvels*, lend credence to many folk therapies. As they state in the introduction, "Our purpose is not to convince the world that folk medicine is the answer. . . . It would be foolish to throw out current practice. . . . Our purpose is to demonstrate . . . that ancient folk medicines have provided so many useful therapies that to ignore this fecund source of knowledge and practice is also foolish."[394]

Modern practitioners are beginning to embrace some of these medicines and therapies, even some that appear to be ridiculous at first glance. For instance, doctors are using sterilized live maggots (larvae of the common fly) to treat pressure ulcers, diabetic foot wounds, venous stasis ulcers, and postsurgical wounds, and to prepare necrotic wounds and ulcers for skin graft.[395] Maggots, which digest dead and infected tissue, have been used to clean infected wounds for centuries. There is evidence

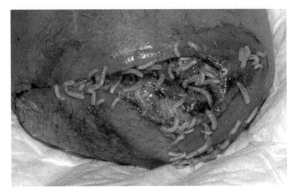

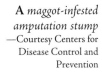

A maggot-infested amputation stump
—Courtesy Centers for Disease Control and Prevention

A PARTIAL LIST OF "GRANNY REMEDIES"

► Oil of goose, wolf, bear, or polecat for rheumatism
► Poultice of slippery elm and cornmeal for burns
► Ointment of crushed sheep sorrel leaves and gunpowder for skin cancer
► Mashed cabbage for ulcer or breast cancer
► Mashed snails and earthworms in water for diphtheria
► Salve of lard and brimstone for itch
► Common salt with scrapings from pewter spoons for worms
► Boiled pumpkinseed tea for stomach worms
► Scorpion oil for venereal disease
► Tea made from dried chicken gizzard linings for stomachache
► Tonic made from half a bucket of rusty nails soaked in vinegar as a blood purifier
► Wood ashes or cobwebs to stanch bleeding
► Brandy and red pepper for cholera
► Mashed potato poultice to draw out the core of a boil
► Mold scraped from cheese or bread for open sores
► A bag of asafetida worn around the neck for a cold
► Fried heart of rattlesnake or skunk meat for consumption
► A rub of green walnuts, bacon rind, or chicken feet for warts
► Carrying an onion in the pocket to prevent smallpox
► Poultice of flaxseed for pneumonia
► Carrying a horse chestnut to prevent rheumatism
► Owl broth for whooping cough
► Scratching the gum of a sore tooth with an iron nail until it bleeds, then driving the nail into a wooden beam, for a toothache
► Boiled toads for heart disease and dropsy
► Burnt sponge for a goiter
► Poultice of soap and sugar for boils
► Gold filings in honey to restore energy
► Rubbing the mouth with a liniment of gum myrrh, golden seal, and red pepper for pyorrhea
► Watermelon seeds boiled in water for kidney trouble
► Blood of a "bessie bug" dropped in the ear for earache
► Wrapping the legs in brown paper soaked in vinegar for muscle ache
► Poultice of a dirt-dauber's (wasp's) nest to remove a carbuncle core
► Sassafras tea to thicken the blood
► Juice of a green walnut for ringworm
► Salve of kerosene and beef tallow for chapped hands
► Two tablespoons of India ink for tapeworm
► Onions boiled in sulphur molasses as a laxative
► Tea made from scrapings of stallion hooves for hives
► Warm brains of freshly killed rabbit applied to a baby's gums for teething pains
► Hot chicken blood for shingles*

*From Robert F. Karolevitz, *Doctors of the Old West: A Pictorial History of Medicine on the Frontier*, 169-70.

that during the Civil War, many undressed wounds became infested with maggots and were thus unintentionally helped. Leeches, today available from special supply houses, are used to reduce the size of large collections of blood (hematomas) in massive traumatic injuries, and to reduce the amount of swelling from hemorrhage in certain kinds of surgical operations. Both of these treatments have been recently rediscovered after having been all but forgotten by medical science.

Research also confirms that honey is a bacteriostatic agent, useful in treating stomach ulcers and burns. The kind of clay frontier folks sometimes swallowed for indigestion finds its counterpart in today's Maalox and Phillips Milk of Magnesia, which contain the same magnesium compounds.[396]

EIGHT

Miracle Cures
Quackery, Fraud, and Faith

Grandpa Murphy, Grandpa Murphy,
Had some trouble with his pee,
Took two bottles of your compound,
Now they pipe him out to sea.
Grandma Murphy, Grandma Murphy,
Had some trouble with her blouse,
Took two bottles of your compound,
Now they milk her with the cows.
—From *Stitches Magazine,* 1998[397]

WHETHER CONSIDERING home remedies, shamanism, faith healing, quack cures, or "real" medicine, emotion plays a role in healing. Trust, faith, and the power of suggestion can be used to exploit the vulnerable, but they can also be used as legitimate adjuncts to treatment. Galen, the great Greek physician and Hippocratic student, observed, "The trust of patients in committing themselves [to a physician] is essential, and he to whom patients entrust themselves cures the most illnesses."[398] The shaman, the hypnotist, and the charlatan all understood the power of suggestion and used it, whether ethically or not.

Ancient medicine men used chanting, ritual, and props to engage the patient and augment the treatment with mental and emotional healing energy. Euro-American physicians had equivalent methods. When a doctor made a house call, he carried with him the ultimate medical prop—the black leather doctor's bag (comparable to the shaman's medicine bundle?). That mysterious, aromatic leather case, filled with technical instruments and vials of potent substances, held, the patient assumed, untold lifesaving power. It was symbolic, this black bag that opened wide at the top and was nearly always scuffed and weathered from use. The bag, along with the doctor's reassuring touch, inspired the patient's trust in the doctor and faith in his own recovery. (For more on frontier doctors' practices, see chapter 9.)

The open-minded modern doctor can recognize the resemblances between the shaman's healing rites, the old-time doctor's black bag, and current medical conventions—the differences are only a matter of degree. Consciously or unconsciously, physicians know the value of atmosphere and accoutrements in stimulating the expectation of wellness: the odor of disinfectants; the hustle and bustle of white coats and uniforms; the stethoscope around the doctor's neck; the hug of the blood-pressure sleeve; the ritual of collecting a urine specimen or a venipuncture; even the ceremony of writing out a prescription. And we must not forget the elaborate, framed certificates—sometimes in Latin—prominently displayed on the walls of the examining rooms. These are the things patients associate with modern medicine and their own well-being.

Most physicians today also recognize the value of suggestion in the use of placebos. Walter A. Brown, a psychiatrist at Brown University School of Medicine, wrote, "I believe that the placebo effect is a powerful part of healing and that more effort should be made to harness and enhance it."[399] Properly and ethically used, placebos are an important tool for managing many conditions. The success of suggestion can be attributed to its ability to enhance the patient's natural resistance through faith and trust.

Unfortunately, this trust can be manipulated and abused by unscrupulous medical con men. Throughout history, swindlers have preyed upon human fear and suffering to sell phony cures and preventatives. In the late nineteenth and early twentieth centuries, the lack of good medical care on the frontier made the West a particular hotbed for bogus healers and medicines. Yet there were also honest and well-meaning doctors, both trained and untrained. The great variation in practitioners of the healing art makes it difficult to make any meaningful generalizations on the ethics of the doctors of the frontier. Furthermore, because the field of medicine was largely unscientific, legitimate doctors often promoted ideas that, viewed from today's perspective, were worthless, if not harmful. In short, in the old West, it was hard to tell a healer from a huckster.

"Little more than the inclination": Dubious Doctors

The use of the derogatory name "quack" was commonly applied by one medical faction against another, sometimes without foundation. The word *quack* is derived from *quacksalver*, a person who claims special merit of his medications and salves. The term generally designates a health practitioner who makes grandiose claims with no medical support. But it is not that simple: one man's quack may be another man's doctor. The quack is often associated with the "snake-oil salesman," a charlatan who sold fake medicines.

In the early days there were no yardsticks to measure doctors by and no laws to regulate their practice. As previously discussed, the amount and quality of education of doctors in nineteenth-century America were highly variable and often inadequate. Students were accepted to medical schools without any formal education. In 1870 Harvard Medical School gave no written examinations because most of the students could not write well enough.[400] As Robert F. Karolevitz put it in *Doctors of the Old West*, "There was a time in America's Old West when becoming a doctor required little more than the inclination."[401] Thus it was impossible to distinguish between trained professionals and medical dilettantes in those days, especially out west.

Some medical schools existed only for profit and turned out nothing more than warm bodies with diplomas, while some healers with no formal training served the frontier commendably. In Turner County, Dakota Territory, a "Dr." A. B. Sage arrived around 1870 with some medical books and a case of homeopathic remedies. Though he had never attended medical school, he was well respected and served the area admirably for many years. During the same era, Dr. William Browner of Jefferson County, Nebraska, was a trained physician who used only one medication, a patent medicine called August flower bitters, which he prescribed for all coughs, colds, fevers, and diseases.[402] It may not have cured much, but it probably did little harm.

Adding to the confusion, for a long time in the United States, many pretenders hung up fake medical certificates purchased from a "diploma mill." Counting on the fact that in sickness, pain, and fear of death, a patient was not likely to scrutinize a doctor's credentials, by the end of the nineteenth century, the diploma-mill industry was flourishing. A "degree" in medicine cost five to ten dollars, depending on whether one wanted "Heavy Royal Linen Paper" or just "Imitation Parchment," on which the buyer's name was handsomely engraved and stamped with a large gold emblem. In *The Golden Age of Quackery*, Stewart H. Holbrook noted, "These [certificates] were not too expensive even for the most poverty-stricken quack."[403]

On the frontier, one need not even bother with a phony license to practice medicine. Westerners generally had a skeptical view of both education and regulations anyway. Many frontier folk were poorly educated themselves and not worldly enough to judge the good from the bad. This fact, coupled with the pioneers' often acute need for medical care, made western soil fertile for quackery to flourish. During the late nineteenth and early twentieth centuries, numerous mystical healers, picturesque Indian-medicine specialists, snake-oil salesmen, and a myriad of other dubious doctors abounded. A 1900 American Medical Association editorial noted, "A Newspaper before us contains four columns of advertisements of clairvoyants, palmists, trance mediums, etc. . . . A third of the advertising space of the same paper, and it is one of the best in Chicago, is taken up with advertisements of quacks and quack medicines."[404]

Two such hucksters, E. W. Davis and B. Robinson, came to Helena, Montana, in 1866, claiming they had been trained in the best hospitals in London. Their advertisements in the local newspapers warned that newcomers to the area "are liable to be affected by absorption of a poison called 'Malaria' which pervades the atmosphere" and that "poisonous salts in the water" caused "Nervousness, Headaches . . . pains in the Chest,

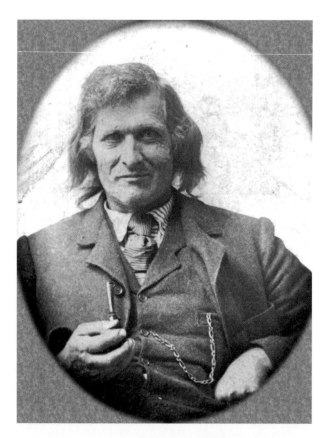

One of many traveling faith healers, herbalists, and quacks, Jacob Derringer, a.k.a. "Indian John," practiced folk medicine along the Kansas-Nebraska border in the late 1800s and early 1900s. His methods and concoctions were credited with miraculously curing countless illnesses.
—Courtesy Kansas State Historical Society

weak Back, Ringing in the Ears, Blushing, Bashfulness . . . the forerunners of those rapid and sometimes fatal fermentations of the blood known as . . . Bilious, Typhoid, Lung and Mountain Fevers."[405] In spite of their outlandish hyperbole, the two men were quite popular. As late as 1871, both "doctors" were still doing brisk business in Helena.

One of the most successful medical hucksters was John R. Brinkley. With a purchased diploma, a little bit of medical knowledge, and a great deal of self-confidence, Brinkley became one of the best-known personalities in America during the 1920s and 1930s. Known far and wide as "The Goat Gland Doctor," he gained a reputation for "curing" impotence by surgically implanting goat testicles beneath the skin—or claiming that he had. He not only made millions, but he was also nearly elected governor of Kansas. Riding on the success of his "rejuvenation through gland transplanting," he wrote books, built hospitals, and controlled radio stations. So successful was Brinkley in his public relations that he eclipsed two contemporary frauds, Norman Baker and Harry Hoxsey, who claimed to have discovered cures for cancer.[406]

In some places, the climate of medical mayhem grew grave enough to inspire a public outcry. As early as 1864, Virginia City's *Montana Post* called for "legislation to check medical quackery."[407] The following year, the city council passed an ordinance that required a "surgeon" to buy a license for ten dollars every six months. Unfortunately, this was more likely a way to add to the municipal coffers than an effort to rid the community of charlatans. A few years later, the first law affecting physicians in the Dakota Territory was passed by the first territorial legislature. It stated that a physician was guilty of a misdemeanor if he poisoned a patient—but only if the doctor did so while intoxicated. If the patient died, the drunken doctor was guilty of manslaughter in the second degree.[408]

Drunk or sober, doctors began to come under more scrutiny. The *Butte Daily Miner* reported in 1885 that "more children have been killed in Butte by empirics–than from all other causes."[409] Furthermore, the newspaper said, people used "less care in selecting a doctor than they would if they had carpenter work to be done." According to the article, "Only 'one-half' of the city's twenty-eight doctors were graduated from regular and recognized medical colleges."[410] Earlier that year, a grand jury had ordered every physician in Butte to appear before it and produce a diploma. This resulted in the blacklisting of a few pretenders.[411]

During this period, many states in the Midwest and West established medical associations to set up some rules and regulations. By 1879 so many quacks had appeared in Montana that a corps of "orthodox" physicians was organized. The Territorial Medical Association became instrumental in the development of much-needed licensing legislation.

In 1889, when Montana received statehood, the Medical Practices Act was passed and a Board of Medical Examiners was created by the legislature. Now only those with proper credentials were supposed to receive a certificate to practice. But there were still loopholes. "Dr." E. J. Leonard was admitted to practice by the Board of Examiners in 1890 based on his claim of a medical degree from Harvard and a practice at Bellevue Hospital in New York. After inquiry, both of these institutions denied any knowledge of Dr. Leonard, and he withdrew his application. Nevertheless, in 1893 Leonard was listed in Polk's city directory as the county physician for Silver Bow County.[412]

Carpetbaggers and Cure-Alls

Along with the settlers, medicine salesmen came west by wagon, by stagecoach, and eventually by train, their carpetbags loaded with bottles of "Indian" tonic guaranteed to cure "secret masculine diseases" or ease "female troubles." They pushed nostrums with names like "Sharpshooter's Liniment" and "Kinkaid Salve," certified to cure ingrown toenails, bunions, or psoriasis. Peddlers of these "cure-alls" became known as "snake-oil salesmen" because some boasted their products contained snake oil. Most of these hucksters were itinerant, stopping at various locations for short periods to collect their spoils, then moving on to other pastures.

Someone once said that the major difference between humans and lower animals is that humans take medicine voluntarily. Perhaps one reason is that the standard ingredient in most "patent medicines" was alcohol. Packaged in fancy bottles, with coloring and flavoring added, these so-called cures were nothing more than second-rate booze. During this period of American life, after the Civil War and through the turn of the century, it was estimated that "more alcohol is consumed in this country in patent medicines than is dispensed in a legal way by licensed liquor venders."[413]

Newspapers of the day carried ads for these potions and creams, and the claims of the charlatans who sold them made news, giving them free publicity. Stewart H. Holbrook in *The Golden Age of Quackery* wrote that snake-oil peddlers "awaited the end of the Civil War, the completion of the first continental railroad, and the rapid settlement of the West.

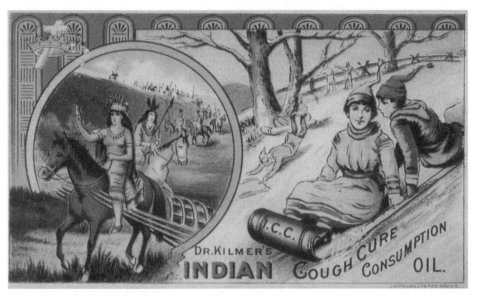

Dr. Kilmer's Indian Cough Cure and Consumption Oil, one of many patent medicines
—Courtesy National Library of Medicine, History of Medicine Division

Above all [they] awaited the coming of the popular press, the basic medium to spread the word of new elixirs, balms, and cure-alls."[414]

Advertisements targeted a vulnerable market. Many men, then as now, were preoccupied with doubts about their sexual potency, and ads for many different products contained discreet but seductive suggestions of miraculous rejuvenation. Likewise women, who in those days had no one to turn to with their "private" complaints, believed that any medicine labeled specifically for them was worth a try. Westerners were particularly attracted to miracle cures of all kinds. Many frontier residents suffered from undiagnosed ailments, and hard labor brought on a variety of aches and pains. Furthermore, the division between the legitimate and illegitimate medical purveyors on the frontier was not so clear-cut, and some of the questionable medicines did in fact do what they were purported to do.

In 1863 one of these patent medicines was touted by no less a personage than Granville Stuart, the famous Montana prospector, rancher, and frontiersman. Stuart wrote, "My hand and arm are much swollen and very painful. Worden and Company's store has a bottle labeled Merchants Gargling Oil, a liniment good for man and beast, and this morning I went for it and wrapping my hand in several folds of cotton cloth kept them soaked in it." "Gargling oil" was one of the most popular patent medicines available. There were two kinds, both laden with alcohol. If the bottle had a white wrapper, it was for human consumption; the one with a yellow wrapper was for animals. Three days later Stuart's hand was much better. "Had it not been for the oil I suppose I would be dead now."[415]

By the late nineteenth century, Americans were being bombarded with ads for medicines. Daily newspapers, magazines, and even catalogs, a favorite reading matter of frontier folk—the leaves of which sometimes served another purpose in western outhouses—promoted nostrums and carried questionable medical advice. The Sears & Roebuck catalog contained twenty pages of medicines, trusses, and other products guaranteed to cure everything from cancer to the common cold. Not satisfied to give all the profit away to their advertisers, Sears had its own brands. One product that was particularly attractive to housewives was the Sears White Star Secret Liquor Cure. Women concerned about their husband's drinking were encouraged to surreptitiously drop the stuff into his coffee. The Secret Liquor Cure was in fact a "Mickey Finn," containing enough narcotic to knock a man out. Needless to say, this product made good on its promise to control the recipient's urge to drink and keep him at home. It is interesting to note that, should the husband became a narcotic addict from this sly therapy, the same catalog advertised a Sears Cure for the Opium and Morphine Habit, which contained—you guessed it— alcohol. With hubby taken care of, Mom could calm that fussy baby with Sears's "soothing syrup," which contained both alcohol and opium.[416]

The world-famous soft drink Coca-Cola began as a not-so-soft quack medicine. Mostly colored water and sugar, it was originally spiked with cocaine. On March 10, 1885, the *Atlanta Journal* called it "A Wonderful Medicine." Atlanta was the first major city in the United States to ban alcohol, which greatly enhanced Coca-Cola's popularity there. The cola was concocted by a country pharmacist who was aware of the hugely profitable coca wine that had been quenching European thirsts for thirty years. The inventor's luck was not to last, however. Bad management, legal wrangles, and bad press due to dependence in customers left the company almost broke. Another druggist bought Coca-Cola in 1889 for $2,300. It is not known when the narcotic was removed from the recipe, possibly not until 1914, with the passage of the Harrison Act, which forced narcotic patent medicines off the open market.[417]

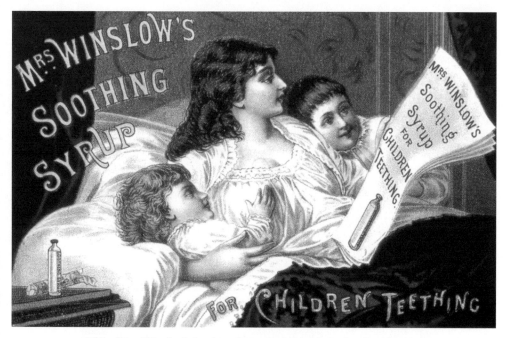

Ad for Mrs. Winslow's Soothing Syrup. Patent medicines such as this usually contained alcohol and sometimes opium and other narcotics. —Courtesy National Library of Medicine, History of Medicine Division

Coca-Cola was only one of hundreds of patent medicines in the United States. Throughout rural America, medicine shows and pharmacies sold these nostrums, all of which were expensive and mostly worthless. One writer in the heyday of patent medicines noted, "When the average American sets out to buy a horse, or a box of cigars, he is a model of caution. But see him when he is seeking . . . 'sound health.' . . . Anybody's word is good enough."[418] The trade in these concoctions was immense. Patent medicine was an eighty-million-dollar-a-year industry in the U.S. in 1906, when President Theodore Roosevelt signed the Pure Food and Drug Act.

In addition to medicines, charlatans sold hundreds of magnetic and electric belts, electric stimulators, breast enlargers, prostate warmers, and gadgets that reportedly analyzed a drop of blood—the test was only good, however, if the blood was drawn in a dim light while the patient was facing west.[419] Promoters, called "toadstool millionaires" by some, were free to make any claim they wanted about their products. Even federal laws passed in the early twentieth century didn't slow the fraudulent medical industry. As late as the 1920s, William J. A. Bailey, a brilliant college dropout, was selling a radium-laced elixir he called Radiothor. Enthusiasts of this radioactive tonic claimed that it benefited dyspepsia, high blood pressure, and especially impotence. Finally the death of a well-known person from radiation toxicity led to an investigation. In the meantime, hundreds or perhaps thousands of lives were shortened from using this so-called medicine.[420]

"All you need's a little nerve": The Medicine Show

In addition to catalog and newspaper advertisements, American promoters of cure-alls used a more colorful and exciting sales method—the medicine show. Using catchy names like Bill the Healer, John "Doc" Healy, Texas Charlie Bigelow, and Dr. "Nevada Ned" Oliver, and accompanied by theatrical displays that resembled a Wild West extravaganza, flamboyant pitchmen sold curative salves, cough syrups, worm killers, and tonics of every description.[421] A lot of the remote and not-so-remote points on the map welcomed these vagabonds as a break in the routine of frontier life, though the shows toured in the East as well. The "doctors," selling their patent medicines and "Indian tonics," furnished entertainment in the form of sideshows, music, slapstick routines, and "blackface" acts. People came by wagon, on horseback, or on foot to enjoy the

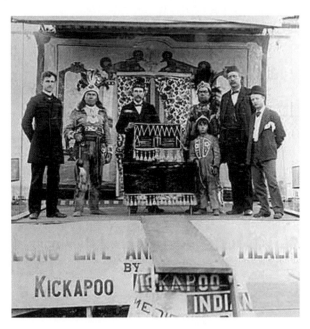

Kickapoo Medicine Show in Marine, Minnesota. On the frontier, traveling troupes provided entertainment and sold "cure-alls." Promoters frequently used an Indian motif.
—Courtesy Minnesota Historical Society

158

performances. If the show delivered, many hard-earned dollars would be dropped into the vendors' palms for worthless concoctions.

Psychology played a large part in these sales. The medicine show was always interrupted at midpoint with the pitch doctor's "lecture," similar to today's television and radio commercials. During "the preachin'," assistants moved rapidly through the crowd, selling all-purpose Swamp Root or Sure Consumption Cure or whatever it was. The assistants' cry of "All sold out, Doctor" and the pitchman's response, "Bless you, my friends" became legendary in the trade.[422] Then as now, not everyone appreciated the commercial break. As one rural youngster said, when asked if he was enjoying himself, "The show's all right but I don't like the preachin'."[423]

The content and theme of the medicine show varied depending on the audience and the talents of the producers. Each huckster had his own gimmick. Take for instance "Dr." N. T. "Nevada Ned" Oliver, based in New Jersey in the 1880s. Known as "the Shakespeare of medicine show personalities," Ned featured an Oriental motif. He himself wore a fancy buckskin outfit, but he had two Syrians and a Hindu magician as pitchmen. The showstopper was a live elephant.[424]

Popular in the West was the long-haired, buckskin-clad Indian pitchman, typified by J. I. Lighthall, known as the "Diamond King" or the "Great Indian Medicine Man" of Peoria, Illinois. As he traveled from town to town in the Midwest and Texas, Lighthall's charismatic personality attracted thousands. He began his show by offering to pull teeth at no charge, whereupon a line immediately formed to take advantage of this service. He must have been skillful at this dental procedure since he advertised a record of "fourteen teeth in nineteen seconds without pain." After the extractions, the Diamond King began the spiel about his medicine, Nature's Remedies, derived from "roots, barks, leaves, and flowers," acquired, he claimed, from Indian doctors. The medicine was described by one customer as a brown liquid that smelled like a mixture of "turpentine and whiskey." Lighthall's business was exceedingly prosperous, even though at times there was a great deal of competition. In San Antonio, the Diamond King's rivals included a blind phrenologist; "the Wizard Oil Chief"; a doctor with special "psychometric" powers of diagnosis; and many others. But Lighthall's popularity remained untouched. The local newspaper said, "The Diamond King is a great character. He amuses the healthy, heals the sick and infirm, and creates happiness out of misery."[425]

Owen Tully Stratton was another famous medical huckster. Bored with college, he began his career during the gold rush to the Klondike in 1897. For a time, he was successful at gambling if not at finding gold. Eventually he landed in Yakima, Washington, where he met Dr. J. L. Berry, who had "starved out" as a doctor and turned to selling patent medicine. As an apprentice of Dr. Berry, Stratton learned the basics of the medicine-show business. He described his mentor as "a sight to behold": six feet tall, with a long, black beard, and always dressed in a Prince Albert and a silk hat. Berry's medicine consisted of salts allegedly derived from a secret mineral spring in Mono County, California, marketed as curative for "whatever ails." The customer had only to add water or whiskey and drink the mixture to get the full value of his investment.[426]

Young Stratton was an apt pupil, a natural showman who loved the limelight. He had also had some medical and pharmaceutical training before he launched himself on the fraud circuit. He sold Dr. Berry's Mineral Water Salts dressed as a Quaker, in a borrowed velvet suit decorated with yards of gold lace. In America, Quakers were generally considered honest and trustworthy, so con men often used Quaker garb and logos as camouflage, sprinkling their speeches with "thees" and "thous."[427] Later Stratton extolled herbal mixtures prepared by "Old Dr. Josia Baker, a Quaker . . . one hundred and four years of age, as hale and hearty as the average man of forty." As further proof of his vitality, Stratton claimed, the centenarian Dr. Baker had recently sired children.[428]

Onstage, Stratton displayed jars filled with worms of all kinds, long tapeworms and coiled masses of roundworms—specimens acquired mostly from slaughterhouses—as evidence of the nasty parasites unwary families might be suffering from. These seeds of suggestion planted in the minds of fastidious mothers were bound to sell a few bottles of worm medicine. At the turn of the century, intestinal worms were a common complaint, especially among transplanted Europeans who ate uncooked meats. In his memoirs, Stratton described the trick used to dupe people into thinking they had been cured of a large tapeworm. After administering a strong cathartic to the customer, a pickled tapeworm many feet long was slipped surreptitiously into the container with the stool evacuation. This repulsive specimen, shown to the "patient" and to the audience, served as a vivid testimonial.[429]

For a while Stratton toured Montana with an alcoholic doctor called Dr. Park and continued successfully to unload all kinds of nostrums. As Stratton advised in his book, "Learn a spiel, and get yourself a banjo plunker, and you can make some real money working watertank towns around here. All you need's a little nerve."[430] Stratton finally quit the grifter circuit in 1904 and went to medical school in St. Louis, later practicing in Idaho and Montana.

The cure-alls sold in medicine shows even extended to veterinary medicines. Jack Healy from Broadwater County, Montana, was described as a "mesmerist of horses" and other animals, and there were numerous local witnesses to back up the claims. It was reported that "he herded sheep without a dog. . . . Without bridles he drove an eight-mule team." One day an enterprising medicine showman passing through Broadwater County hired Healy to work for him. The show advertised for ranchers to bring in their meanest, wildest horses. During the performance, Healy massaged the animal all over with the "medicine," then mounted it, apparently having "cured" it of its orneriness. The "doctor" sold great quantities of the magical liquid before it became obvious to some of the purchasers that they had been hoodwinked, whereupon the pair escaped on the first freight train they could catch.[431]

Being on the medicine-show circuit involved a certain amount of physical risk. While on a tour through the mining communities of Arizona, one well-known huckster, Oscar Dalton Weeks, was punched in the face by a disgruntled customer in Clifton and threatened at gunpoint by another in Globe. Even though the gunslinger was arrested, Weeks left Arizona, never to return.[432]

How's the Bowels?

One category of medicine that deserves special emphasis is the cathartic. Since ancient times, humans have been preoccupied with bowel activity. The theory of autointoxication from stasis (slowdown of passage) in the intestinal tract has been expounded by mothers, neurotics, and even trained physicians for centuries, and it was fair game for quacks as well. It stood to reason, so it was said, that if anything as foul as human feces remains too long in the body, poisons can be absorbed. Advertisements convinced some that "a clean bowel was as vital as a clean home" in the prevention of ptomaine poisoning and other diseases.

This internal cleansing could be accomplished with Jamison's Eager Colon Cleanser or the Kolon-Motor, enema devices mounted on the bathroom wall and used daily by some of the more fastidious. Popular cathartics became household names: Sal Hepatica, Pierce's Pleasant Pellets, and Excelsior Mineral Waters led a field of hundreds.[433] Spas and clinics developed around colonic irrigations. Physicians always asked about the bowels during house calls and stood ready to prescribe their favorite purge to help a patient with sluggish elimination. A far more egregious treatment for the unproven theory of autointoxication was surgery. During the first decade of the twentieth century, a well-educated and properly credentialed surgeon named William A. Lane performed over one thousand colectomies, primarily on women.[434]

Many years of clinical observation have shown no evidence that lethargic bowels can result in illness, yet the belief survives, as illustrated by today's advertising for laxatives and the fashionablity of high colonics in some circles. This statement by Josh Billings, a humorist of the late nineteenth century, is perhaps timeless: "I have finally come to the conclusion that a good reliable set of bowels is worth more to a man than any quantity of wisdom."[435]

"No telling how many people that madstone cured"

Any discussion of questionable cures would be incomplete without mentioning madstones. Stones of one description or another were used for centuries as an antidote to snakebites, insect stings, and especially bites from rabid animals. The popularity of the use of the madstone in the prevention and treatment of rabies continued in the "civilized world" until 1885, when Pasteur's vaccine became available. We now know that rabies, which is always fatal, does not always develop in those who are bitten by rabid animals. In the prevaccine period, about thirty percent of those bitten developed the disease. Nevertheless, most victims saw the bite as invariably fatal, and the fear of such a horrible end led many exposed people to seek any possible cure. The "magic" of the madstone gave some hope—hope being the only thing it provided.

Rabies (hydrophobia), though rarely contracted, was among the most dreaded illnesses on the Great Plains. The terror it inspired was due to the agonizing death throes its victims suffered. Two-thirds of rabies victims develop the furious, or encephalitic, form; the remainder develop the paralytic form, so-called dumb rabies. Victims with furious rabies usually live no longer than seven days, but it takes longer for the paralytic form to kill. The frightful symptoms of furious rabies in humans were similar in most ways to those in animals, including the increased salivation known as "frothing at the mouth." States of agitation, confusion, morbid fear, and sometimes aggression alternated with lucid intervals until the victim finally succumbed to coma and death. People with rabies were shunned, and it was hard to find anyone to care for them, though human-to-human transmissions are virtually unheard of. On occasion, raging, demented victims of hydrophobia were locked in jail or otherwise isolated until they died.

It was generally believed that a bezoar (madstone) would prevent rabies. Madstones are not rocks but concretions, sometimes found in the stomach or intestines of mammals, composed of hair, vegetable material, a variety of minerals, and other foreign material. Arabic physicians also applied the name "bezoar" to gallstones and kidney stones and attributed the same magic to them. Madstones were objects of reverence for their imagined power against toxins and especially as a preventative to rabies.

By the Middle Ages, madstones were kept like heirlooms by families, passed through from generation to generation, or sometimes sold. The ritual of using madstones came with the Europeans as they crossed the Atlantic. The Spaniards introduced the practice to Native Americans, and other European immigrants were already versed in it. In America, madstones were often identified by the name of the family that owned them. The Pointer madstone of North Carolina was handed down from Captain Pointer to his son Samuel, and Samuel's will read, "I give and devise to my four daughters my ¾ interest in the madstone."[436] Owners sometimes charged fees as high as one hundred dollars, a fortune in early America, to use their madstones.

So seriously were the madstone's powers taken that someone's acquisition of one was a joyous public event. In 1848 a North Carolina newspaper wrote, "We are happy to learn that Mr. Elijah Pope, Sr. . . . has succeeded in procuring a Mad-Stone . . . that will cure any poisonous bite. . . . Mr. Pope has been called upon several times to apply the stone . . . and has been successful in every case."[437] Miss Cornelia Roney had a stone that supposedly came from the stomach of a deer. Allegedly only one person treated with her madstone died: "A very small Negro boy went mad because his mother took him away with her before the treatment had time to draw out the poison." This bezoar was still in use in 1904.[438]

Traditionally the madstone was cleansed in warm water or fresh milk and then placed on wounds from rabid animals to "draw out" the poison. When the stone fell from the wound, it was again cleansed and reapplied. One early American described the procedure: "When they would come for the madstone, dad would prick their wound and make it bleed. . . . Then he would apply the stone to where the blood was. If it stuck, that meant that there was poison there. . . . No telling how many people that madstone cured."[439]

Obviously there were failures, and some victims died of rabies after a madstone treatment. But widely circulated "success" stories kept the faith alive. According to one believer, "Father's two Negro boys, bitten by mad dog, were cured, but hogs bitten by same dog died from poison." Another writer said, "They used said stone about one hundred and fifty years, and said no case was ever lost."[440]

Even after the Pasteur vaccine became available, a few people refused to submit to injections and clung to their belief in the madstone. In one famous story, a man from Arizona was on his way to Chicago for the Pasteur rabies treatment when he stopped in Kansas City, where someone talked him into using a madstone instead. A few weeks later he died of rabies.[441] With stories such as this, before long, vaccination became the treatment of choice.

"She appeared as an angel personified": Faith Healing

Organized religions, then and now, have strived to aid the sick with prayer and liturgy. Christians accept the use of the cross and the Bible to give comfort and as symbols of healing, and few question the symbolism of bread and wine as the body and blood of Christ. Some religious groups, such as Christian Scientists, help the ill to gain serenity and an improved sense of well-being from rituals and readings of the doctrines of their creed.[442] The therapeutic value of this kind of support depends entirely on an individual's beliefs and culture.

Faith healing in one form or another has been around for centuries. It was and still is often a last resort for the chronically and seriously ill. Whether faith healing is by definition quackery is a matter of profound debate, but it is unfair to condemn all spiritual healers as frauds. We cannot erase the heralded success of some faith healers who practiced in America. Francis Schlatter, for example, known as the New Mexico Messiah, the Healer, and *El Gran Hombre* during the 1890s, startled observers with his miraculous results.

Schlatter was a Christlike figure who went barefoot and survived on donations. One of his methods included waving a copper "healing rod" in the air. During his career he was lauded by many, including the *Denver Post* and the *Santa Fe New Mexican*. On one occasion, reporters from the

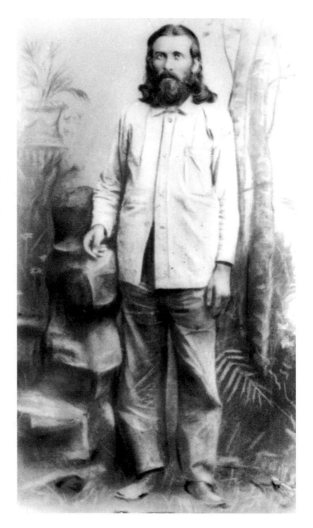

Francis Schlatter, circa 1859. This faith healer wandered across the western United States for two years performing "miraculous" cures. —Courtesy Museum of New Mexico

Albuquerque Morning Democrat witnessed his work and reported, "There is something in his touch which seeks to heal the sick. What you have heard of him is true to the letter."[443] Then one day the famous healer simply disappeared. He died in Mexico just a few years after the peak of his popularity.[444] We are left with the question, did this man actually cure the sick, the blind, and the lame? Hundreds of claims were made, but we will never know for sure.

Other faith healers were obviously frauds. One story of misplaced faith involved a rural Montana family whose mother began to lose her eyesight from optic nerve degeneration. It was about 1921, and none of the few eye specialists in Montana was able to help. The family traveled to California to see Aimee Semple McPherson, a well-known faith healer who preached from her temple in Los Angeles. The woman's daughter described what happened:

> She [McPherson] appeared as an angel personified as she seemingly floated out on stage dressed in a flowing white robe with a background of maroon velvet curtains and soft music. After many quotations from the Bible and more music, she invited the afflicted to come forward and be healed. Mom started down the aisle along with quite a few other people. About two-thirds of the way down they were stopped by some of her attendants and told only the ones who had completed an extensive training course with a substantial fee were allowed to come forward and be healed. . . . We never went back.[445]

NINE

Homestead Doctors

House Calls on the Great Plains

It was a certain kind of people who came.

—Daniel N. Vichorek, *Montana's Homestead Era*[446]

THE HOMESTEAD ACT OF MAY 20, 1862, made it plausible for ordinary folks to secure some land of their own. Many settlers had already put down roots in the West in the wake of the gold rush. The thousands of men digging for precious metal in the mining camps had little time to garden or tend livestock, but they still needed food, a need that enterprising small farmers sought to fill. Crops were soon growing in the valleys near mining settlements, and cattle ranchers spread their "outfits" all over the flat grasslands and foothills, where water and good grass were plentiful.

With the government's encouragement, the trickle westward became a flood. Towns sprang up along the emigrant trails, places where supplies could be restocked, livestock could be rested, and whistles could be wetted. As these outposts became permanent, and as more and more homestead farms and ranches crept over the landscape, the Great American Desert described by early explorers began to fill up.

As settlement grew, doctors followed. Many came west for the same reasons others did—to invest in land or dig for gold. Some of them accompanied the great migration of immigrants to the mountains and Great Plains during and after the Civil War. Others sought their fortunes at the gold camps or joined the army as contract surgeons during the Indian campaigns. As a group, frontier physicians were peripatetic, going where they were most needed and could make the most money. Consequently it wasn't unusual for a doctor to work in several different places before putting down roots.

Though the practice of medicine held little prestige in the 1800s and the profession was not very lucrative, by late century medicine had begun to seem more promising, and many people wanted to be doctors. Medical schools in the East were turning out a surplus of graduates, and the profession was becoming crowded. In 1889 Chicago journalist William G. Eggleston remarked, "There are from 1,500 to 2,000 physicians in the state of Illinois, more than are necessary to supply the legitimate demands for professional services, and who are not earning a comfortable livelihood."[447]

Due to this glut, young graduates of medical school often had to support themselves by entering business or farming or some other endeavor. Thus many moved west. There was also another, lesser-known category of physicians who came west for their health. Tuberculosis was a common disease, and many doctors, exposed to it almost daily in their work, became infected. Because there were few treatment options available, the usual prescription was to move west, where the clean, cold mountain air was thought to ease the unrelenting symptoms of this chronic pulmonary disease.

The movement west continued throughout the nineteenth century and into the twentieth. Government incentives and advertisements from the railroads, established western businesses, and land sellers enticed thousands more homesteaders, sometimes pejoratively called "honyockers" (a term probably derived from "hunyak," a racial slur for Slavic immigrants), to the western prairies. The first few years of the twentieth century were good and wet, producing bumper crops and good publicity. In 1909 the Enlarged Homestead Act doubled the amount of land allowed for individual claims, from 160 acres to 320 acres. Meanwhile Great Northern Railroad, building farther and farther into the frontier, offered cheap transportation to "promised land." Boxcars disgorged newcomers at remote depots on the plains of Kansas, the Dakotas, and Montana, leaving them standing with their meager belongings, disoriented and contemplating their questionable future.

Many homesteaders had little farming experience, but they were convinced by the propaganda that anyone could be successful. The would-be farmers included doctors, lawyers, teachers, preachers, merchants, bankers, and others who were used to having clean fingernails. Soon after their arrival, many of these greenhorns began to see their new home in a different light. During World War I, after a decade of plenty, the rain stopped falling, crops stopped growing, and many farm families fell into debt. In some places, as many as half lost their homesteads. Ranches and farms became, as Joseph Kinsey Howard wrote, "fenced deserts where trapped tumbleweed spun and raced nowhere all day. The little houses stood slack-jawed and mute, obscenely violated by coyotes, rats, and bats, finally faded into the lifeless fields."[448]

Even those with enough resources, determination, and luck to persevere had a rough go of it. Grit and sand penetrated food, water, cabins, and lungs; lightning, hail, and hordes of insects destroyed meager crops; blizzards and subzero cold chilled man and beast to the core. Some claimed that the wind blew four ways at once. With only primitive transportation and rough roads, families were isolated for long periods. Anyone familiar with seemingly endless western winters can sympathize with the Montana rancher who wrote on May 5, 1927, "Weather man still turning loose a lot of snow. You'd think the son of a bitch would run out of stock some time."[449]

These were the people the homestead doctor served, and the conditions in which he or she served them. In the early days, some doctors rode a regular circuit to visit isolated settlers. Later, as mining, ranching, and railroad communities formed, many physicians established a permanent practice. The small-town doctor faced a unique challenge. Not only was he responsible for the lives of his neighbors, friends, and family, but because he lived in the community where he practiced, he saw his successes and failures face-to-face every day. As those in the legal profession say, *Res ipse locutor.* Or as some legal wit might add, the corpus delecti speaks for itself. The bad result of, say, a fractured-leg reduction limped up and down Main Street for all to see. Some doctors, however, were blessed with plain luck or earned respect early in their practice that insulated them from too much criticism. A young doctor's reputation could be made or broken with a single case. A few successful results usually assured a community that the new doc could be trusted.

Even for doctors who had offices in town, the majority of medical visits were house calls. Mostly by horse and buggy, later by automobile, country doctors rode out to see their patients, some of whom might live fifty-plus miles away, at whatever time and in whatever weather the call came.

Heeding the Call

The house call is a medical service that few modern folks remember. Since about the 1960s, doctors have practiced almost exclusively in hospitals and clinics. But there were few such facilities on the frontier, and doctors usually went to see their patients rather than the other way around. In those days, even in the East, almost all health care took place in the home. Because doctors' services were expensive, most families tried to take care of their own medical needs and called in a doctor only when it was unavoidable. For most ailments, the care of a mother or a neighbor seemed adequate. But if a family member was suffering or appeared to be near death, the call went out, "Get the doctor!"

A house call could last for hours, even days. Good doctors spent a lot of time at the bedside. When their patient was desperately ill, they were expected to stay in the sickroom for long periods. Since no specific treatments were known for most ailments, a comforting presence was about all a physician could offer. Sometimes the doctor had to sleep in a strange, uncomfortable bed in a small, crowded shack; occasionally bedbugs or lice made the doctor's experience even more memorable. A country doctor seldom knew what to expect when he or she left on a call, so they had to come prepared for almost anything.

The doctor's saddlebag or leather handbag served as a mobile clinic. Doctors' saddlebags were often fitted with compartments for bottles and instruments, ready to carry to the bedside. It is remarkable how much the doctor's bag contained—numerous vials of powdered and liquid drugs, antiseptics, syringes and needles, sutures, tourniquets, plasters, stomach pump, and other instruments needed for diagnosis and treatment of most injuries and illnesses a physician was likely to encounter. For everything from a sore throat to a broken leg, the bag contained the answer.

Dr. Urling C. Coe, who came to Bend, Oregon, in 1905, carried in his hip pocket a little leather case containing scalpels, artery forceps, scissors, needles, and some sutures. On long calls he packed an assortment of drugs and instruments in five canvas bags. In the bags were bandages, splints, antiseptics, soap, basins, sterile towels and dressings, surgical instruments, and fifty-four different drugs.[450]

If, as often happened, the physician was far out in the country without some essential piece of equipment, he had to improvise. Once while on a duck hunt, Dr. George Kellogg of Nampa, Idaho, was called on to treat a middle-aged woman bleeding profusely from the uterus. On the spot he designed a "Sims speculum from a stirring spoon, a Burnay packer from the bail of a lard pail, used strips of linen from a table-cloth for sponges and packing, and had two pillow cases for drapes." He boiled everything on the kitchen stove, packed her uterus to stop the bleeding, then sent her to the nearest town by wagon with a note to the local doctor. "I was back in my blind for the afternoon shoot," he recalled.[451]

A typical house call went something like this. The doctor sat by the patient's bed, never standing menacingly over him, and visited with the family (all of whom usually crowded apprehensively into the room) about the state of the weather or the crops or other things important to rural folks, putting everyone at ease. Then, with practiced formality, he removed a large gold watch from his vest pocket, grasped the patient's wrist, and looked earnestly at the watch while counting the radial pulse. This clinical ritual is ageless. The ancient Roman physician William of Saliceto said, "The physician should seem very intent on the pulse, because this builds up a lot of confidence in the patient, which will be very useful."[452] This protocol not only inspired trust and allowed the doctor to compose himself, it also allowed time, on cold days, for him and his instruments to warm up.

A wise practitioner consulted the elders in the family about the patient's condition; their experience with illness and knowledge of the particulars of the case could be helpful. Then the doctor laid his hands on the sick one's forehead, cheeks, and neck. This part of the ceremony was performed with great concentration, both to help make the diagnosis and to reassure the patient and onlookers. Thermometers were rare outside the medical centers of the East. If frontier doctors carried them, they usually got broken in saddlebags. Physicians, like mothers and grandmothers, became very adept in determining the presence of a fever by touch.

A good practitioner recognized the therapeutic value of touch. The "laying on of hands" was once an important tool for the family doctor, but it seems to be losing favor with modern physicians. The warm immediacy of the human touch says, "Trust me; we're in this together, and I'm going to get you well." As mentioned in the previous chapter, trust and faith aid natural healing.

After the doctor felt the patient's face and forehead for fever, his hands moved to the patient's abdomen to feel for masses, tender areas, and enlargements of organs such as the liver or spleen. The doctor then listened to the heart and lungs with his stethoscope, telling the patient to breathe deeply each time he moved it. If the patient had respiratory symptoms, the doctor tapped on the patient's chest with his fingers, inclining his head to listen for any abnormal resonance. Then, using a tongue depressor, he examined the tongue and lips to determine the degree of dehydration and whether or not the patient was anemic. Telling the patient to say "ahh," he then looked at the throat. The most up-to-date physicians might also use a sphygmomanometer to check the blood pressure, an otoscope to look at the eardrums, and an ophthalmoscope to examine the eyegrounds.

Once the physician arrived at a diagnosis, he prepared a prescription. Although a few tablets were available as early as 1872, most medicines were powders contained in vials and painstakingly compounded at the bedside. Using the tip of a pocket knife, the doctor would select from several vials the proportions he needed. He blended the powders and folded each dose into a square of newspaper, so the medicine could be easily transferred to a teaspoon or a glass of water.

Doctors on the frontier were expected to have a cure for everything from cancer to worms. Here are a few prescriptions from Dr. Marion DeKalb Steele's 1855 diary. —Courtesy University of Arkansas Libraries, Special Collections Division, Fayetteville, Arkansas

Vermifuge

℞ 4 oz Best Castor Oil
1 " Oil Wormseed
½ " Spts Turpentine
½ " English Calomel   Leave this out
½ Drachm Oil Linen
Shake these well together three or four times
a day for four days.
Children under a year old may take three
doses a day of half a teaspoonful each—one
hour apart
   Those between one and two may take ¾ teaspoonsful
Those between two & three may take a teaspoonful—
Those between three & four may take one teaspoonful &
a half and for older persons the dose may be
increased in portion In all cases three doses
a day should be taken one hour apart and
continued three day If the medicine does
not produce a slight purgative effect a small
quantity of Castor Oil may be taken several
hours afterwards

In cases of pneumonia, when a patient was very sick and no experienced nurse was available, the doctor remained by the bedside, thumping the chest to loosen up phlegm and changing the position of the patient until the "crisis" occurred—a sharp drop in fever and a sudden improvement in the patient's breathing that usually foretold recovery. It could take days for the crisis to come, if it came at all. Before antibiotics, the treatment of pneumonia was an art, and there were some practitioners who deserved the title "pneumonia specialist."

Before he left, the doctor instructed the members of the household on the patient's care. He might recommend that the windows be opened for fresh air and that the room, bedclothes, and fomites be cleaned with soap and water. Depending on the patient's condition, he might explain how to prepare a nutritious soft or liquid diet and suggest a proper fluid intake; demonstrate the application of a mustard plaster or the fitting of a quilted pneumonia jacket; or show caretakers how to thump the chest to loosen congestion and encourage a productive cough.

Many times, the homestead doctor was helpless in the face of overwhelming illness or a diagnostic enigma. But most conscientious and honest physicians knew their limitations and dealt with their patients and the families straightforwardly. For this they were greatly admired and became pillars of their communities.

From Mare to Motorcar

Even doctors with offices in town were often willing to travel to smaller communities. Many doctors spent much of their time on the road. On horseback, by horse and buggy, occasionally by train, and later by automobile, the doctor might spend days traveling on one trip. Practitioners going to see patients encountered perilous weather, rough terrain, even dangerous strangers. Sometimes it took so long to get there that the doctor arrived too late.

For many frontier doctors, house calls began in the barn. The doctor on horseback or in a buggy was a familiar scene, clop-clopping along the narrow roadways of rural America. Moving from house to house at all hours and in all weather, this picture of American medicine was a sustaining influence on folks of all ages—there was comfort and reassurance in knowing that the doctor was on the job. The doctor's posture told a knowing observer a lot. If he sat slumped casually with the reins held loosely, the trip was routine, but if the doctor was erect and spurring his faithful horse with urgency, it was an emergency call. Much was lost on the American landscape when the country doctor replaced his horse and buggy with a reciprocal engine—a symbol gone forever. There are still a few, very few, who can remember when "Doc" rode up, tied "Ol' Dolly" and the wagon out front, extracted a scuffed black bag from beneath the seat, and strode confidently into their family's house.

Horse travel on isolated and hazardous roads and trails, complicated by unpredictable weather, was risky, and all frontier doctors who made house calls were imperiled at times. Historian Francis Niven reported that Dr. Jakes Robinson of Manhattan, Montana, lost his life in June 1865 while attempting to cross the West Gallatin River at flood stage.[453]

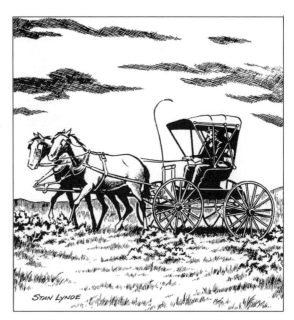

*A country doctor
making his rounds
by horse and buggy*
—Courtesy Stan Lynde

Bad weather brought risks of all kinds of accidents, but one of the biggest dangers of horse-and-buggy travel was the possibility of a runaway team. Dr. Lemuel Line, who came to Columbus, Montana, in 1895, experienced five separate runaway incidents in his early practice. In one of these mishaps he dislocated his shoulder.[454] George W. Beal, a well-known frontier doctor, was killed when his team ran away. According to the *Butte Miner*, "His team had taken an unused road . . . went over an embankment nearly 20 feet high. The Doctor landed back of the wagon which was found bottom-side up."[455]

Fording high rivers was another hazard. Dr. Winifred Braine Reynolds and her husband, Dr. William F. Reynolds, practiced in the little mining town of Aldridge, Montana, in the early twentieth century. One afternoon the Doctors Reynolds were summoned to Gardiner, on the other side of the Yellowstone River, with an urgent message: "Come quick—my baby is burned bad." Ordinarily on a trip to Gardiner, the Reynoldses would leave their team and buggy on the west side of the river, cross a flimsy footbridge, and travel on by rented carriage. But a ford across the river would eliminate many arduous miles. It was an extremely dangerous decision, but the doctors chose to take the chance.

Before we were halfway across, the water was rushing under the seat, but there was no going back. We crawled up on the back of the seat, and I clutched the medicine bags under my arm. The horse got beyond his depth and started to swim, and the buggy swung down stream with the current. Then the horse began to go out of sight. The doctor [William] laid the whip on her. . . . She plunged violently forward and struck bottom and in just a few minutes had scrambled out on the other bank.[456]

Certainly country doctors never knew what they might run into on a trip. Winifred Reynolds recalled another dangerous house call she and her husband made by team and wagon. (For more on Dr. Winifred Reynolds, see chapter 10.) Riding to Cooke City, they passed through the corner of Yellowstone Park, where they encountered a bear:

Just as we passed a little group of underbrush and bushes, out slipped Mr. Grizzly and rose on his hind legs! I don't know how tall he really was but he was the biggest bear I ever saw. He closed his jaws with a snap that we plainly heard and the froth from his mouth flew all

Dr. William P. Reynolds, medical school graduation picture, 1900; Dr. Winifred Braine, medical school graduation picture, 1899 —Courtesy Dr. William A. Reynolds, Missoula, Montana

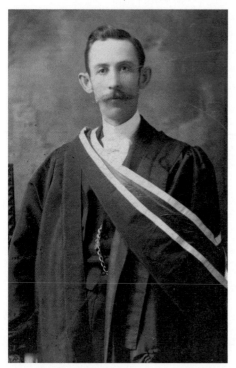
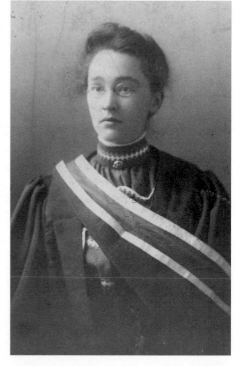

over the horses; and the horses simply took their bits between their teeth and ran away, and such running for about a mile over rocks and stubble! When finally the Doctor got them pulled in, I felt as if I could never get a breath again and were the horses in a lather![457]

Naturally, when a physician received a call, he or she had to weigh the circumstances and the dangers. The decision depended on the distance, the weather, and the roads. Sometimes he chose to go regardless of the risk, and only luck prevented tragedy. The *Billings Gazette* reported on January 24, 1892, a trip made by Dr. Henry Chapple to D. W. Slayton's ranch: "The call was urgent or the doctor would have hesitated to set out in the face of the storm then prevailing. He lost the road several times on the return trip but made the journey there and back in about 36 hours. Mr. Slayton's family increased by one good healthy eight-pound boy, whose arrival was the occasion of the doctor's sleigh ride."[458]

Dr. Chapple made many more trips during his practice, but one extremely difficult journey led to his premature death two years later from Addison's disease, a complication of tuberculosis. "Traveling in the midst of a cold spring rain and heavy roads consuming 30 hours' time, the long tedious trip in such inclement weather, together with a weakened constitution caused him a sickness from which he never recovered."[459]

Not all misadventures had such serious outcomes. One early practitioner in Broadwater County, Montana, was on a house call about twelve miles from home when his faithful horse, Dobbie, became bored waiting for his master and started home without him. When the doctor finished his visit, he discovered he had been left to get himself home on "shanks' mare." He ran, carrying his bag, for four miles before he caught up with old Dobbie.[460] Another country doctor related an early experience on horseback when the weather was far below zero. The cold air coming through the opening beneath the pommel of the saddle threatened to freeze his gonads. He rode using one hand to guide the horse and the other to warm and protect his "vitals."[461]

The passage from horse to automobile was a gradual process. There were times and places and conditions in which the new "flivvers" did not function. If the operator of a Model T forgot to raise the "spark" lever before attempting to crank the handle, the motor would backfire, which could result in a fractured arm. Furthermore, in many ways the early motorcar was a fair-weather device. Thick mud cleaved to helplessly spinning automobile wheels, and tires were easily punctured. Where a horse could break through crusted snow, the auto was paralyzed. And while horse travel had inherent dangers, the automobile was hardly safer.

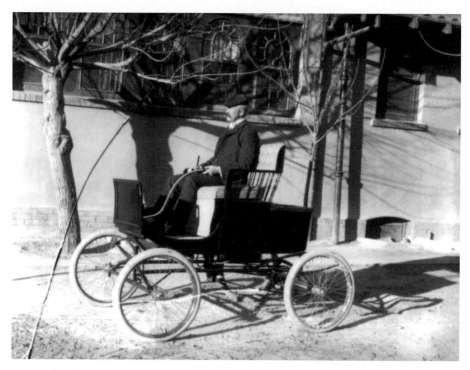

Dr. Hiram W. Fenner, an Arizona physician, in one of the first "horseless carriages," a 1900 Locomobile Steamer. Doctors in the West were among the first to switch from the buggy to the automobile. At first the automobile seemed safer, but this assumption was premature. —Courtesy Arizona Historical Society

Most of the early car accidents weren't fatal, but the roads were treacherous and unsuitable for the breathtaking speed of fifteen to twenty miles per hour. Men and women who were competent driving wagons couldn't always manage a car. Dr. G. W. Gilham of Townsend, Montana, purchased a "high-wheeled International" in 1905. When he failed to make a turn on a rough road, he was dumped down a steep incline. Fortunately he was unhurt, but it was his distinction to have caused the first automobile accident in Broadwater County.[462]

Many doctors hired "pilots" (people who knew the area well) to drive, especially at night. On one trip, Dr. Daniel McKay of White Sulphur Springs, Montana, had a driver who navigated a Maytag automobile up a mountain road through a blizzard. These early cars were topless and powered by a two-cylinder chain drive, and were equipped with carbide lights that flickered badly and had a habit of going out just when they were most needed.[463] The pilots who assisted doctors were of inestimable value. Not only did they know the roads, but during the trip the doctor might relax, rest, and even sleep. In winter in the 1920s, Dr. J. T. Bradbury of Willow Creek, Montana, frequently stopped by the local pool hall to find a pilot to drive and help him push his car through snowdrifts on house calls. On one trip to rescue a miner with acute appendicitis, Dr. Bradbury's driver was so cold that he swore he'd never do it again.[464]

Dr. Lindsey Baskett had a house call up the Boulder River one winter that lasted seven days. It was snowing so hard that as he pushed his car through growing drifts, the snow filled in his tracks. He made his destination and delivered a fine baby, but, weathered in, he couldn't leave for days.[465] While early automobiles were not much of an improvement over the buggy, in time the machine and the roads improved, sparing country doctors hours of travel.

Progress Out of Reach

The automobile wasn't the only sign of progress during the early twentieth century. Advances in medical education, microbiology, anesthesia, and antiseptic and aseptic surgical methods enhanced many patients' chances of survival out West. Better-trained physicians arrived, and a few hospitals sprang up in remote places. During World War I, a great deal was learned about shock, infection, fluid balance, blood loss, and the use of blood transfusion. Some of the advances were available on the frontier, but not all. There were still many pioneers living in far-flung locations, with little access to a doctor, much less a hospital.

Isolated Montana pioneer Henry Bierman recorded an agonizing episode in his journal in 1895:

> I was alone. The pains got so hard I began to think it was my last. I wrote a short farewell note to Ida. . . . I began to vomit some awful stuff, the color of liver and ropey which eased me. I sipped a little water. The pains would come on every few hours and then I would vomit. Dr. McDonald [from Kalispell] sent out some medicine and by degrees I got back on my feet. The sick spell left a lump in my side low down. . . . It was about the size of a hen's egg. I was later examined by Dr. Duncan who said it was from a ruptured appendix which had walled itself off.[466]

That Bierman survived is amazing. Though it ended all right, this story is a reminder that medical care in the West was not distributed equally. In spite of medical advances, many people remained out of reach for years. Without a hospital and if the local doctor was not a surgeon, isolated homesteaders could only be diagnosed with appendicitis and other internal conditions, not treated. Many curable conditions proved fatal. Even when the diagnosis was obvious and treatment was understood, transportation to a place where surgical treatment was available could take many hours, if not days. Autos and motorized ambulances were hardly faster or more reliable than wagons—they were sometimes worse. Later in the twentieth century, small airplane ambulances were sometimes used when available.

Injured and ill people in remote areas sometimes suffered incredibly in trying to get help. One rancher who was bucked from his horse and fractured an ankle on a windy, subzero day crawled about two miles to a grove of cottonwoods, where he fashioned a crutch. He eventually reached his house and drove his truck thirty miles to a hospital. Another man, with a ruptured appendix, rode a full day by horseback to Great Falls, where he was successfully treated.[467]

On the frontier, the transport of patients was a slow and sometimes difficult process. In communities with a hospital, a horse-drawn ambulance such as this was quite progressive. —Courtesy Gallatin County Historical Society, Bozeman, Montana

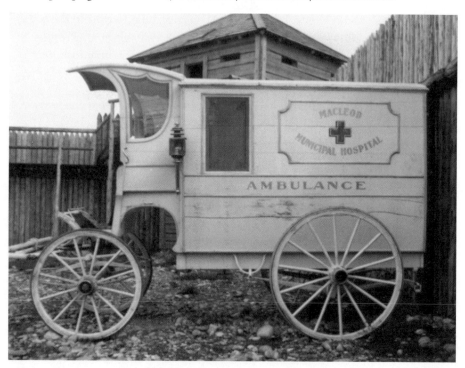

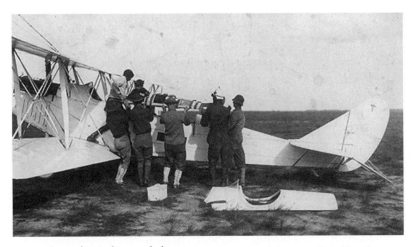

An early airplane ambulance —Courtesy National Museum of Health and Medicine, Armed Forces Institute of Pathology, Washington, D.C.

On the frontier, death from acute appendicitis was common. Because of this risk, the doctor was forced to operate in appendicitis cases or to send the patient to a place with a surgeon. Time was critical, as delayed treatment was often fatal. Farmers and ranchers frequently neglected the early symptoms and arrived for surgery too late. In small communities, most patients with abdominal complaints were transported to a town with a hospital whenever possible. Unfortunately this took time, sometimes too much time. One Montana pioneer wrote, "I will always remember being at the depot in Belmont.... A man by the name of Perry Farmer was there with his [fifteen-year-old] son . . . waiting for the train to Billings. The boy apparently had a ruptured appendix [but] they had to wait. The boy didn't make it."[468]

Money Down

Most homesteaders were so poor that they put off asking for medical help until all else failed. Fees charged by a physician might be ten dollars plus two dollars a mile for a house visit. When farm income was less than five hundred dollars a year, this expense was daunting. A few doctors gouged their patients, which led to the frontier expression, "M.D. stands for money down." For this reason and others, physicians were not generally respected. One popular saying was, "The boy who goes into medicine

181

is too lazy for farm or shop, too stupid for the Bar, and too immoral for the pulpit."[469]

Very few doctors, however, deserved this criticism. Most of them certainly did not get rich practicing medicine. Dr. Lindsey Baskett, who practiced in Big Timber from 1917 until he died in 1962, never sent out a bill. He relied on his patients to come forward and pay him. Many of them did, but just as many didn't. Baskett's son Dr. Lindsey M. (Mac) Baskett shared an anecdote about his father. A number of children were admiring Dr. Baskett's new car, which was parked in front of his office. When he came out of the office, one of the children said, "Gee, Doc, that's a swell car. Didn't it cost a lot?" The doctor replied, "Yes, it did. And it's paid for. That's more than I can say for most of you!"[470]

Like nearly all early physicians, Dr. Baskett was willing to take payment in any form. One farmer promised to give Dr. Baskett a pig as soon it got large enough to butcher. A long time passed. When the doctor asked the farmer about his pig, the man replied sadly, "Well, I meant to tell you . . . yours died."[471]

Dr. Ludwig F. Lubeley of Ryegate, Montana, delivered a lot of homesteaders' babies in the Big Coulee. On one occasion, after the successful delivery of a fine boy, the proud father asked Dr. Lubeley how much he owed. The doctor said, "Twenty-five dollars will be enough." A short time later, the doctor's car was stuck in the mud, and the new father had to pull him out with his team. When Dr. Lubeley asked the man how much he owed him, the father replied, "Twenty-five dollars will be enough."[472] This homesteader was fortunate to be able to pay off his debt so soon.

Fevers, Flu, and Fractures: All in a Day's Work

The homestead doctor might be called upon to treat a fracture, a burn, a miscarriage, or a life-threatening fever. One of the more common conditions requiring medical care was pneumonia, a potentially fatal lung infection. During the influenza epidemic of 1918, pneumonias and empyemas (an accumulation of pus in the chest cavity) were ubiquitous. Some survivors could relate in detail how "old Doc" had saved their lives.

Before antibiotics, the course of lobar pneumonia had several stages. The victim had a good chance of recovery if he reached the stage called the "crisis," a sudden improvement in the patient's condition. But reaching the crisis did not mean the danger was over. Days later, the doctor might have to return to treat an empyema. In this serious complication, if the doctor drained the abscess too soon, it could cause sudden death, yet he could not wait too long either. The doctor decided when to do the procedure and where to make the incision based on physical diagnosis alone, using a stethoscope and percussion with his hands.

In his autobiography *The Horse and Buggy Doctor*, Arthur E. Hertzler recalls an empyema case he examined after a three-hour, eight-mile buggy trip through deep and tenacious Kansas mud. The patient was nearly moribund, so without anesthesia, he stabbed through the chest wall with a scalpel. Foul pus under great pressure sprayed all over the doctor, the bed, and the floor. The patient recovered, but the memory of that "pus bath" lingered in the doctor's memory for a long time.[473]

After their invention in 1896, X-ray machines helped doctors make decisions on the proper type and timing of treatments for pneumonias and empyemas, as well as for bone fractures and other injuries. But in the West, even medical centers had few X-ray facilities until well into the twentieth century. In the little community of White Sulphur Springs in the late 1890s, Dr. Daniel McKay was one of the first doctors to use an X-ray for diagnosis in Montana.[474] A few years later, when Dr. Lemuel M. Line moved to Columbus, Montana, he bought an X-ray machine to help him locate bullets in his patients' bodies. Dr. Line said he encountered a gunshot wound at least once a week. Because there was no electric plant in town, he purchased a "static" machine, "a marvel of the age," to run the X-ray.[475]

In the early years, doctors tested X-ray machines by taking images of their own hands and used fluoroscopy while manipulating fractured bones. In so doing, their hands were exposed to high doses of radiation. Consequently some physicians of this era developed scaly, warty premalignant changes on their hands, and a few developed skin cancers. Although these cases were usually not fatal, Dr. C. F. Watkins of Missoula, Montana, had so much exposure that he had to have an arm amputated for cancer and eventually died from metastasis.[476]

It is remarkable what good results frontier doctors obtained without fluoroscopy or X-ray in treating fractures and dislocations, which were very common. The doctor located the deformity by touch and ascertained the relationship of the bone fragments, then with traction and manipulation tried to realign the fragments. If the alignment was satisfactory, he or she would splint the affected part with whatever materials were handy.

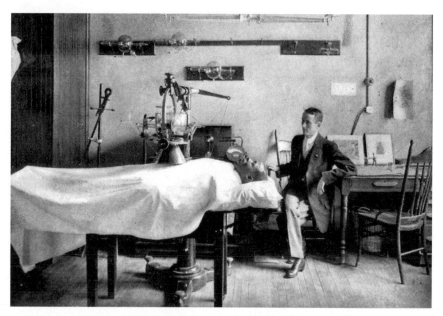

Early X-ray machines and fluoroscopy enhanced the diagnostic accuracy of physicians and helped the surgeon to locate foreign bodies and to align fractures. —Courtesy National Library of Medicine, History of Medicine Division

It is particularly surprising how well an inexperienced practitioner could fare under such trying circumstances. In one incident in 1911, after Alfred Johnson accidentally shot himself with his shotgun, a friend, Oscar Bjoerneby, made a record ten-mile horseback ride to Ryegate, Montana, to fetch the new doctor. Dr. Ludwig Lubeley, only a few weeks on the job, was driven to the victim's bedside in a neighbor's automobile. The young doctor knew the case would make the headlines of the *Ryegate Weekly Reporter.*

Using only manual examination and superficial probes of the gaping wound in Johnson's flank, Dr. Lubeley had to find the answer to the following questions: Had the shot or wadding penetrated the peritoneal cavity, which would result in peritonitis? Were any major blood vessels or nerves injured? Was the kidney damaged? How energetically should the wound be debrided of shot, powder, wadding, foreign material, and devitalized tissue? Should the patient be sent to Billings or Great Falls, where X-ray and more experienced surgeons were available? In the end, Dr. Lubeley treated the wound successfully, Johnson recovered, and a brick of confidence was laid in the foundation of the young sawbones's reputation.[477] Soon he would be indispensable to the little ranching and railroad community.

Fevers, a common complaint on the frontier, could be a challenge even to the most experienced physician. Many fevers were serious and difficult to treat, such as typhoid, cholera, measles, scarlet fever, malaria, and diphtheria. Fevers often presented a diagnostic dilemma, too, as the different types were difficult to distinguish. The better-known conditions could usually be recognized by the symptoms and signs, but there were some mysterious maladies. One baffling condition confronting frontier doctors was known as "mountain fever," a remittent fever that seemed to affect newcomers to the mountains. The disease is still a mystery. It could have been a transient virus that is no longer active, or it may have been Colorado tick fever. Perhaps it wasn't an entity in and of itself, but a name applied to various illnesses. Some cases of mountain fever may have been recurrent malaria, brought west in an already infected patient and precipitated by the effects of high altitude.

Sometimes nature took its course regardless of medical diagnosis or intervention. In his autobiographical book, *The Youngest Science*, Lewis Thomas tells a story about his father's practice in upstate New York in the early twentieth century. One of his dad's first patients was a man with blood in his urine. Unsure of what to do until he could bone up on hematuria, the young Dr. Thomas gave the patient a bottle of Blaud's pills, an iron preparation that was popular at the time for anemia. A few days later, the patient returned with a specimen of crystal-clear urine. Word of the apparent cure rapidly spread through the small community, and the young doctor's reputation was made. In reality, the patient had probably quietly passed a kidney stone.[478]

Kitchen-Table Surgery

The tragedy of the Civil War presented the medical profession with the opportunity to develop better surgical techniques, which continued to be improved and refined through the early 1900s. Even after hospitals reached the frontier, there was still a place for doctors who could provide emergency surgery in the home. For one thing, many people did not want to go to a hospital even when there was one nearby. More often, distance, rough roads, and sometimes weather made getting to a hospital impractical.

Contrary to its image, kitchen-table surgery was not a blood-and-guts nightmare carried out by a drunken doctor wielding a butcher knife. A great deal of knowledge of anatomy, anesthesia, antisepsis, asepsis, and healing was required by the operator. Some frontier doctors became extremely skilled at operating in the home and were able to do major procedures with very little help, often by lamplight or even the dim glow of tallow candle.

Some procedures done in the home included reduction of fractures, treatment of gunshot wounds, amputations, lancing of abscesses, thoracotomy in treatment of an empyema, appendectomy, incarcerated hernia, and, rarely, craniotomy to release a subdural or epidural clot or drain a brain abscess. One of the most frequently performed kitchen-table procedures was a tracheotomy. In cases of diphtheria, an inflamed membrane commonly obstructed the larynx or windpipe. During diphtheria epidemics, tracheotomies were commonplace.

Diphtheria victims were usually children. Because a patient with a blocked windpipe could asphyxiate within minutes, the physician had to take charge immediately. Tracheotomy was not simple surgery; some essential arteries, veins, and nerves lie in the neck near the trachea, and

A tracheotomy is a surgical opening in the trachea (windpipe) to make breathing easier. A tube is inserted into the opening (stoma) to keep it open. —From *The Science and Art of Surgery: A Treatise on Surgical Injuries, Diseases, and Operations* by John Eric Erichsen, 1884

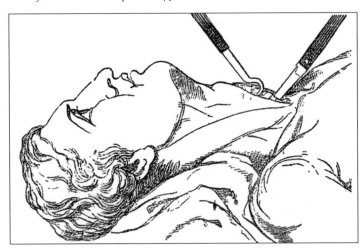

a slip of the knife could be fatal. Often the doctor had to enlist the help of the family. The assistant, usually the mother or father, sat at the head of the table and held the child's head back as far as possible. With the patient in position, the doctor made a longitudinal incision over the midline of the windpipe and through the cartilaginous fibrous wall of the trachea. The gush of inflowing air into the lungs of a cyanotic child must have been a glorious sound to the family and the doctor. But the surgeon wasn't done. Very often, bloody mucus, pus, and pieces of the diphtheritic membrane continued to partially obstruct the windpipe and the tracheotomy stoma. This material had to be removed, and there was only one way to do it. The doctor sucked the material into his mouth and spat it out. This crude method of aspiration had the advantage of giving the doctor an excuse to wash out his mouth with whiskey.

Another operation performed in the home was the mastoidectomy. Mastoiditis is a complication of common ear infection. The bony plate over the mastoid space was drilled open to allow the accumulated pus to drain away, avoiding a possible fatal brain abscess. A generation of young people left with scars and surgical deformities over the mastoid area, veiled by locks of hair, were testimonials to this period of surgical progress. Dr. Camilla Anderson, recalling her early-twentieth-century Montana homestead childhood, described a mastoid operation performed on a little boy in her family's home. A doctor was summoned from Glendive, she remembered, and the patient was laid on the Andersons' dining room table and sedated with chloroform. During the surgery, the little boy's body was kept warm with hot flatirons wrapped in cloth. One of the child's heels was burned by the irons, but "the operation was a success other than that."[479]

The anesthesia most often used in those days was chloroform, administered by a nurse or sometimes a member of the family, often using the "drinking glass" technique. A wad of cotton was packed tightly in a water glass, then saturated with chloroform. The patient held the inverted glass over his or her mouth and nostrils. When the anesthetic took effect, the unconscious patient's hand fell away with the glass, thus avoiding an overdose. Chloroform was very toxic to some, however, and many physicians would use only ether.

By mid-twentieth century, simple laboratory procedures had been developed to aid rural physicians. Blood transfusions, sometimes lifesaving, could be done away from a hospital, with blood from close relatives that was cross-matched with the recipient. Intravenous solutions were prepared by hand—the saline and glucose weighed, mixed with water, and sterilized in a pressure cooker. These preparations could take hours. Moreover, rural doctors who were put on the spot often had to be resourceful in coming up with substitutes for unavailable medical equipment and supplies.

In an anonymous account, Dr. S. A. remembered his Depression-era practice in Shelby, Montana. His ingenuity was challenged when a man was brought in after an accident that had avulsed a large part of his scalp. Much of the scalp was missing, and the skin could not be stretched to cover the defect. The doctor borrowed an electric drill from a garage (not, he emphasized, a variable-speed drill, but a "damned fast one"), and in lieu of a hospital OR, he used a room in a hotel next to his office. Here he sat the man on a chair and began drilling. "The gyrations of the drill, of course, made us both nervous," he said. Luckily the drill holes were made without perforating the inner table of the skull. In about ten days, granulation tissue grew over the drill holes, forming a base for a skin graft. A large portion of skin from a hairy place on the patient's leg was then used to cover the raw area. The result was "good," the doctor reported.[480]

If a surgical case was uncomplicated, the result was usually successful, but sometimes a physician only guessed at the diagnosis, and more serious conditions were discovered after the patient was "opened." Acute gall bladder disease, ruptured gastric or duodenal ulcers, and unsuspected tumors were not easy to treat on kitchen tables. However, many satisfactory outcomes followed just such surprises, attesting to the skill of frontier surgeons.

Not all doctors performed surgery. From colonial times, only a few men had the courage and instinct to be surgeons. Dr. John Jones, professor of surgery at the University of Pennsylvania in 1769, told his students that a surgeon must have "firm steady hands, & be able to use both alike . . . a strong clear sight . . . & above all, a mind, calm & intrepid, yet humane, & compassionate."[481]

One extraordinary homestead surgeon was Arthur E. Hertzler, whose autobiography, *The Horse and Buggy Doctor*, was published in 1938. After attending Northwestern University, Hertzler practiced many years as a country doctor in Kansas and trained himself as a surgeon. Years later he studied under the finest scientists in Europe, built a hospital, helped establish a medical school, and taught pathology and surgery. Of his years as a kitchen-table surgeon, Dr. Hertzler wrote:

> I did operations on the road for conditions I would not think of doing even in hospital now. . . . I operated on patients I had never seen before

and, of course, they had no preparation of any sort. . . . The majority of the operations I did on the road were the usual operations done in any hospital . . . pelvic operations for tumors, as well as the repair of lacerations. Breast operations for cancer, and resection of cysts. . . . I drained four brain abscesses on the road, and did many mastoid operations. . . . Many of the trips were terribly arduous. . . . I look back on those days of kitchen surgery with unadulterated pleasure. . . . I saved many lives. . . . Those days are gone forever. The coming generation of surgeons will not have a like experience. . . .

The story of kitchen surgery should not be lost. . . . It presents many lessons . . . of value today. . . . [Modern doctors] will have to accept the word of the old kitchen surgeons that all that is needed for a good operation is a good surgeon and a patient.[482]

Special Deliveries

One of the foremost medical problems on the frontier was not a disease—it was pregnancy. Most homestead women had several deliveries. The death rate for children was high on the frontier, so women had a lot of babies to make up for the ones who didn't make it. It was a matter of practical need. Children of both sexes helped with the endless work in the home, in the fields, and with the livestock. Children raised in these circumstances became self-reliant at an early age, and without their help, many struggling families would have failed entirely.

The babies usually came normally, but many homestead mothers' lives were shortened by complications before, during, and after childbirth. Western women depended on their neighbors, their family, and, if one was available, a midwife to help with a delivery. Few births were attended by physicians, and some babies were delivered by the father. Some towns had hospitals or maternity homes attended by midwives and doctors, but most western women didn't have access to such advanced facilities. Rural women looked out for one another. As one frontier woman put it, "That [pregnancy] was where we learned what neighbors meant."[483]

Pioneer women had essentially no prenatal care. Little was known about this important time in a woman's life, even in the East. Because pregnancy was viewed as a natural phenomenon, even trained and competent physicians often did not offer prenatal care. A pregnant woman's health was mostly a matter of luck and heredity. Certainly a lack of exercise wasn't a problem with most farm and ranch women, who worked at their numerous tasks until labor pains began. After delivery, the new mother was expected to be back at her duties as soon as possible: cooking, cleaning, caring for her children and her husband, even working in the fields.

The lack of proper medical examination of pregnant women and the often cavalier attitude toward their condition are illustrated in an anecdote about an old doctor in Miles City. On one occasion, after delivering an infant in the home, he left a nurse to care for the afterbirth and other details. A short time later, he was sent word from the frantic nurse that another baby came after he left. The doctor's response for the nurse was, "Just keep count of them and I'll be there in a minute."[484]

When a serious complication during pregnancy or childbirth was discovered, long distances and inadequate transportation to medical help made the situation even more critical. But many maternal deaths were caused by simple neglect and ignorance. One especially egregious tale from an article by historian Mary Melcher deserves to be repeated:

> One woman plagued with hemorrhages and weakness for several months of her pregnancy, also suffered from a severe unrepaired laceration from a previous confinement. During the sixth month of her pregnancy, she saw a doctor who said she needed hospital attention. Her husband, however, was unpersuaded that the natural function of childbirth could be dangerous. During her confinement, she had no labor pains, but she hemorrhaged excessively. They sent for a doctor, who arrived after a twenty-four-hour journey of thirty-five miles. With instruments, he delivered a stillborn baby that had been dead for at least four days. When the mother also died seven days later, the doctor said he believed her death was caused by blood poisoning from the dead fetus.[485]

While there are numerous stories like this one, unassisted home birth during this era had some advantages. As more women delivered in hospitals and maternity homes, the incidence of postpartum infection increased. The mother who had a baby in her own home with no instrumental manipulation and surrounded by bacteria that her immune system had accommodated to had a much better chance of avoiding infections, which were often fatal. Also, the forced early ambulation of a frontier mom prevented vascular disorders such as clots in the legs and emboli. In maternity homes and hospitals, women were sometimes kept in bed for long periods.

For assisting with home births in the country, midwives were indispensable. A midwife could usually be found nearby, and they charged very little. Most women who worked as midwives were not formally trained, and their degree of experience varied. By the early twentieth century, some had nurse's training or specific midwife training. Sometimes they worked with doctors. Most were efficient, knowledgeable, and trusted. Indian women were much in demand for this function. Although probably myth, some people thought Indian midwives were more skilled than white ones.

One Finnish midwife, Aino Hamalainen Putio, came to America in 1911 and practiced in Butte and later in Red Lodge, Montana. She gave her clients instructions on prenatal diet, rest, and physical activity. Her knowledge was so advanced that she sterilized her instruments, used disinfectants, and dropped silver nitrate into the newborn's eyes to prevent an infection from gonorrhea, a frequent cause of blindness. During delivery, she made sure that someone was available to run for a doctor in the event of a serious complication. She also stayed with the new mother and infant during the critical postpartum period, when unexpected crises could and often did occur. For all this care, she charged fourteen dollars.[486]

No matter how qualified the midwife, however, when severe complications occurred, the doctor had to be called. Sometimes the physician was able to handle the crisis, though not always. Medical schools of the era did not offer much practical experience in obstetrics: some physicians had witnessed only one or two deliveries during their training. Most doctors knew, however, that if the mother was dying, a Cesarean section might save her and the infant. Among the indications for a section were a breech presentation in a woman's first delivery, a maternal pelvis too narrow to allow the baby's head to pass, cervical obstruction, and maternal exhaustion during labor.

Because there was seldom any examination of the mother before labor, problems were usually not discovered until delivery. A woman might have a uterine tumor or cancer of the cervix that went completely unrecognized until prolonged labor or bleeding or both made it apparent to the midwife or doctor. Without intervention, a placenta praevia—an abnormal implantation of the placenta—almost always resulted in a fatal hemorrhage. Even when a Cesarean section was done immediately, forty percent of the mothers died.[487] Few practitioners were prepared for this operation, certainly not in the home without any assistance. Other serious abnormalities also occurred that resulted in the mother's and/or infant's death.

One of the first Cesarean sections performed in Montana was reported in the *American Journal of Obstetrics and Diseases of Women and Children* in 1893. Dr. Henry W. Foster of Bozeman was called to treat a Mrs. D., age twenty-eight, in labor with her first baby. At the time of surgery, the young woman was exhausted from prolonged labor in her attempt to deliver a large infant, who had since died in utero. Another physician had attempted a craniotomy on the dead infant (opening up the skull and aspirating brain tissue in an attempt to diminish head size) to allow passage. When Dr. Foster stepped in, the woman was "very much exhausted, pulse 135 and very weak. . . . She was put in as thorough an antiseptic condition as was possible, considering her condition and poverty, the family living in two small rooms. . . . I made an incision in the median line, commencing two inches above the navel and extending almost down to the pubis."

Dr. Foster described how he opened the uterus and removed the ten-and-a-half-pound infant's body. But while he was removing the placenta, his assistant urged him to hurry, "as the patient was sinking." Because of this urgency, Dr. Foster elected not to remove the uterus (called a Porro section, which was thought desirable at the time), but rather to sew up the incision in the uterus and the abdominal wall, which he did using chromized catgut. All this on a kitchen table! "She rallied quite well," he observed. Postoperatively Dr. Foster irrigated her vagina and uterus with bichloride of mercury and sterilized water. She was sedated with hypodermic injections of whiskey. By the third day, Mrs. D's temperature and pulse were normal, and her recovery was uneventful.[488]

Some babies came amid all the modern facilities one could ask for and didn't even need them. A doctor of my acquaintance in Meeker, Colorado, Virgil Gould, told me the story of a delivery that was so easy it was actually funny. It was 1950, and the Meeker Memorial Hospital was nearing completion. One of Dr. Gould's obstetrical patients was anxious to have the first child born in the new hospital. And sure enough, only a few days after the place opened, she went into labor.

Things were moving fast, and the patient was soon fully dilated and was moved from the labor room to the delivery room, which was equipped with all the latest gadgets (none of which the doctor was familiar with). Since this was a historic event and because there were no other patients in the new hospital, nearly the entire staff—nurses, technicians, kitchen workers, everyone—gathered in the hall and watched the procedure through the large double doors.

The nurse was busy arranging her tray of instruments and Dr. Gould was about to rinse his gloves in disinfectant when both of them heard a squishing sound. They turned back to see, laying on a pile of linens that was covering a tray at the end of the brand-new obstetrical table, a full-term infant. The baby was healthy and screaming like hell. The doctor, realizing that the scene had been witnessed by quite a few people, acted as if this was normal procedure. With neither haste nor hesitation, he lifted the child from the tray and performed all the procedures necessary to ensure that the infant was breathing well and functioning normally. The cord was severed, the afterbirth was delivered, and all was well. Only Dr. Gould and the nurse knew that the baby had slid from the uterus to the tray without escort, and that this wasn't the intended use of the tray.

While this story shows that Mother Nature didn't always require assistance, expectant mothers living in or near towns with hospitals were lucky. In rural areas, medical services were less accessible. The advent of telephones, electricity, and other technologies, however, helped improve emergency care in remote places. A doctor in northern Montana related an experience with a serious complication during a delivery that occurred after telephones had just been installed in the area. A midwife called from a Hutterite colony to tell him that a woman in labor had a prolapsed cord—a manifestation that could cause the infant to die in the uterus from diminished blood supply.

Over the phone, the physician told her to keep the baby's head high to prevent pressure on the cord. Then he rushed to the patient's ranch. When he arrived, the cord was prolapsed but pulsating slowly—the baby was alive but weak. Examination showed the infant was in a transverse position, a bad sign. The doctor had one option in the best interest of the mother and child: turn the baby and bring it out feet first, a breech extraction. This procedure is difficult even in the best of circumstances. Without anesthesia, the country doctor, with two women holding the patient's legs, delivered an essentially normal little girl.[489]

"I did not want any more children"

The lack of social support for birth control in the nineteenth and early twentieth centuries prevented most homestead women from getting reliable information. Margaret Sanger's crusade to educate women about contraception, beginning in the 1910s, made little progress in the East, and had even less influence in the West. A few frontier women may have learned some birth control methods from a doctor, nurse, or midwife, or—far more likely—a relative, friend, or neighbor. But most women of that era were taught to accept whatever fate brought them. One Helena woman wrote in 1877, "I did not want any more children, and there have been times in the last few months when I have felt utterly unreconciled to the state of affairs and even now I sometimes think I cannot care for any more little ones; but I try to recall the old proverb that 'the back is fitted to the burden' and come to believe that strength will be given for every duty."[490]

Stoicism aside, if the situation was desperate, there was one last, risky option: abortion. Since ancient times, women have resorted to abortion when they had an unwanted pregnancy. Prior to the mid-1800s, most governments and communities closed their eyes to this activity. Abortions, if they were accomplished before the time of quickening (when the mother feels fetal movement), were tacitly allowed. But beginning in 1857, the American Medical Association and others pressured the government to criminalize abortion, and by 1900 all states had complied. The laws were hard to enforce, however. In 1904 in Chicago, roughly twenty-five percent of pregnancies were terminated by illegal abortions; in 1920 it was estimated that eleven percent of maternal deaths were directly related to illegal abortions.[491]

Many physicians who were publicly opposed to abortion privately sympathized with women who wanted them. Some performed abortions secretly, and others referred their patients to doctors or midwives who did them. Because of this practice, midwives were often attacked in the press as abortionists, and they were scorned by many. In truth, only a few midwives performed abortions—probably no more than licensed doctors. Some doctors did go public in support of allowing abortion, or at least of looking the other way. In 1912 a prominent medical leader said in an address, "The public does not want, the [medical] profession does not want, the women in particular do not want any aggressive campaign against the crime of abortion."[492]

What was a woman on the frontier to do if she wanted to rid herself of a pregnancy? The average doctor seemed blind to the problems of women who had numerous children living in substandard conditions. Hundreds of babies were brought into poverty and disease to suffer from malnutrition and worse. Even of the few women who could find a reliable practitioner to give them an abortion, only the most financially fortunate ones were able to avail themselves of the service.

With so few options, women were forced to try to end their own pregnancies or to rely on uneducated and unskilled strangers, quacks, and charlatans. Secret home "recipes" and potions offered by traveling "medicine men" were often tried. A drug called ergot, though easily obtained, rarely did more than produce a few uterine cramps. Women rode horses, jumped off porches, and threw themselves down stairs, but these "accidents" almost never worked to release the conception from the inner lining of the uterus. Desperate women, blindly and with little knowledge of anatomy, inserted knitting needles, sticks, or other such items into their uterus in an attempt to dislodge the conception. Unsurprisingly, this method resulted in many serious infections and deaths.

Prospects were equally bad for women in the hands of quacks and back-alley "grannies." Bleeding and infection were common complications. Though rare, sudden death could occur from air emboli to the heart and brain during the manipulation, but bacterial infection was the usual killer. It was a slow, painful death as the bacterial poisoning spread inexorably throughout the system. If the woman survived, she was often left with chronic, debilitating pelvic infection and sterility. During the early twentieth century, hospitals witnessed an unremitting stream of patients who were sick and sometimes dying from septic abortion. It was not until the discovery of sulfa drugs and antibiotics, circa 1940, that such women stood a good chance of recovery.

Helena, Montana, had two well-trained doctors who were willing to do abortions. The better known was Dr. Edwin S. Kellogg, whose wife, Delia A. Kellogg, was an open proponent of women's rights and reproductive freedom. Dr. Kellogg came to Helena sometime around 1880. He was trained as a homeopath, but he gained a reputation as a surgeon. Evidently his activity as an abortionist was widely known—the Montana Medical Association refused him a certificate to practice in 1889. He never gained a certificate, but that didn't stop him from practicing.[493]

Kellogg was sued so many times by the medical society that a judge was heard to say, "We are having our annual Kellogg Trial."[494] In 1900 two of his patients, Sophie Hrella and Addie Bromley, died of sepsis after abortions. Kellogg's rivals attacked him, and he was tried on two counts of second-degree murder. He was acquitted. Dr. Napoleon Salvail came to Helena about the same time as Kellogg and was associated in general practice with Dr. William L. Steele. Salvail, trained at McGill University in Montreal, performed abortions but, unlike Kellogg, apparently avoided any prosecution.[495]

In general, women doctors were more sympathetic to the problem of unwanted pregnancy than men. Some of the early women practitioners performed abortions, at least under certain circumstances. For instance,

Nevada's first woman doctor, "Doctress Hoffman," who arrived in the territory in 1865, treated only women and children. She advertised that she offered confidential treatment of "female complaints."[496] Another woman doctor who braved the stigma of being called an abortionist was Sadie Lindeberg. During a sixty-year career that began in 1908, she had a general practice in Miles City, Montana, where she delivered more than eight thousand babies, usually in the patient's home. Most of her abortion cases were referred to her by male colleagues who didn't have the courage to do the deed themselves. Eleanor Mast, a social worker in Gallatin County during the 1950s and 1960s, said Dr. Lindeberg had an "excellent reputation."[497]

Out of necessity, Dr. Lindeberg was discreet. Although her activities were common knowledge, she was never prosecuted. After Dr. Lindeberg's death, a leading physician in the town rather sheepishly said, "I couldn't verify it [that she was performing abortions] but we were all sure it was happening. There were a lot of coat-hanger abortions being done and we ran into a lot of problems with that, infections and all sorts of things. We decided Sadie was doing a good job [and agreed] 'Let's let her do it, rather than all these quacks.'"[498]

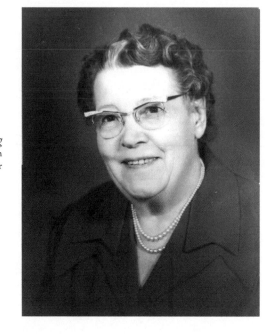

Dr. Sadie Lindeberg
—Courtesy Malcolm
and Beth Winter

Country Doc

Dr. Theodore J. Benson was the quintessential country doctor.[499] He began his practice in Fromberg, Montana, a small but busy community of coal miners and railroad builders, in 1907. His parents were Swedish immigrant farmers in Minnesota who encouraged him to attend college. By alternating his studies at the University of Minnesota with working on the farm every other year, Benson was able to finance his education. Once, when asked why he entered medicine, Benson said he had always been interested in machinery, and "the human body was the most marvelous machinery in the world."[500]

Dr. Benson's horse and buggy traveled the lonely roads and trails within a fifty-mile radius of Fromberg, an area that included most of the Clark Fork Valley. He also visited patients on the Crow Indian Reservation, which took him as far south as Chance, Wyoming. His horse knew by rote the way to Bridger, Joliet, Edgar, and Pryor. In 1911 Benson replaced his faithful horse with a Model T Ford—a one-seat runabout with a magneto and a crank.

From memories half a century old, a former patient, Genevieve Buchanan, paid tribute to Dr. Benson:

> I recall as a child the fascination his little black bag held for me. . . . Hundreds of vials of mysterious looking pills and potions. . . . I can see him measure out some pills in the palm of his hand—then ask Mom for a dish to put them in—or perhaps a glass of water in which to dissolve them. Next he would give her instructions how the medicine should be administered. Then, the sick child having been attended to by the usual examination of tongue, temperature, pokes and soundings—and already improved from the health and strength his being seemed to exude—he would chat and josh with the folks before he went tirelessly on his way. Then the tension and feeling of uneasiness and apprehension always lessened.[501]

Benson's nurse, Alma Claus, wrote:

> His office was typical of the country doctors at that time—a small frame building with an inner office, outer waiting room, and no running water. . . . He had his supply of wooden slats from which he fashioned splints for broken bones. One interesting piece of equipment was a device for suctioning mucous and blood from patients' throats during the removal of tonsils, fashioned from an old automobile tire pump. . . . We used boiling water for sterilizing instruments and quantities of alcohol for antiseptic. . . . It was a common sight to see his office and lawn outside filled with Indians in every kind of dress and description.

. . . His office walls were hung with Indian lore . . . spears, bows and arrows, hides and headdresses given by Indians in payment.[502]

Dr. Benson's skills as a country doctor left an indelible imprint on his community. Though he died in 1959, as recently as 1990, Benson was still remembered by his community. The Clark's Fork Valley Museum honored his memory by moving his little two-room office building, built in 1907, to its grounds and opening it to visitors, allowing them to see how a frontier doctor practiced.

Many Hats

Pioneer doctors often did more than practice medicine. Some owned businesses such as hotels or drugstores. Others invested in gold mines, land, and cattle. Dr. William Lee Steele of Helena, for example, made a fortune in mining, and he also raised mules to sell to the homesteaders.[503] A respected leader, he was elected president of the Fairweather Mining District of Alder Gulch in Virginia City. In most places, doctors,

Dr. William L. Steele at St. John's Hospital, Helena, Montana, 1897. He came to Bannack in 1863 from South Carolina, becoming successful and popular as both a businessman and a doctor. —Courtesy Montana Historical Society, Helena

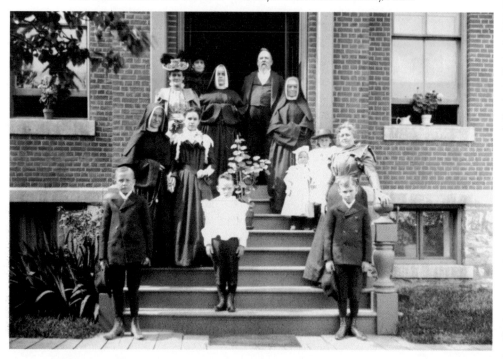

along with lawyers, newsmen, and judges, were members of the educated elite. Many were active in community affairs and acted as leaders in their towns.

In the early homesteading period, doctors found many ways to contribute to their developing communities. After Dr. William Whitwell came to Salmon, Idaho, in 1889, he became instrumental in getting the town to pipe water from a clean stream in the nearby mountains. A member of the school board for twenty years, he helped plan a new building; he also served Lemhi County as state senator for three terms. His death during the flu epidemic in 1918 cut short his productive career.[504] Another Idaho doctor, George Kellogg, also rendered a nonmedical service to his community of Nampa. During his rides he carried a repair kit, climbers, and test set to check the telephone lines along the way. He could get the central line from any pole in the backcountry. Kellogg also carried his shotgun, rifle, and ammunition in case he saw any wild game along the trail.[505]

Another doctor who helped build his community was Dr. Urling Coe. When he arrived in Bend, Oregon, in 1905, the town was in its infancy. In addition to his grueling practice, the young doctor was involved in the social issues of the day, such as women's suffrage and public health, and he served as the town's second mayor. By 1911, when the railroad arrived in Bend, newcomers found a stable and prosperous community.[506]

Dr. Maria Dean gave much to her town of Helena, Montana. Arriving about 1885, she was the first licensed female doctor in the state. Her large practice served primarily women and children. During her career, she was on the school board and was chairman of the Helena Board of Health. Dr. Dean helped to establish a YWCA in the town, and she was very active in the woman suffrage movement in Montana. She died in 1919, at age sixty-one.[507] (For more on Dr. Dean, see chapter 10.)

Women doctors on the frontier were especially remarkable given their additional burden of overcoming prejudice. We will examine this subject and meet some of these intrepid women in the next chapter.

TEN

"No Prejudice Against Women"

Female Physicians in the West

Dr. [Helen C.] Roberts's large practice bears witness that Montana has no prejudice against women in professions—when they are successful at all events.

—From a short biography of Helen C. Roberts, M.D., circa 1894,
in "History of Montana," Montana Historical Society Archives[508]

THE FIRST DOCTORS on the frontier were men. Army surgeons traveled with expeditions and staffed the forts. During the gold rush, the vast majority of those who came to California, Montana, and other gold-fields were men. Some of the miners claimed to be doctors, and some of them were, but few had come west to care for the sick—most of them were infected themselves with a condition known as "gold fever." Women came west to settle and to enjoy freedoms that were repressed in eastern society. Among the westering women were doctors. Nearly all the female doctors who came west arrived after the Civil War. No doubt there were female healers before then, both Indian and white, but women were not even allowed to attend medical school until the 1840s.

A prejudice against women doctors weaves like a thread through the history of the world. Even the area of gynecology, which had not always been the province of male physicians, shifted from female control to male involvement over the centuries. Before the fifth century B.C. and the advent of Hippocratic medicine, childbirth had been entrusted to the mother's female kin and neighbors, some of whom earned the informal title of midwife. But eventually, traditional female control of care during pregnancy and childbirth started to break down, and male doctors became increasingly involved in gynecological cases. Male anxiety about a woman's potential for sabotaging her husband's production of an heir made men, physicians included, suspicious of women's reproductive autonomy.

Since antiquity, women have shouldered much of the responsibility for health care. History is filled with tales of women nurses, herbalists, and healers throughout Europe and the Holy Land, and it seems that most were tolerated as long as they didn't step on the toes of their male counterparts. If they did, their activities were promptly curbed. According to Lois Magner's *A History of Medicine,* a woman practitioner named Jacoba Felicie of Paris was prosecuted in 300 B.C. for "illegally visiting the sick of both sexes, examining their pulse, urine, bodies and limbs, prescribing drugs, collecting fees, and worse yet, curing her patients."[509]

Even in modern times there was a distinct separation of caregiving according to gender. Women were nurses, and men were doctors. It is an enigma why men who were born of women and cared for by women through injury and sickness still held the female to be inferior in the lofty fraternity of the medical profession. Progress for women continued in fits and starts throughout the 1900s, but it was late in the century before attitudes changed appreciably toward the female medical student.

The first American woman to graduate from medical school was Elizabeth Blackwell, who earned her medical diploma in 1849. Turned down for admission by many schools, Blackwell was finally accepted to the Geneva College of Medicine in Geneva, New York. An outstanding student, she later studied in France and England. After returning to the United States, she established a clinic for poor women and children in New York City.

The Boston Female Medical College, later called New England Medical College, founded in 1848, was the first medical school in the world exclusively for women. But few women in the United States went to medical school until the end of the Civil War. One stunning exception was Dr. Mary E. Walker, who graduated from medical school in 1855 and served in the Union Army during the Civil War as a contract acting surgeon. She was awarded the Congressional Medal of Honor for her service. Her medal was revoked for a time because she had not been a combatant, but it was reinstated in 1977. The U.S. Postal Service later produced a stamp in her honor. Dr. Walker, a humanitarian and patriot, fought for women's rights throughout her life.

Between 1880 and 1910, the percentage of women doctors increased nationally. In 1880 two thousand women had medical degrees, and by 1900 seven thousand women physicians were practicing in the United

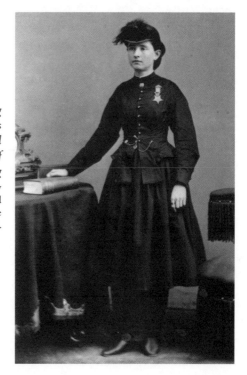

States.[510] Still, women represented only a small proportion of practicing physicians. The barriers to women in the elite colleges of the East were slow to come down. In 1890 Johns Hopkins agreed to admit women, but only after a women's group raised half a million dollars in endowment money. The American Medical Association refused to accept women as members until 1915.

The turn-of-the-century trend of women training as doctors did not last. Between 1900 and 1926, the number of females graduating from medical school diminished.[511] As established medical schools began to admit women, schools exclusively for women closed down. Yet the men's schools discriminated against women students, sometimes covertly and often overtly. The conservative, male-dominated medical profession was threatened by women participating as equals, and society in general frowned on women pursuing professional careers, especially married women.

Women medical students were demeaned and intimidated by their classmates and faculty alike. A woman who wished to become a physician needed luck, courage, and a very thick skin. In 1919, when Montanan Jessie Bierman entered the University of Chicago to study medicine, the dean said, "I want you to know, young lady, that you are getting the place of a man, and we have a rule here that we try to keep the percentage of women, niggers, and Jews to a minimum."[512]

Because they had to prove themselves, most women aspiring to medicine worked extra hard and were outstanding students. Dr. Caroline McGill of Butte, Montana, graduated first in her class at Johns Hopkins medical school in 1914. At the University of Pennsylvania in the 1920s, the esteemed Dean William Pepper said slyly in an address to the interns, "Now, girls, you will have to be three times as good as the boys here. But that won't be hard, will it?"[513]

Go West, Young Woman

On the frontier, the "weaker" sex was less of a threat to men, and women were more likely to be treated as partners, assisting the men in manual work on the farm or ranch as well as caring for the children and home. The restrictive rules of eastern society were bent if not abandoned. One reflection of the more progressive attitude is the fact that female suffrage was passed in the western states earlier than on the eastern seaboard. Thus it is unsurprising that the frontier West attracted professional women, including doctors. According to Linda Peavy and Ursula Smith in their book *Pioneer Women*, only four percent of the nation's adult women lived in the West, but a greater number of them were professional. In 1890 ten percent of American female doctors practiced in the West.[514]

Nevertheless, the treatment of women in the nineteenth and early twentieth centuries was far from equal, even in the West, and many women doctors had to struggle for acceptance in their communities. Their acceptance was hastened, however, by the urgent need for medical care on the frontier. The growing population and rough conditions of the plains and mountains meant that doctors, whether male or female, were in demand. Homesteaders suffered from conditions we no longer fear today, such as scurvy, measles, smallpox, diphtheria, whooping cough, scarlet fever, erysipelas, typhoid, cholera, and tuberculosis. The harsh climate, physical danger, and prevalence of disease on the frontier was especially hard on women and children. Women during this era had many pregnancies, and due to lack of prenatal and postnatal care, the mortality of mothers and infants was considerable.

The Mormon community in Utah was one of the first to embrace women as medical practitioners. At first, Mormon leader Brigham Young rejected sectarian medicine and encouraged ministration by the Mormon brethren. Young believed in Thomsonian medicine, which relied on steam-baths, enemas, cayenne pepper, and a variety of herbs. Thomsonian physicians, like most doctors of the day, were generally men. Then in 1868 Young did a complete about-face and encouraged Mormon women to become trained in "anatomy, surgery, chemistry, physiology, the preservation of health, the properties of medicinal plants, and midwifery."[515] In other words, to become doctors. We can only speculate about the reason for this change of heart. One of Young's wives, Zina, was a midwife and delivered all her husband's children as well as hundreds of other babies. Her work could have influenced his thinking.

Romania Bunnell Pratt, a Mormon wife and mother, heard her leader's call for women to enter medicine and became the first Utahan to go to medical school. She attended the Women's Medical College in Philadelphia and began her Utah practice in 1877. However, the first woman physician to practice in Utah was Dr. Ellen B. Ferguson.[516] In 1873 Young suggested that women's classes in physiology and obstetrics be offered in Salt Lake City and asked the bishops to "see that such women be supported."[517] Nine years later, the Women's Relief Society in Utah founded Deseret Hospital, directed by Dr. Ferguson. Here women learned nursing and obstetrics. Before the century was out, Utah had about twenty women doctors, giving the territory the highest percentage of female physicans anywhere.[518]

"Doctresses" of the West

Regardless of their profession or primary purpose in coming west, women were civilizers. Wherever women settled, home and hearth became the norm, and schools and churches pushed out "dens of iniquity." Men understood this, and most saw their lives improve with a more stable community. Women doctors had such an effect, if less obviously, on the profession of medicine as practiced on the frontier. Most female doctors demonstrated an interest in public health and the diseases of women and children, subjects that had been sorely neglected before they came.

One of the first female physicians in the West, known only as "Doctress Hoffman," came to Comstock, Nevada, in 1865. Her practice was restricted to women and children. Another early woman doctor was Susan E. Bruce, a pioneer in public health in Idaho. Born in Canada, Dr. Bruce graduated from the Homeopathic Medical School of Chicago in 1880. After moving west in 1905, she was appointed to the Idaho State Board of Health and later became the Public Health Officer for

Lewiston, Idaho. On several occasions during her career, she was able to isolate outbreaks of smallpox. Her department was described as "arduous and exacting."[519]

Most women doctors came with the homesteaders around the turn of the twentieth century. Some of those early women physicians were specialists. Among these in Montana were Dr. Dora E. Walker, the first radiologist in the state; Dr. Caroline McGill, Montana's first pathologist; Dr. Anna Adelaide Cook-Owens, an ophthalmologist; and Dr. Mary Babcock Atwater, an early proponent of public health who helped to develop Galen State Hospital for the treatment of tuberculosis.[520]

Montana's first woman doctor was Maria M. Dean. She was licensed to practice in 1889, the same year Montana became a state and the year the Medical Practices Act was passed by the Montana Legislature. Focusing on diseases of women and children, she was the first woman physician on the staff of St. Peter's Hospital in Helena and served as chairman of the city Board of Health. In addition to her busy practice, she was involved in community affairs and women's suffrage activities.[521]

Dean graduated from the University of Wisconsin Medical School in 1880, received further training in Boston, then went to Germany for even more training. In the late 1800s and early 1900s, Germany was considered the center of western medicine, and Americans who wished to study with the best teachers went there.[522] While Dr. Dean was there, the Berlin Opera House burned, and she was assigned to care for some of the most severely injured victims of the fire.

Her youngest sister and her husband having recently moved to Helena, Montana, Dean decided to practice there. Tragically Dr. Dean's career and life were cut short in 1919, when she died of cancer. In testimony to her national importance, after she became ill during a visit to Washington, D.C., President Woodrow Wilson allowed her to use his private railroad car for her trip home to Montana.[523]

The remarkable medical career of Mary Babcock Moore Atwater deserves a prominent place in Montana history. After graduating from Women's Hospital Medical College in Chicago in 1887, this intrepid young woman rode horses and buckboards to care for the sick and injured in the roaring mining town of Bannack, Montana. She made it her personal mission to achieve better medical care for Montana's growing number of tuberculars, and in 1900 Dr. Thomas D. Tuttle, Secretary of the State Board of Health, joined her in her efforts. Together they convinced the legislature to fund Galen Hospital, completed in 1913.

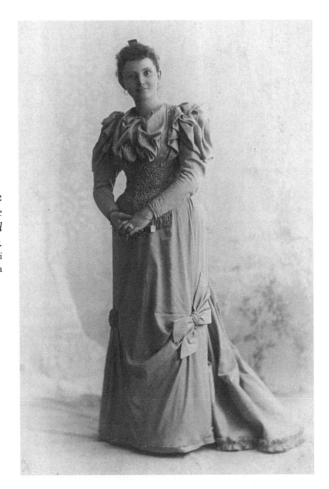

Mary Babcock Moore. She later married Ben Atwater.
—Courtesy Mari Graña

Even though the first patient admitted at Galen Hospital was a woman, it took three years for Dr. Atwater and her campaigners, along with the Montana Federation of Women's Clubs and the Montana Tuberculosis Association, to raise enough funds to provide separate accommodations for women.[524] Eight more years would pass before a building was provided for infected children. By this time, it was estimated that five hundred of Montana's children had the disease.[525] Soon after this, Dr. Atwater retired; she died in California in 1941, at age eighty-two.

Dr. Susan Anderson became an icon in the community of Fraser, Colorado. Shortly after graduating from the University of Michigan School of Medicine in 1897 and setting up practice in the flatlands of Colorado, she discovered she had tuberculosis. She promptly moved to the mountains, where the cold, clean air was thought to be beneficial.

She ended up in Fraser, about eighty miles west of Denver, high in the Rocky Mountains. Here at nearly ten thousand feet elevation, she began a practice that would last more than half a century. "Doc Susie," as she was affectionately known, lived a spartan life of service to the miners and families of this cold, forbidding place. She died at age ninety in 1960 in a Denver rest home. She is listed in the Colorado Women's Hall of Fame.[526]

Mary Canaga Rowland was another remarkable doctor, born in a Nebraska sod house in 1873. Her mother was a midwife, and early in her life Mary witnessed her mother deliver babies and peeked at her mother's books on obstetrics. At the age of eight, hidden in the attic of her home, she watched an autopsy being performed. These extraordinary experiences guided the young girl toward a career in medicine. She graduated from a women's medical college in Chicago in 1901 and later attended classes at Creighton University.

Dr. Susan (Susie) Anderson graduated from medical school in 1897. She practiced in Colorado, mostly in the mining community of Fraser. "Doc Susie" was an institution unto herself. —Courtesy Denver Public Library, Western History Collection

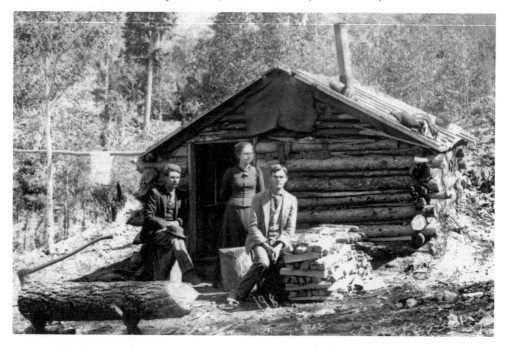

Mary married another doctor, J. Walter Rowland, and the couple practiced together for a short time until he was murdered. Left to carry on a busy practice with little experience, she rose to the occasion. By the time of the great flu epidemic in 1918, she was practicing at an Indian reservation in Salem, Oregon. She and her daughter were struck down by the virus, but both survived. In 1927 she went to study at the DeLee Lying-in Hospital in Chicago. She died in 1966, at age ninety-three.[527]

Dr. Caroline McGill was one of the most prominent people in Montana.[528] Montana State College president Dr. Roland R. Renne, presenting her an honorary degree of Doctor of Science in 1955, called her an "eminent Montana physician, diagnostician and pathologist, long-time student of Montana history and geography, and generous personal benefactor."[529] Years after her death, medical historian Dr. Pierce Mullen said, "Dr. McGill represents in her own persona the new practitioner … respected—indeed held in awe—by her patients, community, and peers."[530]

Born in 1879, McGill spent her early life on a tenant farm, but by seventeen she was teaching school. She earned a Ph.D. in anatomy in 1908 at the University of Missouri and spent a year in Europe as the first recipient of the Sarah Berliner Fellowship for Scientific Research for Women. She continued her medical training at Johns Hopkins medical school, graduating first in her class in 1914, then set up a practice in Butte, Montana. For the next forty-five years, Dr. McGill was a significant force in the progress of medical care in Butte and the state. Her work, a mixture of the didactic and the practical, gained her wide recognition among her colleagues. As laboratory doctor she helped educate her peers in miner's lung, tuberculosis, syphilis, streptococcal infections, and other diseases common at the time. She also treated patients, caring for the poorest of the poor, and she was known for her kindness.

In the boisterous mining camp of Butte, Dr. McGill served patients in saloons and prostitutes' "cribs," as well as in fine houses in the best districts. She was there to help in 1917 at the disastrous Speculator Mine fire, when 165 Butte miners died. A year later, as president of the Silver Bow Medical Society, she ushered the community through the great flu epidemic of 1918, a time fraught with death and politics.

In addition to her medical service, Dr. McGill was a local history enthusiast and collected historical artifacts. Her collection served as the basis for the McGill Museum at Montana State College in 1955, which later evolved into the Museum of the Rockies. She also donated part of her ranch on the Gallatin River for public use and to the U.S. Forest

Service for the betterment of the Gallatin elk herd. Her biographer, Margaret Woods of the Museum of the Rockies, said that McGill "had a true passion for the people and material culture of Montana. Her collecting accomplished two things: it provided a diversion from her strenuous practice and also preserved those objects that represented something of our Montana heritage."[531] Caroline McGill died in 1959, at the age of seventy-nine.

Preceding Dr. McGill as a woman physician in Butte was Dr. Olive Violet Brasier Cordua. She did not feel particularly welcome when she opened an office there in 1907. Although she had received special training in anesthesia, a skill that was greatly needed, Butte wasn't ready for a "lady doc." After a year of seeing few patients come through her office door, she applied for a job in the remote mining town of Elkhorn, using only her initials, O. V. Brasier, M.D., against the probability of sex discrimination. Upon meeting the mining superintendent, she convinced him she could do the job—later she said that she may have been the only applicant.[532]

For ten months, Dr. Brasier made her rounds in Elkhorn. Her small figure on horseback, with her black bag tied to the saddlehorn, became a common sight. She delivered babies, treated pneumonia and mining injuries, and, since there was no dentist, pulled teeth. When she returned to Butte, her training in anesthesia paid off. She won a contract at Murray Hospital for "a magnificent $1000 a year." She also accompanied the surgeon at the hospital on trips into the country, where the "kitchen served as an operating room."[533] She married Henry M. Cordua in 1913. After moving to California, in 1922 she became chairman of the first San Diego County Public Health Committee, a position she held for thirty-four years. She died in 1970 at age eighty-seven.

Another Montana woman doctor was Dr. Winifred Braine Reynolds. When Winifred's patriarchal father was reluctant to allow her to attend medical school, she convinced him she wanted medical training because she intended to be a missionary. As a strict Methodist, he could not reject this argument. She attended Dalhousie Medical School in Nova Scotia, married one of her classmates, William F. Reynolds, and moved to Montana. She and her new husband worked together as frontier doctors in the isolated mining community of Aldridge. When the Reynoldses lived there, Aldridge was a thriving town with over 280 miners and their families. It even had a hospital. Until 1908, "Mr. Doctor" and "Mrs. Doctor," as they were called, treated victims of dynamite explosions, crushed bones from falling timbers, and other traumas inherent in the ever-dangerous mining occupation. In 1908 William became ill, and the pair eventually moved to Stevensville in 1917. William died in 1936, but Winifred continued to practice until she died in 1941.[534]

The stories of the courageous, stalwart, and resourceful women physicians who helped turn the West from a frontier into a comfortable and healthy society are little known. As Dr. Mabel Tuchscherer wrote in *Petticoat and Stethoscope*, "Women physicians established a shining record in coping with the hardships . . . the difficulties of travel . . . the lack of hospitals and other facilities and the general lower standard of medical resources which made practice frustrating."[535]

Now at the beginning of the twenty-first century, women comprise approximately fifty percent of students admitted to medical school, and more than twenty percent of practicing physicians are women. In 1998 Dr. Nancy W. Dickey was named president of the AMA, the largest doctor's group in the United States.[536] It is more than coincidence that she is a westerner.

Part Two

Public Health and Health Education on the Frontier

ELEVEN

Early Western Hospitals

A quiet home with pleasant surroundings for invalids and those desiring Surgical Operations.

—From an advertisement for Dr. Henry Foster's Bozeman Sanitarium, 1896[537]

IT TOOK A LONG TIME for humankind to respect the value of the hospital. There were many reasons for this, not the least of which was a bad reputation. Hospitals evolved from pesthouses and almshouses, where the contagious or hopeless were brought to die out of sight of the public, and it was a slow process for hospitals to become accepted as places for ordinary folks to be treated for illness. The situation was not unique to the American frontier; it was worldwide.

For most of the nineteenth century, there was no clear understanding of hygiene and public health, and in general, hospitals were unhealthful places. Most patients, admitted for whatever reason, would have been better off at home. In the last two decades of the 1800s, however, germs, contagion, and sanitation were better understood, and hospitals gradually became safer, cleaner places for sick people. British surgeon Joseph Lister's discovery of antisepsis, a strategy that relied on a carbolic acid spray to prevent infection during surgery, revolutionized the field.[538]

In addition to this medical advance, another development credited with spurring the evolution of the hospital was the burgeoning of the nursing profession. The seeds of this noble calling were planted during the Civil War, where the cleanly habits and compassionate support of field nurses had a significant, if undocumented, impact on wounded soldiers' recovery. Wartime nurses were the forerunners of the professional hospital nurse. Without the pragmatic efforts of these dedicated women, the quality of hospital care would not have progressed as it did. (For more on the contributions of nurses, see chapter 12.)

From about 1870 to 1910, the hospital evolved from a repository of the dead and dying to an establishment vital to public health care

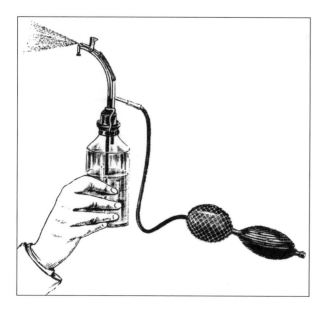

Surgery was revolutionized with Joseph Lister's discovery in 1867 that carbolic acid spray could prevent infection during procedures. The disinfectant was sprayed on the patient and the surgeon's hands with an apparatus such as this. —Courtesy National Library of Medicine, History of Medicine Division

and eventually the center stage for medical education and innovation. Progress in the fields of anesthesia, antisepsis, and asepsis led to surgical techniques that were best performed in a hospital setting. Hospitals also began to provide laboratory and X-ray facilities, which greatly enhanced practitioners' diagnostic capabilities. In time many communities organized to build hospitals, and physicians practicing in remote locations eventually saw these places, no matter how humble, as the best venues for their knowledge and skill. As the tide of knowledge surged, the hospital became a center for procedures such as blood transfusion, fluid replacement, immunizations, and other cutting-edge technology. Today's magnificent institutions are the direct result of these modest beginnings.

Military Hospitals

Hospitals at military posts were the first medical institutions on the western frontier. During the gold rush and subsequent western settlement, the United States Army established forts to protect the emigrants. Nearly all of these posts had a hospital of some sort. These facilities were just as important to the opening of the West as the soldiers and artillery. They provided an oasis of civilization for weary pilgrims and medical care for the sick and injured among them.

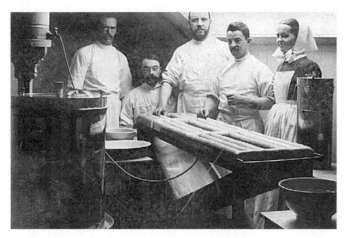

Doctors and nurse in the operating room of a St. Paul, Minnesota, hospital, circa 1890 —Courtesy Minnesota Historical Society

The size and quality of army hospitals varied. Some were simply converted barracks, while others were specially constructed with kitchens, laundries, and bathing facilities. Fort Yuma, one of the earliest military posts, was established in 1849 near the confluence of the Gila and Colorado Rivers in Arizona. It was a precarious, poorly supplied fort subject to frequent raids by Indian warriors, Mexican soldiers, and American desperadoes. The hospital, described as "well adapted," consisted of two tents covered with brush and a vegetable garden tended by the doctor.[539]

As hastily built outposts became permanent establishments, the medical facilities tended to improve. For the first year at Fort Halleck, near Elko, Nevada, the hospital consisted of a single tent, but the next year, 1868, an adobe structure measuring forty-by-thirty feet was completed. The same year at Fort Harney, in southeastern Oregon, a hospital of logs and mud was constructed. Depending on their location, some military hospitals were busy and others were not; as times changed, some posts were abandoned and new ones were built.[540]

In 1875 the Surgeon General's Office issued *A Report on the Hygiene of the United States Army*, which included descriptions of military posts. Included in the report was Fort Ellis, three miles east of Bozeman, Montana. The account gives insight into the kinds of problems military hospitals of that period faced. Over a four-year period (1870-74), the

Fort Ellis Hospital treated 134 fevers, 71 cases of rheumatism, 39 cases of syphilis, 101 cases of catarrh and bronchitis, 71 cases of dysentery, and 28 cases of gonorrhea. There were 400 accidents with only 1 death. Detailed evaluation of these statistics is difficult, however, due to differences between period and modern terminology. In addition, some of the most common complaints doctors treated at Fort Ellis were lumped under "other local diseases."[541]

The first Fort Ellis Hospital, established in 1867, consisted of three small rooms. The post surgeon, Dr. Clarence Ewan, complained that this thirty-by-forty-foot space was inadequate. It was shabbily built, insufficiently heated, poorly lit, and underventilated. It had no laundry or bathing facilities, and the latrine was too far away. The bedding consisted of bags of straw for mattresses covered with blankets and buffalo robes. "Earth boxes" were used in severe weather and for immobile patients. Apparently Dr. Ewan convinced the army brass of the fort's inadequacies because, in 1871, a larger and better building was erected. The new two-story structure accommodated twelve patients, staff, and storage. Water from the East Gallatin River was put in barrels and delivered each morning. By all reports, the food supply was good, with fresh vegetables, meat, and fish from the river.[542]

Mining-Town Hospitals

In May 1863 gold was discovered in Alder Gulch, Montana, and more mineral discoveries soon followed. Scattered throughout the territory, camps with descriptive names like Hog'em, Beat'em, and Cheat'em came and went with the metal. As the golden prize they sought played out in one place, the miners moved on. With this boom-and-bust attitude, community developments such as schools, hospitals, water systems, and sewage disposal didn't seem important. As populations grew and stabilized, hospitals became an important mark of a community's progress. In the early days, however, public medical facilities were created only in the face of urgent need.

One gold find, labeled Last Chance Gulch, blossomed into the city of Helena, Montana. Helena was an unruly place. "Like other mining camps," says Paula Petrik in *No Step Backward*, "Helena was founded on the principle of impermanence; its inhabitants never intended it to be a permanent settlement."[543] Nevertheless, after the severe winter of 1865–66, public-spirited citizens of Helena donated money for a hospital. The Miners' Hospital was probably the first such institution in Montana.

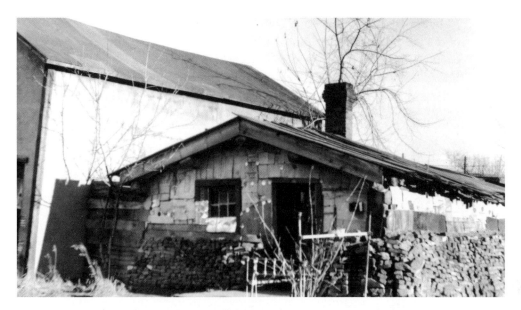

Miners' Hospital in Last Chance Gulch (Helena), Montana, 1928. This hospital, probably the first one in Montana, opened in 1866. —Courtesy Montana Historical Society, Helena

The hospital was created to take care of an unusually high number of miners suffering from frostbite and starvation. The desperate situation was brought about after John McClellan, an exceptionally lucky prospector, left Helena for the Sun River Country. Hundreds of men followed him, expecting "Lucky John" to find another mother lode. The miners, hurried and ill-prepared for the trip, never caught up with McClellan and floundered back to Helena through deepening snowdrifts. The influx of frostbitten, sick, and starving miners created a crisis.

The local newspaper editor urged the four hundred residents of Helena "to contribute fifty cents or one dollar each per week to support of the valuable project. I will head the list with a subscription of one hundred dollars, and will double it if necessary."[544] The original hospital was little more than a deserted cabin with a roof, but in a few years the community raised enough money to provide accommodations for 163 county patients, and the old building was eventually replaced by a better structure.[545]

In Nevada, it took epidemics of smallpox to convince most Nevadans of the need for medical facilities. In Watson's Mill, an 1862-64 smallpox epidemic prompted local leaders to levy a twenty-cent tax on each one hundred dollars of property value to build and run a hospital. Similarly in Elko, after a smallpox outbreak a few years later, the town constructed a hospital for the sick and injured and a "pest" hospital at the outskirts of town to isolate infectious patients.

These hospitals were sorely needed. In addition to the many diseases that affected western communities, mining accidents were commonplace. In Comstock, Nevada, at least one person a week died in the mines, and many more were injured by falling rock, explosions, and scaldings. Eventually the miners formed a Miner's League to improve working conditions. The organization also collected money from each miner for the care of their injured and sick. Ten years later, some people who had "made it big" from mining donated funds for a three-story, seventy-four-bed hospital, an institution that also provided room for the insane in the basement. The Virginia City facility attracted nurses from Maryland's Daughters of Charity as well as some better-trained physicians.[546]

The mining town of McCarthyville, Montana, had a hospital in 1890. The building was a low, log structure with no floor, and the only window was a hole covered with a canvas flap. Many men developed pneumonia that winter, and the hospital was the busiest place in town. Unfortunately most patients who went to the hospital came out dead. According to one observer, "It got so that every morning just at daylight a big Swede that was a kind of nurse ... would come outside with a hand-sled. He'd have a body wrapped in a two-dollar blanket.... Then he'd start off up the creek and perform the obsequies by digging a hole in the snow and rollin the corpse off the sled."

The citizens of McCarthyville were soon fed up with the failure rate of the hospital's "doctor," who had come from Great Falls, "where it was understood he had built up a fine reputation as a veterinarian." A committee of citizens went to the hospital and knocked on the door. "The Swede opened it part way and then when he saw who it was he tried to shut it again, but Hardy [one of the men] reached over and tapped him with the butt of a gun. He dropped like a leaf.... Then the men cast a glance about for the doctor, just in time to see his heels following him through the window.... McCarthyville never saw him again."[547] According to the story, another doctor came, and the death rate declined.

Catholic and Philanthropic Hospitals

Many early medical institutions in the West were established by Catholic nuns. In 1864 the Sisters of Charity of Providence from Montreal, Quebec, came to St. Ignatius, Montana, and set up a an "infirmary," where they cared for Indians and white people alike. There were no physicians in the area, but in a simple room the dedicated nuns diagnosed illnesses, prescribed treatments, set broken limbs, and performed some surgery. In the strict sense, the sisters practiced medicine, and their work filled a void of medical care in western Montana. Raising donations during excursions to more populated and prosperous areas of Montana, by 1914 the nuns had acquired enough money to build their first hospital, the Holy Family Hospital. In time, with the support of Father Laurence B. Palladino, the same order of sisters established other institutions in Missoula, Fort Benton, and Great Falls.[548]

Around the time the St. Ignatius infirmary operated, Father Pierre-Jean DeSmet requested nurses from the Sisters of Charity of Leavenworth, Kansas, to serve in Helena, Montana. Five sisters and a lay woman from Leavenworth responded to the call, and by 1870 they had formed St. John's Medical Center in Helena. By the end of the century, the women of this order had established both schools and hospitals in many Montana communities, including Billings, Butte, Virginia City, Anaconda, and Deer Lodge.[549]

In Billings, after St. Vincent Hospital was built in 1898, the town's Protestants decided they wanted their own place. Due to World War I and a prolonged drought in the area, it was 1922 before enough money was raised. The Billings Clinic, an independent organization founded by Drs. H. H. Bridenbaugh and A. J. Movius, formed the cornerstone for the Protestant hospital, Billings Deaconess.[550]

The town of Havre, Montana, spawned by the Great Northern Railroad and homesteaders lured by the propaganda of railroad tycoon Jim Hill, had two doctors, but no hospital. Neither the doctors nor the citizens saw any need for a hospital until an incident in 1909, when a young man died of appendicitis en route to Great Falls for treatment. This and similar stories paved the way for four Sisters of Saint Francis from New York to open Sacred Heart Hospital in 1911.

Two years later, Sacred Heart suffered a disastrous fire. Sister M. Mericunda, who was among the founders of the hospital, went into the burning building to make sure that no patients had been left behind.

Although she had been assured that no one was in there, she found a man with a cast who could not walk, a pneumonia patient too ill to get out of bed, and a third invalid. The brave nun called through the smoke for help, and as she and the others escaped with the last patient, the staircase and part of the flooring caved in. Sister Mericunda continued nursing at Sacred Heart Hospital for fifty-three years.

After the 1913 fire, Sacred Heart was rebuilt just in time to treat patients during a typhoid epidemic in 1916 and during the terrible scourge of influenza a couple of years later. By 1925 Havre had a Methodist hospital, Kennedy Deaconess, bringing additional medical support to the community. Both hospitals had schools of nursing. In 1975 the two pioneer hospitals merged to form the Northern Montana Hospital.[551]

Private Hospitals

In addition to Catholic, Protestant, and other philanthropic hospitals were government institutions such as military veterans hospitals, state hospitals, and Bureau of Indian Affairs and Indian Health Service facilities on the reservations. Big industries, especially the railroad companies, also built and operated hospitals in some communities. Moreover, individual doctors and medical groups founded private hospitals and health centers throughout the West.

Some medical establishments got their start in strange ways. Dr. Henry Foster of Bozeman advertised his hospital, the Bozeman Sanitarium, as "a quiet home with pleasant surroundings for invalids and those desiring Surgical Operations." It was the beginning of what would later become Bozeman Deaconess Hospital. Dr. Foster, who came to Bozeman in 1882, built the sanitarium in 1896.[552] According to Montana historian Dr. Merrill Burlingame, Dr. Foster acquired $25,000, with which he funded the hospital, in a settlement against Nelson Story, the legendary, irascible cattleman who brought the first cattle to Montana from Texas.

Story was an unpopular figure in Bozeman after he took advantage of the 1893 panic to close the bank, threatening the holdings of the depositors. Dr. Foster was vocal in his criticism of Story and even maintained that the man should be hanged. One Sunday morning in downtown Bozeman, Nelson encountered Dr. Foster, and the two men had words. The argument escalated, and Story began beating Dr. Foster with his hickory cane. The bank president happened to see the fight and pulled

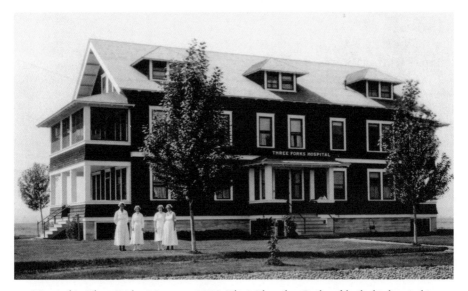

Hospital in Three Forks, Montana, 1928. The Milwaukee Railroad built this hospital in 1915. For several years, it had a training school for nurses. Many early hospitals in the West were built by the railroad companies. —Courtesy Montana Historical Society, Helena

the doctor out of harm's way. After Foster threatened to sue, he was awarded a $25,000 settlement. The sanitarium was subsequently constructed at a cost of $20,000.[553]

Early hospitals accommodated all sorts of illnesses and gave charity and comfort to the homeless, orphans, the insane, invalids, and the aged. In time, separate institutions were created for specific problems. Among these were tuberculosis sanatoriums, mental asylums, homes for the elderly, orphanages, and children's hospitals. The Children's Hospital of Denver was an outstanding example of the last category. Its first annual report in 1910 said, "Operations of many kinds have been successfully performed, and scores of sufferers sent away cured or greatly relieved."[554] Originally housed in a converted residence, Children's Hospital, through the dedicated work of nurses, doctors, and administrators, became one of the foremost research centers in the country. Developed during a golden era of medical progress, the hospital was one of the first to use direct blood transfusion in treatment, to utilize the electrocardiograph, and to adapt X-ray methods for the diagnosis of pediatric diseases.[555] Over the years, many doctors and nurses would train here for a lifetime of caring for sick children.

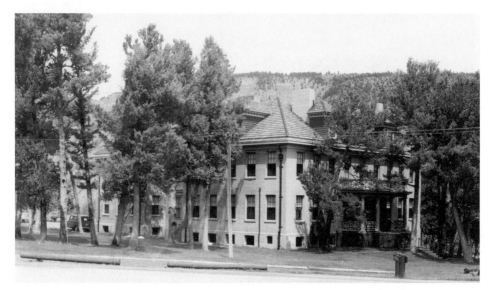

The Yellowstone Park Hospital at Mammoth Hot Springs, circa 1950
—Courtesy Dr. Lindsey Baskett, Livingston, Montana

Hospital in the Wilderness

Even today, the wilderness we call Yellowstone National Park still embodies the frontier. Thousands of tourists come here every year to experience the wild, sometimes for the first time in their lives. Inevitably, some of them encounter illness or injury during their stay. The park has provided medical services for visitors and area residents since the late nineteenth century.

An army hospital was built near Mammoth Hot Springs in 1886, primarily to serve the enlisted personnel of Camp Sheridan. A new hospital was built in 1894 at Fort Yellowstone, which was then replaced by an improved facility near today's Mammoth Chapel in 1911. The new Yellowstone Park Hospital, also known as Mammoth Hospital, served park visitors and local residents until the early 1960s. The new facilities included an early X-ray machine, a rudimentary laboratory, and a large operating room on the second floor. Dozens of lightbulbs in the concave ceiling lit up the room brilliantly during operations, but the hospital had no elevator—patients were carried on a litter up the long stairway to the OR. In 1924 doctors from Livingston, Montana, who had been working at the park hospital took over its management from the army.

The physicians who practiced in the park were kept busy treating a large variety of conditions, especially during the summer. Not only did they see the usual problems, from minor diarrheas to myocardial infarctions, but many injuries were unique to the wilderness. Unwary visitors traveling through the park were gored by buffalo, stomped by moose, and mauled by bears. They were injured in rock-climbing falls, burnt in boiling hot springs, bashed on the rocks of raging streams, or hit by falling trees during storms.

Injuries from bear attacks required special handling. The mostly black bears that wandered throughout the park had numerous contacts with unprepared humans. In addition to potential infection from a bear bite, the animal's powerful jaws can crush the victim's body part and devitalize the muscle and other soft tissue underneath. Dr. Alfred M. Lueck, a

The second floor of the Yellowstone Park Hospital had a large, brightly lit operating room. —Courtesy Dr. Lindsey Baskett, Livingston, Montana

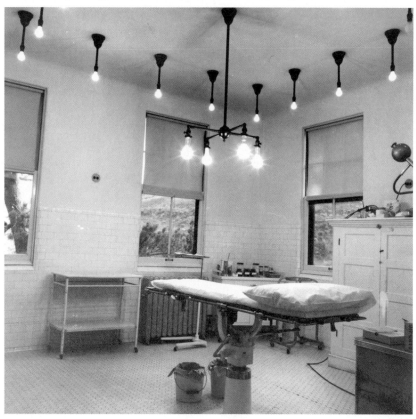

longtime surgeon in Livingston, treated many of these potentially fatal injuries. He discovered that the wound had to be opened up completely and all damaged tissue debrided. This procedure was necessary to prevent serious infection in tissue that could act as culture media for bacteria, especially such pathogens as gas gangrene. In the early 1960s, Lueck reported on a large number of cases he sucessfully managed. The only one that became infected was a patient who, refusing treatment at the old-fashioned park hospital, left for the Mayo Clinic. The delay in proper treatment was fatal.[556]

Another common condition that park physicians treated was acute pulmonary edema from the high altitude. A compromised heart and lung couldn't handle the stress of the diminished oxygen supply above eight or nine thousand feet. Usually this frightening condition developed in older park visitors with a previous history of heart and/or lung disease. Sometimes patients with borderline cardiac function were actually sent to the park for a "rest" by physicians who didn't appreciate the deleterious effect high altitude had on an already compromised cardiovascular system. The treatment was simple: patients were instructed to get in their cars and drive to a lower altitude immediately. Though the method virtually always worked, in today's litigious environment, this type of pragmatic medical advice might backfire.

In the early days, only a few health-care professionals stayed in the park during the off-season, left to face any problems on their own. When nurse practitioner Donna Mae Snodgrass and her husband worked for Yellowstone National Park in the 1960s, she was often the only source of medical care for area residents and occasional tourists during the long, frigid, snow-packed winter. Sometimes she had to hike or ride horseback into the backcountry to assist someone. During medical emergencies her husband drove the ambulance, their children huddled by his side, as Donna Mae attended the patient in the backseat for seventy miles to the Livingston Hospital. Donna Mae was not only the "town nurse" for Gardiner, Montana, but she also helped organize an ambulance service, a well-child clinic, screening clinics for glaucoma and diabetes, and even Red Cross blood drives. Later, Donna Mae's outstanding work as a member of the Montana Nurses Association resulted in a governor's appointment to the organization's board of directors.[557]

Lake Hospital replaced Mammoth Hospital for full-range medical services in 1963, and in 1980 West Park Hospital in Cody, Wyoming, took over the medical concession. Mammoth still operates a year-round outpatient clinic in the park, and Lake Hospital still offers full hospital services seasonally.

From Insane Asylum to Psychiatric Hospital

Much of the history of mental illness and its treatment is not pleasant to recall. Ancient Greece was among the few societies that saw mental illness as a disease and not demonic possession. It was several hundred years before this view was accepted by most cultures. In the meantime, these unfortunate folks were considered witches and were ostracized, beaten, shackled, imprisoned, tortured, and even put to death. Even in the more enlightened eras of the eighteenth and nineteenth centuries, although some hospitals did admit them, many mentally ill people were still being locked in jails, isolated at home or in almshouses, or left to wander without supervision. The problem was largely a question of public perception and a lack of understanding on the part of the medical profession. Until modern times, doctors wanted little to do with the problems of the mentally ill, so it was left to social reformers to help them.

Dorothea Dix (1802-87) was one who met the challenge head-on. This stouthearted lady had witnessed mentally ill men and women incarcerated with criminals; left naked without heat, light, or bathrooms; and sometimes beaten. She dedicated herself to stopping this treatment. In forty years of effort, she helped establish thirty-two state hospitals and even convinced Pope Pius IX to speak out.[558] By 1880 mental institutions, both government and private, were much improved and hospitalization of the mentally ill had garnered wide public support.

At first, therapies at state mental institutions emphasized kindness and restraint, but these principles eventually broke down. Why? Due to their low cost, the state-supported institutions were soon overwhelmed with patients whom families and communities found difficult to care for, including the chronically ill, the senile, and the mentally retarded. Places built with facilities for a few hundred were forced to accommodate several thousand. Naturally, the quality of care suffered greatly.

Nevada's territorial legislature showed remarkable progressiveness in 1867 when it allocated ten thousand dollars for care of the insane. But by 1871 that amount was found inadequate to the demand. It was less expensive to send Nevada's mentally ill to the California State Hospital in Stockton, at a cost of nine dollars per week per patient. This solution served as an adequate stopgap until Nevada built its own mental hospital near Reno in 1881.

In its third year, the Nevada Hospital for the Indigent Insane had 140 patients. The conditions diagnosed were recorded as: "masturbation (20 percent of the men), onanism, heredity, typhoid, religion, scarlet fever, epilepsy, syphilis, fright, intemperance, jealousy, alcoholism, ardent spirits, weak mind, disappointment, loss of money, and solitary life."[559] Although there is a considerable degree of difference between the terminology of the past and that of the present, we do know that advanced syphilis was among the leading causes of insanity in those days. One might also conclude from the conditions listed that many patients were severely depressed. Many people with conditions no longer considered psychiatric illness, such as epilepsy and Alzheimer's disease, were placed in mental hospitals back then. The developmentally disabled were commonly committed to insane asylums under vague diagnoses such as imbecility, idiocy, and constitutional inferiority. The term "heredity" included conditions designated as adolescence, ill health, chorea, and menopause.

Until near the turn of the twentieth century, mental hospitals followed the peculiar custom of exhibiting patients to the public. This form of "entertainment" began in 1770 at St. Mary of Bethlehem Hospital in London, where visitors paid a fee to "laugh at the lunatics." Gradually, as understanding grew, this practice was stopped. In 1895 the Nevada Hospital for the Indigent Insane changed its name to Nevada Hospital for Mental Diseases, and the superintendent prohibited "placing the inmates on exhibition for the amusement of and to gratify the morbid curiosity of visitors."[560]

The mental hospital at Warm Springs in Deer Lodge, Montana Territory, evolved from the well-known spa there. The alleged healing powers of natural hot mineral springs made them a popular treatment for alcoholism and other addictions, and by the late 1800s, spas were recommended as a therapy for many kinds of mental illness. For instance, hot-spring baths were considered effective in calming some psychotic patients. In 1877 two Deer Lodge physicians, Armistead H. Mitchell and Charles Mussigbrod, purchased the Warm Springs Hotel to use as an asylum.

Montana was apace with, perhaps even ahead of, many more-populated parts of the country in the field of mental illness care. By all reports, the new Warm Springs institution met the governor's mandate "that the treatment be of the same character that patients now receive in the best regulated asylums in the States." Each inmate was clothed, housed, fed, and treated for eight dollars per week. Patient care was reported to be "exemplary." Visitors reported that the patients looked "happy and contented."[561]

In 1887 Dr. William L. Steele, Territorial Inspecting Physician, reported to the governor that the 132 patients at the hospital were receiving excellent care. "The diet, medical and surgical treatment and attention, and all other matters pertaining to the welfare of the patients, are beyond criticism." Dr. Steele wrote that the surroundings were "homelike" and that "kindly treatment, constant care and attention" was paid to these "unfortunate" persons.[562]

In 1912 the state of Montana bought the Warm Springs facility from the estate of Drs. Mitchell and Mussigbrod and renamed it the Montana State Hospital for the Insane (later it was called the Warm Springs State Hospital for Mental Diseases, now Montana State Hospital). At the time of purchase, there were already 854 patients. Some were longtime residents.[563] Because of the stigma of mental illness and because recovery was rare, many patients stayed their whole lives. Thus more residents were admitted than discharged every year, and the number grew.

In 1942 the state board of health's biennial report stated that the Warm Springs hospital had "a greater population than all the other State's charitable and penal institutions combined."[564] "It must be borne in mind," the report noted, "that the Montana State Hospital for the Insane receives all public charges afflicted with different mental ailments, as the insane, the aberrated epileptics, imbeciles, idiots, morons, criminal insane, and alcoholic and narcotic addicts."[565] A special committee report the same year found that, among other things, the patients were housed in wooden "fire traps" and were so crowded that one dormitory had fifty-eight women patients with only one "old fashioned" bathtub. The committee was alarmed that the state budgeted only 6.3 cents for each meal.[566]

Overcrowding in mental hospitals was partly due to this tendency to use asylums as catchalls for chronic and difficult patients. People with various forms of senility, depression, a history of substance abuse, or any illness with apparent neurological symptoms were included, as were those with developmental disabilities. Many people suffering from convulsive disorders or any kind of epilepsy were institutionalized. In 1919 Luminal (phenobarbital) was found to prevent convulsions in some epileptics, a major advancement in treatment.[567]

About twenty percent of the admissions to Montana State Hospital in 1919-20 had syphilis, a figure on a par with mental institutions in other parts of the country, and one of the leading causes of death at the hospital was classified as paresis, or advanced syphilis.[568] The treatment for external syphilitic lesions was mercury rubs, and all syphilis patients were given arsenic and mercury salicylate by "deep muscular injections."[569] Until the discovery of penicillin, these were the only therapies available.

It was always difficult to keep physicians at the Montana State Hospital and similar institutions because the responsibility was great, the pay was poor, and the facilities were inadequate. As late as the 1960s, Montana State Hospital's wards were so crowded that shower stalls were used as patient rooms, and sometimes there were no licensed physicians on the staff.

One may logically ask, why aren't mental institutions still overcrowded and understaffed today? Mental illness is just as prevalent now, but modern diagnosis and therapy means fewer people are inappropriately hospitalized. People with conditions such as stroke, congenital disabilities, and convulsive disorders are no longer classified as mentally ill and receive treatment from more suitable specialists. Among patients with true psychiatric problems, drug therapy and counseling allow a large percentage of them, even psychotics, to be treated as outpatients. No less significant is the fact that, thanks to antibiotics, syphilis is no longer allowed to advance to the stage of paresis, whose victims once clogged mental wards.[570]

"Taking the waters": Spas

Since ancient times, natural mineral springs have been used for therapy, and spas predated hospitals as health centers. In many places in the United States, hospitals and other healing institutions evolved from these spas. This makes sense—hydrotherapy has legitimate salutary benefits. Recent research on water immersion by Dr. Murray Epstein and others demonstrated many positive physiologic changes in patients and concluded that bathing at spas had "true medicinal value."[571] While hot mineral baths are not in most instances curative, they do have an established beneficial effect on problems like high blood pressure, renal disease, gout, and arthritis.[572]

People have had faith in the healing properties of hot water for centuries. Hydrotherapy was first used by the Chinese around A.D. 145–208.[573] Up to the early twentieth century in Europe and the eastern

United States, many spas gained renown as resorts and health centers. Out west, however, although the Rocky Mountains have numerous hot springs, entrepreneurial efforts to develop them as travel destinations largely flopped. Such places were considered an extravagance by most locals, and their remote locations made them undesirable to easterners.

Although western hot springs had been used for both recreation and recuperation up to the mid-1800s—first by the Indians, then by white explorers, trappers, gold miners, and early settlers—when the homesteaders took over and natural resources became commercial property, many of these springs were bought up, built up, and eventually abandoned. Most frontier residents were simply too busy, too isolated, and too poor to bask in hot mineral water. Those who could afford it went east to the more celebrated watering holes that catered to the affluent.

Several hot springs in the West were developed by doctors as serious treatment facilities rather than tourist resorts. Most made little money, but some survived, and a few eventually became hospitals. In Montana one of the early entrepreneurs in hydrotherapy was Dr. Andrew Jackson Hunter. In 1864, while traveling west with his family by ox train, Dr. Hunter discovered and claimed Hunter's Hot Springs, on the Yellowstone River about fifty-five miles east of Bozeman Pass. After working at the famous Arkansas Hot Springs, Dr. Hunter became convinced that hot-water therapy was revolutionary, and he believed the springs would be a good investment, even though they were in Indian country.

To keep peace with the Crow tribe until they were moved to a reservation in 1875, Hunter paid the Indians with "bolts of calico, sheeting and ticking, piles of tobacco . . . sugar, coffee, kegs of powder."[574] A reporter described the scene at one of these exchanges: "The beating of Indian drums, singing of the braves and squaws and the barking of dogs . . . form a combination which if praised for its volume could not be termed a sweet concord of harmony."[575]

Dr. Hunter's facility began with a log cabin, but he later constructed a hotel and bathhouses for patients. In this primitive and remote location, a few whites came to relax and bathe away their infirmities among the "savages." Claiming that his water, taken internally or bathed in, "cured or benefitted" rheumatism, gout, paralysis, syphilis, colic, bunions and corns, poor complexions, and "womb troubles," Hunter struggled for twenty years to tempt travelers and patients to his facility.[576] In 1885 he sold the springs and retired to Bozeman. The new owners built a new hotel and made other improvements, but the resort remained a financial

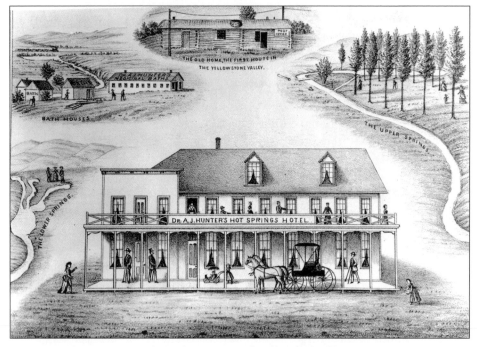

Hunter's Hot Springs. The Rocky Mountains have hundreds of hot springs. Many were developed as resorts or medical centers. —Courtesy Montana Historical Society, Helena

struggle and changed hands several times. The enterprise was abandoned in 1921, and the hotel burned down eleven years later.

In 1877 Dr. William Parberry, whose Montana career paralleled Dr. Hunter's, purchased Brewer's Hot Springs in the Smith River Valley and renamed it White Sulphur Springs. The town of the same name developed around the waters. Dr. Parberry believed that the sulfur water in his springs was particularly beneficial for rheumatism, dyspepsia, skin diseases, and "those afflicted with the harassing cares of business."[577] He didn't mention it by name, but the effects of overindulgence in alcohol, an endemic problem, was another condition thought eased by a soak in the springs. Dr. Parberry also recommended the water as a good sheep dip. Furthermore, some of the guests at White Sulphur Springs claimed that with a little salt and pepper the water made a "first class" chicken soup.[578] White Sulphur Springs never reached the dreams of those who promoted it. Dr. Parberry sold his interest in 1883, and over the years the spa's success has waxed and waned. Today the springs attract mostly local bathers.

One specialized use of hot mineral springs was as therapy for alcoholism and other addictions. This idea was generally supported by the medical profession in the nineteenth century, and the waters were used to treat certain mental illnesses as well. The mental hospital in Warm Springs, Montana, discussed previously, was built around the springs. Another Montana spa, Boulder Hot Springs, near Helena, was developed as a treatment center in 1893 by the Keeley Institute, a national franchise for the treatment of drug and alcohol addiction.

Since about 1880, Dr. Leslie E. Keeley of Illinois had been experimenting with a treatment for addiction that included injectable bichloride of gold. He claimed great success in curing alcohol, opium, morphine, cocaine, and tobacco habits. Neurasthenia and nervous exhaustion were reportedly improved as well. In spite of the fact that the American Medical Association labeled Dr. Keeley's methods quackery, Keeley Institute clinics spread all over the country.[579] By 1904 the facility in Montana had folded, but others persevered for several more decades.

Another resort-turned-hospital was Chico Hot Springs, on the Yellowstone River south of Livingston. Chico was a popular oasis for local people and early visitors to Yellowstone National Park. In 1912 a young surgeon, Dr. G. A. Townsend, opened a hospital at Chico. Touted as "one of the finest hospitals in the west with the best equipped offices in the entire state of Montana," the Chico Institute attracted patients from around the state. The facility boasted twenty-five beds, a round-the-clock staff of eight nurses, and a full laboratory.[580]

Dr. Townsend garnered an excellent reputation as a physician. He journeyed into the wilderness of Yellowstone Park and other remote places to attend patients. In addition to caring for the routine injuries of local ranchers and hunters, the Chico Institute was equipped to treat serious medical conditions and perform major surgical procedures such as appendectomies and cholecystectomies.[581] Dr. Townsend left Chico in 1949 but continued to practice in Livingston until he retired in 1966, shortly before he died. After Townsend's departure, Chico Hot Springs no longer functioned as a medical facility, but it is still a popular resort and dude ranch.

Through the early twentieth century, "taking the waters" was a popular treatment for sore muscles and joints from arthritis and injuries. Self-prescribed hydropathic "cures" were also sought for a myriad of illnesses, and spa owners made great claims about the healing effects of their water.

While hot springs produced no miraculous cures, many people found symptomatic relief in the baths. As medical science progressed, interest in hydrotherapy diminished. After the turn of the century, the popularity of hot-spring resorts steadily declined. Crumbling ruins and deteriorating hotels may still be seen at some spring sites, testifying to their transitory fame. Nevertheless, spas are still of great value in physical therapy.

Medical Innovators in the Middle of Nowhere

If there is any doubt about the challenges of rural medicine, one needs only read Dr. Ron Losee's autobiography, entitled simply *Doc*. The book, packed with anecdotes of his frontier practice in Ennis, Montana, in the mid-twentieth century, is sometimes sad, often humorous, and totally honest. It should be required reading for every young medical student. While carrying the load of a general practice in this small town on the Madison River, Losee became a specialist in orthopedics. He would practice for a while, and when he had enough money, he arranged for other doctors to work for him while he continued his training. After several years, he qualified as an orthopedic surgeon. He did not stay in a population center; instead, he returned to his home and the little hospital in Ennis. According to Losee, the rule of country doctoring was "Anybody, anything, any place, any time, anywhere, anyhow, no matter what, do it. It's your duty!"[582]

Losee did anatomical research at Montana State University, and, capitalizing on his own powerful ability to observe, he developed a unique procedure for treating a kind of knee injury. His innovative surgical technique gained him national fame, especially of interest to those concerned with athletic injuries. He was invited to demonstrate his operation, the Losee procedure, live in surgical amphitheaters for other specialists and medical students, and to speak at orthopedic and coaches' conventions. Taking a cue from the well-known orthopedists who began their talks with a photograph of their hospital, such as the Mayo Clinic, Johns Hopkins, Yale, or some other impressive place, Dr. Losee opened his presentations with a photograph of the Ennis Hospital, a small, one-story frame building that resembled a house. Parked in front of the modest building was a pickup truck with a rifle in the cab and a few bales of hay and a stock dog in the bed.

On one occasion, Dr. Losee spoke to the Gallatin Valley Medical Society in Bozeman, Montana. The physicians who were assembled at the Baxter Hotel were stunned when he presented not his surgical victories, but his surgical defeats. The cases he discussed were not mistakes, however. They were children from the Montana State School and Hospital whose reconstructive procedures had not obtained a result that satisfied Ron Losee. It is this kind of self-scrutiny and intellectual honesty that shines brightly through the years.

Ron Losee's talent and refusal to leave his small town benefited a great number of patients. Among the most helped were the children at the Montana State (Boulder River) School and Hospital in Boulder, Montana. From 1959 until 1975, Losee made the ninety-mile trip from Ennis to Boulder every Wednesday, "Losee's day off." There he assisted Dr. Phil Pallister, the medical director of the institution, in surgically correcting the severe congenital deformities of their patients. Losee's and Pallister's successes were numbered by the score. Most of the patients could not walk at all, and the deformities of some prevented them from even lying flat in bed or being fitted with diapers. The surgeries corrected

Dr. Ron Losee performing orthopedic surgery at Boulder River School and Hospital, 1965 —Courtesy Dr. Ron Losee

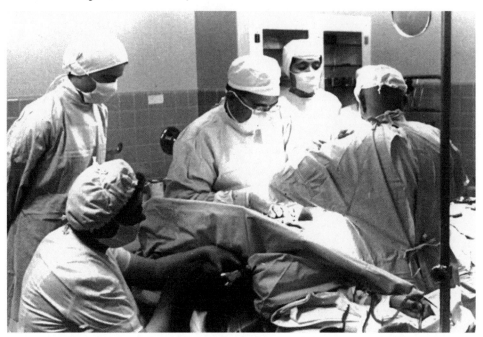

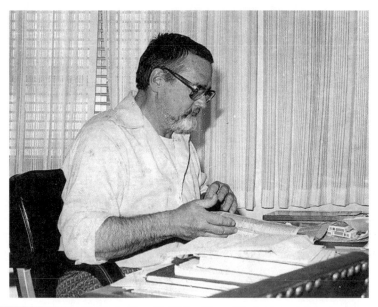

Dr. Phillip Pallister, 1970s —Courtesy Dr. Phillip Pallister

many of these problems in such a way that the patients' comfort was significantly enhanced. In some cases, patients could even achieve a nearly normal life. Harry L. Helton Jr., who worked at the Children's Center in Twin Bridges, Montana, remembered a teenage girl with leg paralysis and contractions from poliomyelitis.[583] She was taken to the Boulder hospital for orthopedic treatment. After Dr. Losee repaired her legs, she returned to school, and, although walking with a decidedly unsteady gait, she was able to cross the stage unassisted to receive her well-earned high school diploma.

Dr. Phillip D. Pallister was a medical pioneer in his own right. Settling in Boulder, Montana, after World War II, he expected to have a quiet general practice in a small town in good fishing and hunting country. Soon after arriving, however, he was asked to be the physician for the Montana State School and Hospital, also called the Boulder River School, for the mentally and physically handicapped. Dr. Pallister didn't anticipate how this institution would affect his life.

The Boulder River School housed children with a myriad of physical and mental problems. Some were totally disabled and bedridden, others were partially ambulatory, and a few were partially self-sufficient. Many were brain damaged. The causes of these problems were not always known, but undoubtedly they included birth injuries or infections, congenital abnormalities, fetal alcohol syndrome, and many other things.

From the outside, the school was a pleasant-looking set of brick structures with a neatly landscaped exterior. But on the inside, "the institution housed a horror, it was a warehouse," Pallister said. Many of the patients had no diagnosis or hospital records, and some had never even been examined by a physician. There was no laboratory and only a tiny, ill-trained nursing staff. Some of the patients were bunched together naked and corralled like animals. Reforming this outrageous care became the challenge of Pallister's life.

Pallister described the first "sick call" he attended, in 1947. The patients who had complaints were lined up in single file and came forward one by one. Regardless of the complaint, a headache or a backache or a sore foot, the "nurse" dipped a large sponge into a vat of the disinfectant Merthiolate, swabbed the area, and called "Next!" Pallister saw to it that his visit was the last time that kind of charade was performed. From then on, under his direction, there was a steady improvement in the medical care at the Boulder facility. No longer would more state monies be spent on lawn and landscaping than on the care of these unfortunate patients.

Little by little and with only modest help from a few unpaid associates from other towns, Dr. Pallister made changes. In time this forceful, principled, and energetic man created a place to diagnose, treat, and comfort many afflicted people, even if there were seldom any "cures." Meanwhile he also worked and studied to become a geneticist.

At the time, the average physician knew little about the genetics behind mental and physical disabilities or about caring for mentally handicapped people. The study of so-called "idiots," "imbeciles," and "morons" held little interest for the profession in general. Furthermore, according to a Montana Medical Association report, "the medieval stigma attached to the mentally incompetent and the convulsive patient probably kept the families of Boulder patients from raising a hue and cry" about their care.[584] Of these early days, Dr. Losee said, "We were privately embarassed. We suffered as we managed our own appalling ignorance, and what is worse, we would sometimes try to hide it behind a hypocritical, juvenile, role playing behavior."[585]

Over time Pallister honed his clinical diagnostic skills and electroencephalograpic expertise and eventually set up a clinical and genetic laboratory that turned the Boulder "warehouse" into a respected teaching facility, now called the Montana Development Center. Later he served as the director of the genetic unit at Shodair Children's Hospital in Helena from 1976 to 1982. Pallister identified many obscure hereditary conditions and described for the first time entities that are now designated by terms that include his name. He published papers, established workshops, spoke out, and faced off bureaucrats. He invited leading geneticists from major universities and hospitals to teach, consult, critique, and help.

A Montana Medical Association report said that the Montana State School and Hospital "reflects the tardy development of enlightened and compassionate patient care."[586] Montana is now on the map in genetics, and the physician largely responsible for this is Dr. Phillip D. Pallister. His own satisfaction and a paltry salary were the only thanks he ever received for removing this grievous blight on the conscience of the citizens of Montana, and most of them never knew it.

TWELVE

The Professional Nurse

With loyalty will I endeavor to aid the physician in his work, and devote myself to the welfare of those committed to my care.

—From the Florence Nightingale Pledge[587]

ANY DISCUSSION OF MEDICAL progress or the emergence of modern hospitals cannot be complete without honoring the nursing profession. The status of both hospitals and the nursing profession developed together. Yet women have served as amateur nurses for centuries. As previously pointed out, tending to the personal care of sick people has always been primarily the responsibility of women. Yet it was well into the twentieth century before nurses began to gain respect as professionals. Yet even in the early days, many young women were drawn to this calling as a way to make their mark in the world. As historian Pierce Mullen pointed out, "As poorly salaried as it was, and as difficult as it was to achieve for many young women, nursing was a move up in status; it was a profession."[588]

Wartime Heroines

During the Crimean War, in 1854, wounded soldiers were dying of infections in military hospitals when British nurse Florence Nightingale came on the scene. By simply improving hygiene, scrubbing the wards and halls from top to bottom, washing the linens, and separating infected patients from noninfected ones, she reduced the mortality rate from infections in British soldiers from forty percent to two percent.[589] She achieved this remarkable feat over the ignorant and arrogant objections of doctors and politicians.

Nightingale, born in Italy in 1820 to British parents, was well educated for a woman of her day. Her desire to work in medicine, in spite of her

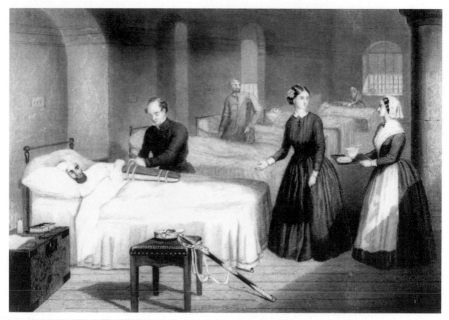

Florence Nightingale (1820–1910). The modern profession of nursing can trace its origin to this remarkable lady. —Courtesy National Library of Medicine, History of Medicine Division

parents' objections, was reinforced when she met Elizabeth Blackwell, the first woman doctor in the United States. Nightingale began her training as a nurse in 1851. After her legendary service in the Crimean War, she published several books and established a school for nurses in London. She lived to be ninety years old.

In America, many army doctors during the Civil War refused to work with the women who volunteered as nurses. It required thousands of deaths in army hospitals before the military hierarchy—especially doctors—accepted nurses and their instincts for cleanliness as a valid way to reverse the trend of death. On the Yankee side, one outstanding nurse, Mary Ann Bickerdyke, would become a legend. This forceful lady from Ohio became known as "Mother Bickerdyke," the "Cyclone in Calico." With only personal experience and a great deal of common sense, she fashioned hospitals on the battlefields, on the decks of ships, and in barns, houses, and abandoned buildings. In all, she set up about three hundred field hospitals for General Ulysses S. Grant's western armies.[590] She nursed, cooked, organized supplies, and arranged transport for her "boys." She gathered herbs and made poultices and medicines. When one haughty doctor asked her where she got her authority, she said, "From the Lord God Almighty." After the war, someone said of her efforts, "Your army record, which was a record of service to the sick and wounded soldiers in camp hospital and on the battlefield, transcends that of all other women."[591]

In general, nursing throughout the 1800s was an art learned at a mother's knee. Nuns of various religious orders also served as nurses during wartime and on the frontier. It is interesting to note that during the Civil War, black women were accepted as nurses, and in this capacity suffered less prejudice. Among African American women serving as nurses in the Civil War was Susie King Taylor, who accompanied her husband to battle with the First South Carolina Volunteers and nursed the sick and injured. Harriet Tubman was also said to have nursed Union soldiers in the hospitals.[592]

While there were few effective treatments available for many of the sick and wounded soldiers, nurses did much to promote their comfort and raise their morale. Louisa May Alcott, a Union nurse, wrote of her experiences in a makeshift army hospital: "[I would] poke up the fire, add blankets, joke, coax and command, but continue to open doors and

Mary Ann "Mother" Bickerdyke worked tirelessly to improve army hospitals during the Civil War.

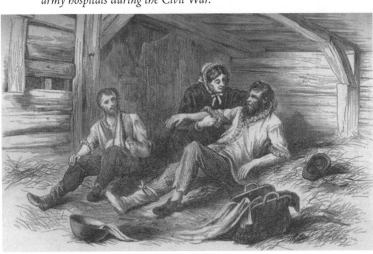

windows as if life depended on it. Mine does, and doubtless many another, for a more perfect pestilence box than this house I never saw—cold, damp, dirty, full of vile odors from wounds, kitchens, washrooms and stables."[593]

Another Civil War nurse described how she went from cot to cot sponging foreheads, talking and reading to the wounded, writing letters for them, bringing them food, and giving them medicine. "We begin the day by getting them all washed, and freshened up, and breakfasted. Then the surgeons and dressers make their rounds, open the wounds, apply the remedies, and replace the bandages. This is an awful hour: I sat with my fingers in my ears this morning."[594]

In the South, well-bred ladies were discouraged from working as nurses, for it was viewed as a degrading occupation. Nevertheless, many of them did volunteer, but because of the social attitude, most remained anonymous. One Southern nurse, Kate Cumming, alluding to Florence Nightingale, said bitterly, "It seems strange that the aristocratic women of Great Britain have done with honor what is a disgrace for their sisters on this side of the Atlantic to do."[595]

Medical care during the Spanish-American War showed little progress. Nurse Anna Turner volunteered for service in Virginia in 1898, where she cared for wounded soldiers returning from Cuba; many of the men were sick with typhoid. She describes the hospital in her diary: "A tent hospital was set up consisting of four tents placed together—this housed 100 men ill with typhoid. Equipment consisted of twenty cots, one hand basin, one water pail and dipper, one bed pan, a stand by each cot, a corpsman, no training."[596] When she first arrived, her commanding officer had told her, "You are not wanted." After weeks of observing her grueling work, he apologized.

By 1917 trained nurses were sorely needed, not only to care for wounded soldiers in World War I, but also to fight another enemy that was killing thousands worldwide—influenza. For nurses who served during this period, whether overseas or stateside, the terrible pandemic dominated their lives. As in other wars, more soldiers suffered from sickness than from wounds, and many hospitals overflowed with influenza patients. The number of nurses volunteering for military service caused a shortage at home. After the armistice, many nurses' tours were extended to care for the men with influenza.

The flu epidemic at the end of World War I resulted in an unintended breakthrough for black nurses. Before the epidemic, most

African Americans were effectively banned from the Army Nurse Corps and the Red Cross. The urgent need for nursing care finally overruled the entrenched discrimination against nurses of color. Yet the struggle for equality was far from over. Black nurses continued to face institutional barriers, both in civilian service and in the military, well into the mid-twentieth century.

Octavia Bridgewater of Helena, Montana, was a pioneer black nurse. Refused admission to the schools in her home state, she attended the Lincoln School of Nursing in New York, one of the few nursing schools in the nation that accepted African Americans. After graduating in 1930, she went back to Montana, working first as a private nurse, then at St. Peter's Hospital in Helena. In the early 1940s, she became one of a handful of black women accepted into the U.S. Army Nurse Corps, where she rose to the rank of captain. Bridgewater died in 1985 at age eighty-two.[597]

It was not until World War II that American nurses really came into their own. During that war, army nurses could achieve full officer status, and all nurses enjoyed an improved public image. It was through wartime service that the women of this humanitarian vocation eventually earned the appreciation of the medical establishment as well as the public. Eighty years after the Civil War, when doctors dismissed the efforts of volunteer women, nurses finally gained acceptance as true partners in the medical profession.

Frontier Nurses

There is little doubt that doctors practicing on the frontier needed the help of a good nurse. Most sick people were bedridden for long periods, and nursing care was the primary treatment for illness. Despite the great scientific and technical progress in medicine and nursing during the twentieth century, many facilities in rural areas remained primitive for years. Hospitals were sometimes merely converted homes or other buildings with minimal equipment. Major surgical cases were usually sent to larger towns, and a nurse would often accompany patients on these uncomfortable trips by automobile, train, or even sleigh. Sometimes the railroad put patients on cots in the baggage compartment.[598] Such was the state of medical care in some remote places.

The first nurse to come to the Montana frontier with formal training was probably Katherine Babbage Carruthers, known in the region as "Miss Babbage." After training in midwifery in Washington, D.C., she arrived by steamboat at Fort Benton in 1864. Doctors were scarce, and Miss Babbage filled the shoes of both nurse and doctor to many frontier men and the few families in the area.[599]

One of the first nurses registered in Montana was Elizabeth Rae, called "Auntie Rae" by her patients, who moved to Livingston in 1889. She had studied her craft at the Provincial Hospital for the Insane in Halifax, Nova Scotia, then earned a diploma in nursing at Boston City Hospital.[600] Rae established a maternity home in Livingston where women from distant ranches and farms could await their birthings in a homelike atmosphere. Premature infants and women with compromised pregnancies were also brought to "Auntie Rae's Maternity Home." With no modern incubators available for premature infants, Rae "put them in a shoebox on an oven door."[601]

Another early Montana nurse was Thora Firming Phalen. She had studied nursing in Minneapolis, where she worked with the physician-inventor of a sterilizer and learned to make the first catgut suture used by the surgeons in St. Paul. Both of these were progressive medical achievements of the era. After serving as an army nurse in the Spanish-American War in 1898, Thora Firming came to Montana shortly after the turn of the twentieth century. She worked for a short time at St. Peter's Hospital in Helena, where her talents were put to good use during an epidemic of typhoid.

After she married Mr. Phalen, she went with him to ranch in the Bear's Paw Mountains north of the Missouri River. This was a blessing for the families who lived in these rugged foothills. Traveling by horse or wagon, Phalen nursed her neighbors through epidemics of typhoid, measles, scarlet fever, and whatever else assaulted the area's homesteaders. There were no doctors nearby, so she was usually on her own to face any misfortune that presented itself, which she did with calm self-assurance.

During her career, Phalen braved many hazards to attend her patients. On one occasion, to reach a child suffering from a severe infection, this intrepid woman traveled thirty miles by horse and wagon in a blizzard. She found the little girl shivering in a unheated shack, with the wind whistling through the cracks in the walls. There was no water, so Phalen started a fire and melted snow. She bathed the child in the heated water, wrapped her in blankets, and made a bed using sawhorses she found in the yard. What other measures she took are not recorded, but they must have been effective, for the child survived.[602]

Perhaps Phalen's most remarkable achievement was the successful delivery of a transverse, arm-presentation birth—a dangerous complication that many physicians practice a lifetime without having to confront.[603] To complete this difficult task, she first had to anesthetize the patient deeply enough to get total relaxation of the skeletal muscles without harming the mother or the infant. Next she had to comprehend, through careful internal examination and palpation of the patient's distended uterus, the fetus's position, when all she could see was an arm extended through the mother's dilated cervix. Today a physician has radiological and ultrasound equipment to help do this. After determining its position, she rotated the infant until its buttocks were in the breech position. She had to do this without disrupting the placenta's attachment to the uterine lining, an injury that could result in massive hemorrhage, sometimes fatal to both mother and baby. Finally and most dangerous to the child was extracting the fetus from the womb without harming its legs or body. What an amazing feat for a nurse alone in the backwoods of Montana.

Hospital Nurse Training in the West

From approximately 1870 to 1910, as doctors and patients began to accept hospitals as true medical facilities, the education of nurses evolved. This blossoming of nurse training was prompted by the need for cheap labor in hospitals. Women, especially female students, fulfilled that need. In spite of the low wages, many women entered the nursing field. In 1873 there were only three nurse-training schools in the United States, but by 1900 there were 432, and by 1910, more than 1,000.[604] Many of these schools were in the western states. Utah may have been the first state in the West to have a training program for nurses. The Deseret Hospital in Salt Lake City opened its school for midwives, where nurses were also trained, in 1884.[605] In contrast, it was 1910 before Phoenix, Arizona, opened its first nursing school.[606]

Montana was among the earliest states to offer nurse training. Columbus Hospital in Great Falls was the first institution in Montana to inaugurate a nursing school. In 1894, with three hundred patients and few people to care for them, the hospital saw a need to train new nurses. The students received most of their training at the hospital, but they were also sent out to practice at private homes. One early student at Columbus Hospital recalled making trips by stagecoach, traveling up to sixty-five miles, the last few miles on foot.[607] In rural areas, home care remained a common service until the mid-twentieth century. Well into the 1900s, nurses practiced primarily in private homes, working round-the-clock, with no time off, for $6 per day plus meals.[608]

Montana Deaconess Hospital in Great Falls began operation in 1898. E. Augusta Ariss served as director of nurses there for thirty years. Ariss was a missionary and trained her nurses for "Christian service." Her colleague, Rev. W. E. "Brother Van" van Orsdel, said that she often "prayed that the Lord would send in the suffering who needed care. . . . They seemed to come from all directions after she prayed."[609] As an educator, Ariss considered it her responsibility not only to train young women as nurses, but also to foster their spiritual lives. Her regimen for the students at Great Falls became the model for all Deaconess hospitals. Each nursing student was required to attend daily chapel, with morning prayer every day at 7 a.m., hymns every evening at 7 p.m., and prayer meetings on Saturday.[610]

Eight young women entered the first nursing program at Murray Hospital in Butte, Montana, in 1909 and graduated in 1912. The population of the state was rapidly expanding, creating a desperate need for trained nurses. St. Vincent School of Nursing in Billings opened in 1913, and others followed. By 1917 there were sixteen hospital-based nursing schools in Montana.

Nurse's training in the first few decades of the twentieth century was not easy. Working twelve-hour shifts with no breaks, students were instructed one-on-one in a hands-on apprenticeship. A nurse and her students were busy throughout their long shift. Among her many nursing duties, the probational student, or "probie," cleaned and scrubbed the rooms, walls, and floors before and after each admission. Because early ambulation for patients was not encouraged as it is today, hospital patients in this era were mostly bedridden and required a great deal of personal care. They needed daily baths, and the sheets were changed daily or more often as needed. Back massage was a daily ritual against the threat of bedsores. The emptying and cleaning of bedpans also fell to the student nurse.

In those days, physicians ordered time-consuming therapeutic procedures that today are no longer necessary. The nurse prepared and applied boric acid solutions and dressings to infected wounds, or injected the solution into inflamed pustular cavities; cleaned, changed, or replaced surgical drains and tubes; gave cold baths to patients with high fevers to reduce their temperatures, and hot baths to chilled patients; assembled and applied flaxseed and mustard plasters to painful chests and joints; and changed and cleaned pneumonia jackets (a quilted vest thought to stabilize body heat). Fluid balance was maintained by proctolysis

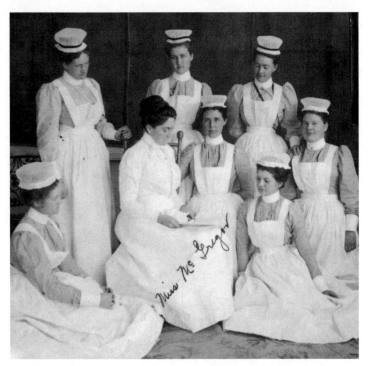

A head nurse with her team of nurses, probably in training. (Unknown location, circa 1900.) Nurse training was grueling work. —Courtesy Montana Historical Society, Helena

(enema) or by subcutaneous injection, and medicinal enemas were also commonly prescribed; nurses were responsible for administering these therapies. Medications had to be administered according to the doctor's sometimes complicated orders, and vital signs such as temperature, pulse, respiration, and blood pressure had to be recorded religiously at four-hour intervals.

In the midst of all this work, when the doctor made his rounds, a nurse was expected to drop what she was doing and accompany him, keeping notes and recording his comments. In addition she had to meticulously and accurately maintain the hospital records and the patients' charts. After twelve hours of grueling duty, the student nurse was required to attend lectures by nursing supervisors and staff physicians. Finally after all this, the exhausted young student could return to her small dormitory room, where she had to make sure her uniform was immaculate and her cap starched and folded, ready for the next day, before she could steal a few hours of sleep.

The nursing student's life was not her own, even when she was not on duty. Student behavior was strictly governed. Nurses in training were not allowed to date or attend social functions. On duty, a student nurse could not enter a room before a superior student or nurse, and she could never precede a doctor. After the three-month probationary period, during which time the student could be expelled instantly for the slightest rule infraction, life became a little easier. Survivors of the "probie" period were paid ten dollars a month. More important, they earned the right to proudly pin a white, cone-shaped nurse's cap to their hair.[611] With this symbol of accomplishment, the student's resolve to succeed was reinforced.

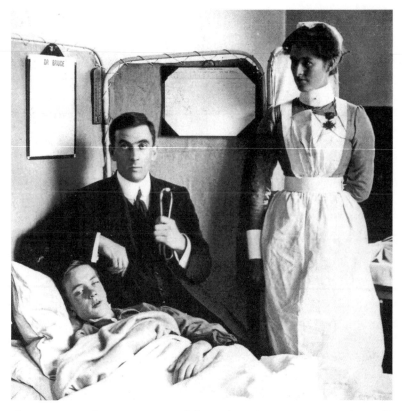

A doctor, nurse, and patient at a British hospital, circa 1904. Sometimes doctors had little to offer, but nursing care could make a difference. Many survivors of illness owed their recovery to good nursing. —Courtesy Wellcome Institute Library, London

By graduation, the nurse had learned her art. She had worked long hours in the operating room assisting surgeons with the procedures of the day—cholecystectomies, appendectomies, hysterectomies, prostatectomies, and other "ectomies." In the obstetrics ward, she shared with expectant parents the hours and hours of waiting, followed by the excitement of delivery. But withal, she witnessed tragedy. By graduation, the young students, some teenagers, had seen the face of death and felt the futility that all professional healers experience with failure. To survive in her profession, a nurse had to cope with suffering.

From the earliest days to the present, the selfless work of nurses has never been truly appreciated. Even doctors who work side by side with them often fail to recognize their invaluable contribution to medicine. Yet physicians, patients, and indeed all of humankind owe a profound debt of gratitude to those professional women and men whose creed declares in part, "With loyalty will I endeavor to aid the physician in his work, and devote myself to the welfare of those committed to my care."[612]

THIRTEEN

Sanitation and Public Health

*What are the lives and health of
our people worth in the State?*
—Dr. Thomas D. Tuttle[613]

IN COLONIAL AMERICA, personal hygiene and sanitation was lacking. A foreign observer noted that "baths are a rarity, the philosophy of personal cleanliness is not understood."[614] In the late eighteenth and early nineteenth centuries, Dr. Benjamin Rush spoke out to encourage better habits of cleanliness, but only gradually did attitudes change. Over the course of time, doctors and scientists learned that certain conditions were contagious and that epidemics could be curtailed through isolation and quarantine. Later research confirmed that diseases such as cholera and typhoid were caused by contamination. By the end of the nineteenth century, sanitation laws began to be passed to guard public health, and health boards were organized. As vaccinations against some diseases were discovered, efforts to immunize the public were launched. Most of the improvements in public health in the 1800s and early 1900s were directly related to the better understanding of germs, sanitation, and disease prevention.

Interest in public health issues became especially focused during the Spanish-American War, which began in 1898. If any good came out of that conflict, it was that medical science was forced to face its inefficiency in disease prevention. Many illnesses plagued the soldiers, but the worst problem was typhoid fever. Epidemics swept through the crowded army camps with a vengeance and left many young soldiers dead or disabled. The reason for this unnecessary tragedy was a near total disregard of preventative health measures such as safe disposal of sewage and garbage and insect control. The mode of transmission for typhoid was well known by this time, but when war was declared, the U.S. was totally unprepared, and the servicemen's health was essentially an afterthought. Those in charge of the camps ignored medical recommendations, and the army doctors were powerless to do anything about it.

More than 20,000 cases of typhoid occurred during the five months of the Spanish-American War, and more than 1,500 soldiers died of the disease, compared to only 280 killed in battle.[615] These disgraceful statistics served as an object lesson for the American people and the profession of medicine, inciting moves toward better sanitation in the future. (For more on typhoid and other epidemics, see chapter 14.)

"Offensive to my nostrils": Sanitation Issues in the West

On the early frontier, public health was not high on the list of the population's concerns. Many people who came west—mostly men—did so in part to eschew the trappings and mores of "civilization." Not until the great migration of homesteaders did disease prevention and health care become a serious consideration. As families put down roots, schools and churches sprang up and values shifted. Soon the desire for clean water, proper disposal of sewage and garbage, and other public health improvements grew.

But there were stumbling blocks to progress in western communities. Most of the hurdles involved politics and money and sometimes a callous disregard for public good on the part of community leaders. Rivers and streams offered ready-made, no-cost sewage and garbage disposal. When drinking water sources became unsafe, local officials often ignored proposals to fix the problem. Not only were the solutions relatively costly and bothersome, they could provoke resentment in citizens and business owners who viewed regulations in general as unwarranted government interference.

Given this attitude, it isn't surprising that throughout the West most of the streams and rivers near settlements became polluted. Some doctors and others aware of the dangers recommended that people boil their drinking water. This simple procedure helped prevent diarrhea and several contagious diseases. Yet in many places, ignorance and apathy triumphed. Rivers and streams continued to be used as sewers into the twentieth century. As late as 1905, an erroneous theory prevailed that a running stream purifies itself every seven miles. To prove otherwise, frontier public health physician Dr. Samuel J. Crumbine of Kansas collected and tested water samples from the Kansas River near Topeka. His experiment established that dangerous bacteria survived as far as twenty-eight miles. Crumbine led a successful campaign to restrict the pollution of streams, and he won support for other public health measures as well.[616]

In addition to river dumping, other unhealthy practices continued in many western towns. Basic rules of hygiene were ignored. Garbage accumulated in piles, and domestic animals roamed freely. Open trenches for human excrement were not unusual. Household water usually came from a well, and many were improperly dug near outhouses, animal pens, and barns. Water contamination was a serious medical problem, and many state health departments tried to educate people not to dig wells where drainage from human or animal waste areas could contaminate them.

One Idaho doctor wrote in 1908, "I have scrubbed up in water that was so offensive to my nostrils that I made them boil it first, yet the

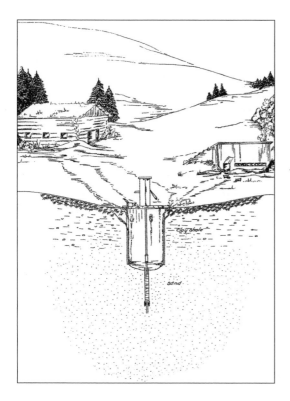

This drawing shows a well that was dug downslope from livng quarters and livestock areas, unsuitably placed for drinking water. A poorly located well was one of the ways homesteaders contracted typhoid and other gastrointestinal infections.
—From State of Montana Department of Health

family was using it for domestic purposes."[617] It is no wonder that gastrointestinal complaints, especially in children, were so common. In addition to contaminated water, unpasteurized milk was a source of tuberculosis, diphtheria, and scarlet fever.

Quarantine

Quarantine—isolating the sick from the healthy—is a centuries-old practice to stop the spread of disease. In American port cities, quarantines were placed on incoming ships to prevent an influx of contagion. Over the years, quarantines of infected individuals were put into effect during various epidemics. Among the diseases that prompted quarantine were Asiatic cholera, diphtheria, influenza, measles, plague, polio, rabies, Rocky Mountain spotted fever, scarlet fever, smallpox, tuberculosis, typhoid, whooping cough, and others. As public health laws were established, quarantines became more institutionalized, but in less developed places, such as the West, the procedures were less structured. The specific methods of implementing quarantines varied according to the nature of the epidemic, what facilities and medical care were available, and the public attitude.

—Courtesy National Library of Medicine, History of Medicine Division

QUARANTINE

SCARLET FEVER

All persons are forbidden to enter or leave these premises without the permission of the HEALTH OFFICER under PENALTY OF THE LAW.

This notice is posted in compliance with the SANITARY CODE OF CONNECTICUT and must not be removed without permission of the HEALTH OFFICER.

Form D-1-Sc. _____ Health Officer.

In some communities, abandoned buildings, empty boxcars, or other isolated enclosures were used as pesthouses. The conditions in these places were usually crude and miserable, and the buildings were often guarded like a prison. In most cases, however, the victim of a contagious disease was isolated in his own home, with a placard hung on the door for all to see. The rules for quarantine of the sick were stringent and firmly enforced. Everyone in the household was confined, and any contact with the outside was prohibited. Nurses and doctors could enter and leave the residence, but they followed strict procedures. Any item removed from the house was washed and disinfected. There were specific directions for laundry, food preparation, and the disposal of bodily fluids. Naturally all this put a great deal of stress on the patient and the family, especially the children. There was a stigma associated with being quarantined, and sometimes, even after the quarantine was lifted, the family was shunned, at least for a while.

While quarantine had some value in guarding public health, sanitation, it was eventually learned, was an even more effective preventative. Early ignorance about germs and infection, and later public and political resistance to change, made for slow progress in this area, however. Even after medical practitioners began to advocate for public sanitation measures, it took decades for laws to be implemented, especially in the West, where the culture of rugged self-reliance stood opposed to regulations of any kind. Communities with this attitude paid a heavy price in disease and human suffering.

The Government Slowly Steps In

By the early 1900s, a few people in Montana, Washington, Kansas, and other western states began to put pressure on state governments to form health boards and develop programs for the prevention of disease. But the governments weren't willing to part with much money at first. In Kansas in 1905, the state's first health department was granted an annual budget of only $3,080.[618] In Montana in 1901, the legislature appropriated even less: $2,000 annually.[619] This paltry sum was meant to fund programs for clean water, garbage and sewage disposal, control of contagious diseases, and other improvements. In addition, the governor asked the secretary of the board of health to "do something" about Rocky Mountain spotted fever. No one foresaw how difficult this task would be. As described in the next chapter, it would take nearly twenty-five more years to develop and distribute a vaccine for this dreaded illness.

Conditions in Montana are a good example of what was happening in most western states. Mining towns and other communities were overcrowded, with filthy streets and living conditions. As populations grew, sporadic outbreaks of infectious diseases were clustered enough to fit the definition of an epidemic. With improved transportation, rural communities were just as likely as more populated places to harbor disease.

Dr. Thomas D. Tuttle of Billings, Montana, was a public-health hero. Elected secretary of the Montana State Board of Health in 1903, he held the post for nine years. His slight form and youthful look belied his underlying strength, courage, and determination. In the board's third biennial report, Dr. Tuttle chastised the state government for his department's grossly inadequate budget, saying, "What are the lives and health of our people worth in the State?"[620] He pointed out that the state appropriated over $175,000 for the cattle and sheep industry and $17,000 for fish and game protection.

A fiery man, Tuttle popularized the need for good sanitation and forced state officials to do their jobs. He lobbied for many things, including

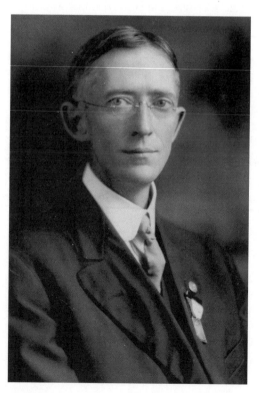

Dr. Thomas Tuttle served as the executive secretary of the Montana State Board of Health from 1903 to 1912. Early health officers struggled against great odds to bring clean water, proper sewage disposal, vaccinations, and many other health measures to western settlements. —Courtesy Montana Historical Society, Helena

registration of births and deaths, clean water, regulations for sewage and garbage disposal, and child welfare. Most of all, he worked to fight the ever-increasing problem of tuberculosis. Of the unsanitary conditions of railroad passenger cars, for example, he said, "The average day coach would turn the stomach of a coyote. . . . The tobacco chewer spits on the floor, the consumptive expectorates on the floor. . . . Then here comes the brakeman with his broom. . . . He brushes this dried filth into a dust. . . . This dust is laden with the germs of tuberculosis the passengers must breathe . . . and the law says they must not kill the brakeman."[621] Lecturing on the importance of meat and milk inspections, Dr. Tuttle quipped, "We cannot teach cows to expectorate in a cuspidor."[622]

Unfortunately some Montana doctors did not cooperate with the board of health. Even those paid by the state as health officers failed to report all contagious illnesses. This behavior infuriated Dr. Tuttle. He fired some of these government doctors and appointed new ones, then redoubled his efforts to win the support of his colleagues. Although Tuttle's efforts and those of other dauntless doctors came to fruition

Dr. William F. Cogswell replaced Thomas Tuttle as Montana's Board of Health secretary, serving from 1912 to 1946.
—Courtesy Montana Historical Society, Helena

slowly, over the years the message got through. Tuttle's successor as secretary of the Montana State Board of Health, Dr. William F. Cogswell, was also a determined public-health advocate, described as "the driving force behind state health policy" during his term.[623]

By the early 1900s, most western states had established health boards and appointed health officials with some legal power. Eventually even the most skeptical critics began to see improvement in public health. This is lucky, because many more challenges to public health in the West were still to come. Many communities would face sporadic epidemics of smallpox, diphtheria, typhoid, scarlet fever, tuberculosis, and poliomyelitis before the century was half gone.

In spite of their success, public-health institutions continued to meet resistance in many places well into the twentieth century. Not only were business interests, politicians, and citizens suspicious of new laws and ordinances, but even some doctors were threatened by health requirements. More than a few private practitioners saw public-health clinics and officials as unfair competition, and they often refused to cooperate with authorities. Among the measures many doctors and others opposed were vaccination efforts. Some thought vaccination should be in a physician's purview exclusively. Others believed vaccination was too dangerous, an opinion with some foundation—death rates associated with inoculation for smallpox in the early years were not insignificant.

This lack of endorsement by the medical profession, carried into government, caused a reluctance to fund vaccination for many diseases or make it a public health requirement. Powerful "anti-immunization" groups put up further resistance, often on religious grounds, throughout the early twentieth century. Eventually, however, vaccination, like sanitation regulations and other public health measures, was accepted as sound policy throughout the United States.

FOURTEEN

Epidemic Diseases in the West

*Sometimes there were two, and once,
three funerals in one day. The mortuary
became short of caskets.*

—Hospital volunteer Jessie Moore, of the
1918 influenza epidemc[624]

THOUGH PUBLIC HEALTH ISSUES were poorly understood until nearly the twentieth century, people had a general awareness that some diseases were "catching." Plague, smallpox, yellow fever, typhoid, and scarlet fever were some of the diseases known to be contagious, and during epidemics victims were usually quarantined to contain the spread. Isolation was of only limited usefulness as a preventative, however. It is often difficult to diagnose the first case in any epidemic, before the outbreak is full-blown. Early diagnosis and swift action were the keys to successful containment.

As medical science learned more about germs and sanitation, doctors began to practice antiseptic methods and communities gradually adopted public sanitation measures. Immunization was another concept that eventually took hold, and scientists worked to develop vaccines against the major infectious diseases throughout the nineteenth and twentieth centuries. It took a few years, however for vaccines to be publicly accepted, and a few more years for them to be distributed to outlying areas. In the meantime, epidemics posed a challenging threat to public welfare on the western frontier and worldwide.

With the white infiltration of Indian lands, natives and whites intermingled and infected one another. The European disease smallpox decimated tribal populations, who had no immunity to it. Later, diseases such as tuberculosis took a heavy toll on reservation Indians. As western expansion moved forward, army camps and mining camps endured various epidemics. Given the unsanitary conditions, close quarters, and limited medical care of these camps, the spread of disease was inevitable. Even into the twentieth century, epidemics of typhoid, smallpox, measles, tuberculosis, influenza, polio, and other diseases scourged hundreds of communities, often hitting hard in the West, where medical resources were scarce and resistance to public health regulations was high. Eventually the toll that infectious diseases took wore down such resistance.

Smallpox

Smallpox, or variola, was one of the first infectious diseases doctors were able to vaccinate against. For centuries throughout Europe, Asia, and Africa, inciting immunity against smallpox by introducing matter from the blisters of infected people into the skin of healthy people through superficial scratches (inoculation) was a well-known technique. Later, milkmaids in Europe learned that if they developed the relatively benign pustules of cowpox on their hands, they became immune to smallpox. In 1796 Edward Jenner experimentally demonstrated what the milkmaids already knew, and soon material from cowpox blisters became the standard smallpox vaccination all over the world. Through the nineteenth century, immunization became almost routine in many places—but not everywhere.

Out west, the government made some attempts to vaccinate American Indians, but few natives received the "matter," and they had no natural immunity. In 1837–38, the plague of "many scabs" ravaged western tribes, especially the Assiniboines, Mandans, Hidatsas, Arikaras, and Blackfeet. The devastation smallpox caused in indigenous populations is discussed in chapter 1. Even among whites, vaccination against smallpox was far from universal. Vaccines were expensive and not always available. In addition, religious groups, skeptical citizens, and even some doctors resisted immunization efforts. Thus many early emigrants to the West were not immunized against the disease.

Smallpox was highly contagious, the symptoms were severe, and the outcome was often fatal. The onset of the illness was characterized by aches, high fever, and delirium during the first week, followed by a rash and pustules that form over the entire body, often worse on the face. Due to severe itching, scratching commonly caused secondary infections. Many survivors of smallpox were left with facial scars from the skin eruptions.

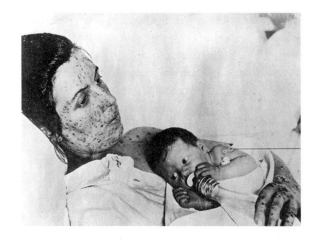

Woman with smallpox with vaccinated infant.
—Courtesy National Museum of Health and Medicine, Armed Forces Institute of Pathology, Washington, D.C.

The persistence of this ugly plague in some western states eventually generated support for public health measures. At first, anti-immunization groups, politicians unwilling to fund efforts for public health, and people with a general distaste for regulations put up more resistance than many local governments and health-minded citizens could overcome. But in time, determined government officials proved the value of vaccination, quarantine, and sanitation in protecting people's health.

In Minnesota, Dr. Henry F. Hoyt, the city health commissioner of St. Paul, 1889-98, challenged the lack of community cooperation in his bustling town. During his service he controlled two smallpox epidemics with quarantine, disinfection, and vaccination. When he closed two hotels in which smallpox cases had been found, the chamber of commerce criticized him for interfering with business and alarming the public. In response, Hoyt used his new Kodak camera to photograph some victims of the disease and placed the pictures in a window at the chamber of commerce. The disturbing photographs attracted crowds unaccustomed to seeing such graphic images. Dr. Hoyt's action silenced his critics, and people were soon standing in line to be vaccinated.[625]

In Montana, the failure of communities to vaccinate against the disease and quarantine victims finally forced the state legislature to create the board of health in 1901.[626] A smallpox epidemic in Billings in 1905 was one of the board's early challenges. In January, twelve days after a masked ball, smallpox broke out in the town. A few cases were also diagnosed in Silesia, Lavina, Livingston, and Bozeman. Some of the organizers of the ball had recently survived the illness and were still contagious. Responding to this outbreak, the state health department began a program of vaccination and quarantine, curtailing the epidemic in Billings and preventing further spread to other towns.[627] Educational pamphlets were distributed around the state, and all new cases were isolated. By June 1906, Montana was nearly free of the disease. In spite of these efforts, smallpox came back with a fury two years later, this time around Butte, where sanitation was poor. Over seven hundred cases were reported. Again the health board instituted timely measures in response. To minimize future epidemics, officials campaigned vigorously for better public health and ultimately won wide public acceptance.

Sporadic cases of smallpox continued to appear over the next two decades, but the numbers had dropped to virtually zero by the 1920s. Vaccination had become a universally accepted, mandatory practice. By 1977 the variola virus was unable to find a victim, and this age-old world plague was conquered. The public health pioneers would have been pleased to know that the war against smallpox was won using the same commonsense public health procedures they themselves promoted.

Cholera

Cholera was a major killer on immigrant ships, on the trails west, in army camps, and in the early mining towns (see also chapters 4, 5, and 6). Epidemics ravaged several eastern cities in the mid-1800s, and the disease spread rapidly along waterways and trails, sweeping through western army posts, mining camps, and settlements. The most deadly of the many types of dysentery that dogged western soldiers and settlers, this dreaded and mysterious illness spread so furiously that it could wipe out dozens of people within days. Asiatic cholera ravaged not only the white population, but also Native Americans who drank from the same polluted sources.

Cholera is caused by the bacterium *Vibrio cholerae*, transmitted in human waste. The disease is characterized by the sudden onset of severe abdominal cramps and diarrhea. The loss of massive volumes of intestinal fluid dehydrated victims to the point of death. Today cholera, rare in developed countries, is treated by replacement of fluids and electrolytes, but that therapy was unknown in frontier times. Also unknown was how to prevent the disease, and cholera killed thousands worldwide before researchers figured out its cause, contaminated water. Discoveries about cholera and other diseases in the late 1800s and early 1900s ushered in a new understanding of the value of public sanitation, especially clean drinking water.

Diphtheria

Epidemics of childhood diseases in frontier communities were common tragedies. The most dreaded of all was probably diphtheria, sometimes called "croup," which struck little ones at random and was often fatal. For ages this dreadful infection of the throat had cursed mankind and was the leading cause of death in children under ten. Frontier doctors did not fully understand diphtheria or how it was transmitted. The antiserum or antitoxin against the disease was not available until approximately 1895. Today, thanks to wide immunization, most physicians have never seen a case.

Frontier parents were well aware of the potentially terrible consequences of "croup." A single case of diphtheria could start an epidemic, and if that happened, townspeople knew they'd have to dig many little graves in the local cemetery. Diphtheria caused death in one of two ways: asphyxiation or heart failure. In the first case, the bacteria created a pseudomembrane in the throat and pharynx that obstructed the windpipe and

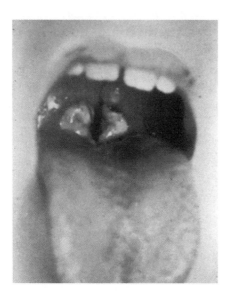

Inflamed throat with white membranous patches from diphtheria. The bacteria that causes this often-fatal infection produced a membrane in the throat that could obstruct the airway.
—Courtesy Immunization Action Coalition

shut off air to the lungs. The reason for the second problem, heart failure, was that the bacteria secreted a potent toxin that specifically affected the heart. Many children recovering from the throat infection died suddenly from an acute inflammation of the heart (acute myocarditis). The second condition was unpredictable and untreatable in that era. The first problem, obstruction of the windpipe, was treatable with surgery, but the procedure, a tracheotomy (tracheostomy), was not well known until the late 1800s.

A tracheotomy involved making an incision into the trachea to let in air. During diphtheria epidemics, some doctors carried a scalpel in their vest pockets so as not to waste time looking for a sharp knife. Death from anoxia takes only a few minutes. But a tracheotomy was a dangerous procedure, especially since the surgery was done in the home, often under very difficult conditions and with panicked family members looking on. Sometimes, to avoid doing the surgery, the practitioner held the child upside down and tickled her throat with a feather, causing her to gag and retch, in the hope that she would dislodge the membrane obstructing the airway and cough it up. If this didn't work, as a last resort, the surgeon performed the tracheotomy. But even doctors prepared to do the operation sometimes arrived too late.

In *The Horse and Buggy Doctor*, Dr. Arthur E. Hertzler describes one difficult and tragic visit from his early practice. "The child is dumpy, listless and feverish. . . . The membrane more or less covers the tonsils. . . . The pulse rate becomes rapid . . . and thready until it is uncountable . . . the effect of the poison produced by the bacteria." As the condition progresses, the membrane extends, often causing air obstruction. If it is not relieved, the awful result is asphyxiation: "Fevered and delirious, [the child] becomes bluer and bluer. . . . He is too busy breathing to cry. . . . The deeply blue face is made more terrible by the bulging, unseeing eyes. Then the entire body relaxes and the face becomes less livid. The child is dead."[628]

In 1878 epidemics of both diphtheria and scarlet fever rendered doctors in Virginia City, Montana, all but helpless, and many children died. Ten years later, after epidemics of scarlet fever and typhoid had already taken a great toll, Elkhorn, Montana, suffered a diphtheria epidemic. Unconfirmed estimates said that over one hundred people (ten percent of the town's population), mostly children, died. Local physician William H. Dudley lost his own infant son in the epidemic.[629]

Burning lime in the rooms of diphtheria sufferers was the main treatment at the time, along with bed rest, but little else could be done but pray and wait. By this time, diphtheria was generally regarded as infectious, and local newspapers urged people to avoid contact with victims. During the Virginia City epidemic, the paper published home remedies such as this one: "Mix with half pint of limewater a teaspoonful of sulphur or finely powdered brimstone. Boil two hours and serve to patient through the nostrils by the use of a quill. . . . This will destroy the germs and prevent their poisonous influence on the body."[630] Of course this recommendation, though well intentioned, was totally useless.

The small comma-shaped bacterium that caused diphtheria, named *Corynebacterium diphtheriae*, was discovered in 1883. By 1895 an antitoxin against diphtheria had been produced by Dr. Emile Roux of the Pasteur Institute in Paris. It was one of the most important medical triumphs of the century. If an exposed person received the antitoxin soon enough, diphtheria was often prevented or at least converted into a less virulent condition. Simply stated, timely injections saved lives.

Problems remained, however. The serum was not always available in remote places. Doctors who did have access to the antitoxin had to employ it as soon as possible to prevent progression of the disease in the individual patient and to keep the infection from spreading to others. But it was difficult to diagnose an epidemic in its early stages, and it was not

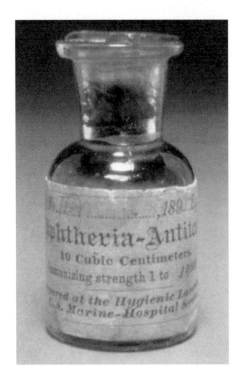

The development of a diphtheria antitoxin was a major medical advance. The injected antiserum neutralized the diphtheria toxin and diminished the disease's morbidity and mortality.
—Courtesy U.S. Department of Health and Human Services, National Institutes of Health

always caught in time. Medicine gained ground in the early 1900s, when scientists learned to identify the bacteria with a culture from a throat swab, eliminating some of the guesswork in diagnosis. Most western doctors embraced the procedure and used it to confirm their cases of diphtheria, but a few, for reasons not entirely clear, did not. Thus many "sore throats" that should have been tested were not properly diagnosed and isolated in time to prevent an epidemic. For example, in rural Montana in November 1904, a dairyman's infected daughter was the source of nineteen cases of diphtheria, of which four died. It was believed that if she had been promptly diagnosed and isolated from the dairy, the epidemic would not have occurred.[631]

Diphtheria epidemics continued to challenge doctors and public health boards in the early twentieth century. In Montana from 1904 to 1906, 806 diphtheria cases were reported to the state board of health, so many that the funds available for throat culture became exhausted.[632] By 1913 a skin test that determined a child's susceptibility to diphtheria, called the Schick test, was available, further enhancing diagnostic practice. Yet as late as 1925, there were still susceptible populations in the United States. Progress in disease prevention was frustratingly slow.

Other Childhood Diseases: Whooping Cough, Measles, and Scarlet Fever

Young children on the frontier were vulnerable to a multitude of contagious diseases, many of which could have serious, even fatal, complications. A good number of these diseases are rare today due to immunization, and improved treatments have rendered others less threatening. But before the development of modern methods, parents knew they could expect at least one of these diseases to attack their children sooner or later. In most cases, there was nothing they could do except hope that the infections were mild. Among the most prevalent, and most dangerous, childhood diseases, in addition to diphtheria, were whooping cough, measles, and scarlet fever. (See table for death rates of diphtheria, measles, scarlet fever, and whooping cough.)

Scarlet fever was a serious streptococcal infection that occurred mostly in children. Named for the diffuse scarlet-color rash that accompanied the illness, it often spread rapidly and could be fatal. It was common for those infected to develop serious complications in the heart or the kidney, so even survivors sometimes had shortened lives.

The early symptoms of the illness, fever and a sore throat, were similar to other common upper respiratory diseases. But soon a high fever, red rash, and severe prostration, along with a white coating on the tongue, distinguished it from less serious maladies.

Measles (rubeola), another common childhood illness with a rash, is a highly contagious virus. It is not usually fatal in itself but can lead to pneumonia, ear infections, and other serious complications. Symptoms include an itchy generalized rash along with fever, cough, runny nose, and conjunctivitis. Frontier mothers dreaded measles almost as much as diphtheria, as it could spread through communities with amazing rapidity.

DEATH RATE FROM SCARLET FEVER, WHOOPING COUGH, DIPTHERIA, AND MEASLES IN MONTANA, 1910-1927

YEAR	SCARLET FEVER	WHOOPING COUGH	DIPTHERIA	MEASLES
1910	16.2	10.9	16.2	4.2
1911	9.3	6.8	7.5	12.3
1912	6.3	13.5	3.1	1.4
1913	27.5	10.6	5.3	12.5
1914	7.3	4.0	8.0	6.0
1915	3.4	7.7	4.5	1.5
1916	3.9	16.2	7.8	7.4
1917	17.1	8.5	7.9	9.1
1918	13.8	12.3	8.6	3.4
1919	10.6	2.4	7.6	3.0
1920	3.9	9.1	5.7	4.8
1921	1.6	12.4	8.9	6.2
1922	3.5	1.3	11.7	0.0
1923	3.5	3.3	9.1	2.9
1924	5.8	4.7	10.2	13.1
1925	3.6	10.4	5.8	0.7
1926	4.6	7.8	2.7	3.5
1927	4.6	2.6	4.2	4.7

State of Montana, Bulletin of the Montana State Board of Health, Special Bulletin No. 37, April 1928.

Whooping cough, a contagious bacterial infection, was more deadly than either scarlet fever or measles, particularly for babies, causing thousands of deaths each year. The infection caused intense fits of coughing followed by a gasp for air, making the "whooping" sound. Very severe coughing could cause apnea (stoppage of breathing) and hemorrhage. Whooping cough frequently led to pneumonia, a common cause of death, as well as brain damage from high fever or hemorrhage. There was no treatment for this condition other than rest and nursing care. Many doctors and family caregivers recognized the value of steam in relieving coughs, and homemade "croup kettles" helped many children with respiratory symptoms.

About the only way to prevent the spread of these diseases during epidemics was with isolation or quarantine. In the early days, however, many physicians simply didn't subscribe to preventive methods and were wary of government health programs. The second biennial report of the Montana State Board of Health said that in one year in the early 1900s, fifty-two children died from whooping cough and twenty-two from measles. In this report, health officials decried the callous attitude of doctors who ignored the rules of isolation and quarantine.[633] In 1909 seventeen hundred cases of scarlet fever were reported in Montana, and in 1910 there were over nine hundred cases, seven percent of whom died.[634] A vaccine for whooping cough was developed in the 1940s, and one for measles became available in 1963. There is no vaccine to prevent scarlet fever, but prompt treatment with antibiotics has controlled the disease and its complications.

Rocky Mountain Spotted Fever

For decades, the condition known today as Rocky Mountain spotted fever was a terrifying mystery. "Black measles," as it was once called, was a serious, often fatal infection. There was no treatment, nor was its transmission understood. The disease, which began with flulike symptoms, often followed a rapid course. The victim usually developed a red rash that turned dark and mottled; the infection could affect the vital body systems and frequently proved fatal.

In the last decade of the nineteenth century and well into the twentieth, the dreaded Rocky Mountain spotted fever became more common, particularly in Montana's Bitterroot Valley. It was originally thought to be restricted to the Rocky Mountains, hence the name, but it was later found to occur all over the United States. Researchers finally discovered that the disease was transmitted by ticks, which were rampant in southwestern Montana due to environmental changes caused by the forest-products and mining industries. These discoveries were a long time coming, however. The effort to identify the disease's cause and to control its spread was a difficult struggle.

Decades before researchers proved that the wood tick was the vector for this disease, some doctors suspected the culprit. One of these was John B. Buker, who established a practice in Missoula, Montana, just north of the Bitterroot Valley, in 1866. One of Buker's patients, whose skin was "spotted like a rattlesnake," still had a tick imbedded in his skin.[635] Buker was sure that the tick was responsible for the man's illness and subsequent death. Buker's experiences were later studied as part of the research that eventually resolved the issue.

In 1901 the governor of Montana appointed Dr. A. F. Longeway to solve the "black measles" problem. Longeway asked his friend Dr. Earl

Rash of Rocky Mountain spotted fever —Courtesy Rocky Mountain Laboratories, NIAID

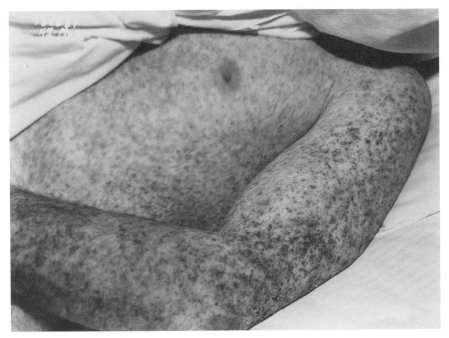

Strain of Great Falls to help him. Dr. Strain had studied with the foremost teacher of medicine in the United States, Dr. William Osler, at the University of Pennsylvania, and had done postgraduate work in London, Berlin, and Vienna. It was Strain who first suspected that the etiology of the illness was not from drinking "snow water" in the spring runoff, a theory favored by most people and some doctors, but rather that it was transmitted to humans by the lowly wood tick.[636]

The insect as a vector of infectious diseases was not entirely unknown in the early 1900s. Microbiologist Dr. Theobald Smith and his associate, veterinarian Frederick L. Kilborne, had found in 1892 that ticks transmitted the bovine disease known as Texas fever, and in 1896 Dr. Ronald Ross, working in India, had discovered that mosquitoes transmitted the malaria parasite.[637] This up-to-date information probably influenced the Montana physicians in their thinking. Strain and Longeway's theory, however, was challenged a short time later by some leading eastern researchers. The doctors had critics outside the scientific community as well—particularly among those with business interests in western Montana.

Montana entrepreneurs and land speculators watched the value of their Bitterroot Valley investments drop precipitously as the deadly disease became more prevalent, and if the cause turned out to be hard-to-avoid tick bites, prospective homesteaders would stay away in droves. The businessmen did their best to divert attention and money toward researching other causes. The mining industry, which was indirectly implicated in the epidemic, also preferred to keep such speculation quiet. During his lifetime, Marcus Daly, the copper king and the Bitterroot Valley's most influential citizen, had destroyed much of the valley's forest to support his mining operation in Anaconda. The process of natural reforestation among the deteriorating stumps and slash of the ravaged foothills provided a favorable environment for insects of all kinds, including the wood tick. Of course, the tick infested wild and domestic animals and before long found its way to humans.

The story of Rocky Mountain spotted fever research and the heroic personalities involved in the project is an epic.[638] In 1906 the U.S. Public Health Service sent the University of Chicago's Dr. Howard Ricketts to Montana to find the cause and method of transmission of the disease. The severely underfunded Montana Board of Health scraped together enough to buy Dr. Ricketts two monkeys for experimental studies. The board's secretary, Dr. Thomas D. Tuttle, commented sarcastically on the state's "extravagant expenditure" of forty dollars to support the research of a disease that claimed the lives of eight to fifteen of its citizens every year.

The following year, the Montana legislature appropriated a somewhat more generous two thousand dollars for the spotted fever program. A year later, from a primitive laboratory housed in a tent, Ricketts found an organism smaller than a bacterium and larger than a virus, transmitted by the wood tick, that caused the infection. The discovery of *Rickettsia rickettsii* was a momentous breakthrough that would soon be applied not only to spotted fever but also to typhus and other diseases. The heroic Dr. Ricketts went to Mexico to study the transmission of typhus based on his research of Rocky Mountain spotted fever. While there, in 1910, the young scientist acquired typhus and died.

The fate of Ricketts's successor in Montana, Dr. T. B. McClintic, is also poignant. In August of 1912 McClintic was bitten by an infected tick. Knowing he would probably die, he boarded a train to Washington, D.C.,

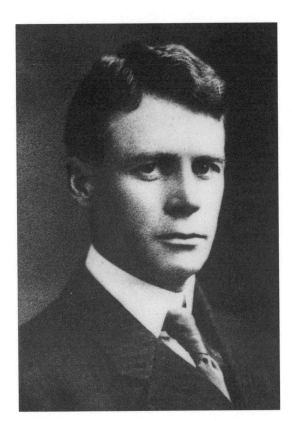

Dr. Howard Ricketts
—Courtesy Rocky
Mountain Laboratories,
NIAID

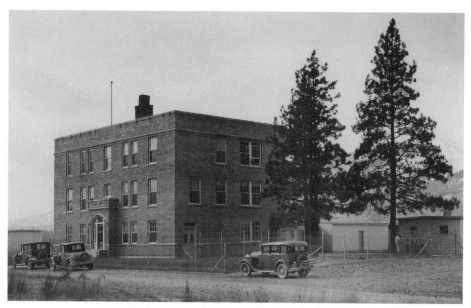

Original Rocky Mountain Laboratories building, 1932
—Courtesy Rocky Mountain Laboratories, NIAID

in the hope of seeing his wife and children again, but he succumbed en route. Four other scientists also died from this infectious disease during the course of their work: Dr. Arthur H. McCray, state bacteriologist, in 1919; William E. Gettinger, a young graduate of Montana State College, in 1922; George Henry Cowan, entomology field worker, in 1924; and Arthur LeRoy Kerlee, laboratory staff, in 1928.[639]

While researchers continued to study spotted fever in an attempt to find a cure or a vaccine, others concentrated on eradicating ticks from the Bitterroot Valley. Dr. Lumford Fricks of the Public Health Service decided in 1917 that introducing large herds of sheep into the area would control the ticks by eating the tall grass in which the insects lived and bred. With this plan in place, the Public Health Service declared the problem solved. But it wasn't. In 1921 state senator Tyler Worden and his wife Carrie died of spotted fever. Because the Wordens were prominent citizens and relatives of the governor, Joseph M. Dixon, their deaths caused a public and political clamor. Under this pressure, the Public Health Service, local physicians, and entomologists renewed their efforts.

Some of the heroes in Rocky Mountain spotted fever research survived to tell the tale. In 1924 Dr. Roscoe R. Spencer and Dr. Ralph R.

Parker developed a vaccine, but their budget was so limited, they had no primates but only guinea pigs on which to test it. No ill effects in the guinea pigs resulted from the vaccine, which was a chemically treated solution of ground-up infected ticks. On the morning of May 19, 1924, Dr. Spencer bypassed further animal tests and proceeded to inject himself with the tick emulsion. Fortunately he suffered no harm from this potentially fatal preparation, and the vaccine was deemed safe for the public.[640]

The results of the Spencer-Parker vaccine were impressive. Public vaccination began in the spring of 1925. Between 1927 and 1940, half a million people in the Rocky Mountain region were vaccinated. Of these, only sixty-one developed spotted fever, with three deaths. The demand for the vaccination exceeded the supply in the very first year, so the state built the Rocky Mountain Laboratory in Hamilton, Montana, to manufacture it. Though the vaccine was eventually taken off the market, the few cases of spotted fever seen today are usually treated effectively with antibiotics. In 1934 the federal government purchased the Hamilton laboratory, and it continues today as a fine institution for research.

Typhoid Fever

Typhoid fever is a diarrheal condition caused by the organism *Salmonella typhi*, which damages the lining of the small intestine. The typhoid bacteria sometimes enters the bloodstream and spreads throughout the body. Before the development of antibiotics, most victims of this complication, called septicemia, died. The disease spread through the ingestion of contaminated water or food. The contamination was caused by contact with the feces of an infected person; transmission could occur when an infected person handled food without washing his hands, for example, or if sewage leaked into a water supply. Houseflies could also carry the bacteria.

Not all people who harbored the bacteria in their intestinal tract became ill. Some were asymptomatic carriers, able to transmit the infection to others, especially if they were food handlers. In some cases, known carriers were ostracized. The most famous example of this was Mary Malone, who became known as "Typhoid Mary" in the early twentieth century after it was discovered that she was a typhoid carrier. She was associated with forty-seven cases of typhoid, three of them fatal. After being forcibly removed from her home and subjected to medical procedures against her will, she was later banished for twenty-six years to North Brother Island in New York's East River.[641]

Epidemics of typhoid flared up from time to time in crowded eastern cities, as well as in army camps, as with the terrible epidemic during the Spanish-American War, discussed in the previous chapter. But the West also saw its share of the disease. It was common on emigrant passenger ships and wagon trains, in army camps, and in mining towns. Typhoid fever was a severe illness on the frontier. Whole communities were laid low by diarrhea and the resultant dehydration. Children, especially infants, were the most severely affected and often died. Patients who developed complications, such as septicemia or a perforated intestine, also died. There was no treatment other than good nursing care, rest, and fluids. Early doctors sometimes purged their patients with calomel, others prescribed enemas, some probably used blistering, and a few might have given ipecac to induce vomiting. All of these "treatments" would have added to the torment of feverish, nauseated, and dysenteric typhoid sufferers. Fortunately most doctors and caregivers, especially after the mid-1800s, avoided these methods. If they administered anything, it was the narcotic laudanum, which gave the patient pain relief and induced sleep.

By the late 1800s, many people rightly suspected that contaminated water was usually the source of this disease, though food and milk could also harbor the causal bacteria, which was identified in 1892. Dr. William Treacy, a well-respected Montana physician, reported in the journal *Times and Register* in 1890 that an epidemic in Helena was the result of seepage from toilets getting into the town's water supply.[642] Due to underdeveloped sanitation and lax public health standards, typhoid continued to plague western communities well into the twentieth century.

The West was vast, and there was plenty of room to dump things. It was easy to discharge the filthy contents of spittoons and slop jars, refuse, and unwanted substances of all kinds into flowing rivers and streams, to be carried downstream. Rotting carcasses and a variety of garbage could be tossed out of sight. But this offal was not hidden from the common housefly. During the warmer seasons, swarms of these insects carried the bacteria everywhere. In 1905 in Bend, Oregon, an epidemic of typhoid was observed to wax and wane with the number of flies. Families who were able to screen their living quarters and protect their water sources were not exposed.[643]

In 1908 there were over fifteen hundred cases of typhoid in Montana. Forty percent were people who lived along the contaminated Yellowstone

River. The secretary of the state's board of health, Dr. Thomas D. Tuttle, faced an uphill struggle to get the legislature to institute sanitation and clean-water regulations. Industry, politicians, and the public all put up resistance. Local health officials seldom provided much support.

A Fergus County epidemic illustrates some of the difficulties Tuttle encountered. After taking the train to Lewistown and driving twenty miles, a long trip in 1903, to Judith, the site of the epidemic, he found that the Fergus County health officer had performed virtually no investigation into the illnesses at the Norris ranch, where the problem was centered. Dr. Tuttle found twelve active cases of typhoid at the ranch, and the wife of the ranch manager had died the day before. The conditions at the ranch were appalling: "The 'boarding house' was run in a most filthy manner. The swill was thrown on the ground. . . . The house was about as filthy inside as it was outside. . . . It is utterly impossible to free that house of disease germs except by the process of fire."[644] He ordered that the sick be taken to a hospital and instructed the other workers to move into tents, then he indeed had the house burned.

The feisty Tuttle battled for Montana's public health right up to the end of his tenure. In his 1911 bulletin, Tuttle used humorous rhyme to educate the public on the danger of houseflies:

> The dirty rascal plants his feet on filth . . .
> He gathers poison with his toes, and leaves it on the baby's nose
> He's on the friendliest of terms with all the death dealing germs
> One dirty, nasty little fly can spoil a whole day's milk supply . . .
> Make friends if you wish, of a rabid dog, a rattlesnake, or a slimy hog
> But every time you see a fly, biff him squarely in the eye.[645]

Dr. John C. Docter said that one of the first calls he made after moving to Drummond, Montana, in 1915 was to the Thayer ranch, where there were seven cases of typhoid. As a conscientious young doctor, he called the county health officer, who refused to respond. It was determined that the carrier was the cook, whose husband was the first to get the disease and had already died. Soon after this event, Dr. Docter himself became the county health officer of Granite County, a position he held until he left Montana in 1920.[646]

It is still possible to contract typhoid today. As recently as the 1970s, a number of cases of typhoid fever appeared in Gallatin County, Montana. All the victims had eaten at a certain popular restaurant, and the state health department determined that one of the cooks was an asymptomatic carrier of the typhoid bacillus. While complications can now be

treated successfully with antibiotics, civilization will never be free of typhoid and other diarrheal maladies as long as some food handlers refuse
to wash their hands and public health officials do not require routine
stool cultures from food-service employees.

Venereal Disease

Venereal infections were and still are common worldwide and of great
concern to health departments everywhere. Sexually transmitted diseases
have resulted in untold misery and disability for both sexes. The types
of venereal diseases and their transmission and treatments have been
discussed previously: the spread of VD between explorers and Indian
women was examined in chapters one and two, and the infection of soldiers and miners from prostitutes, in chapters five and six. Early efforts to
control VD were mostly limited to the crusades of "upright citizens" to
shut down local brothels and red-light districts. The rise of public health
movements in the twentieth century brought government-sponsored campaigns to control sexually transmitted diseases.

In 1905 the spirochete that causes syphilis, *Treponema pallidum*, was
discovered. The following year, scientists developed the Wasserman
blood test, a laboratory procedure to diagnose syphilis even after the external symptoms had disappeared. The Wasserman test was an important step in finding cases so doctors could treat them and isolate them
to prevent further spread of the disease. Though some public campaigns
emphasized education and advised early treatment, many focused on abstinence and fueled their message with fear.

Montana's board of health secretary Dr. Thomas D. Tuttle closed
brothels, prepared strident educational pamphlets, and instituted other
unpopular measures to control syphilis. He complained that "even the
slightest move toward checking this disease" resulted in "a great howl
from the 'liberty-loving batchelor' and I regret to say, some of the 'liberty-
loving married men.'"[647] The pamphlets he wrote to be distributed by
physicians were graphic and filled with stern warnings about syphilis.
"If it does not kill him it may blind him, rot his bones, or make him insane."[648] To those already infected, he counseled, "Keep away from women,
do not even let your mind approach the immodest." Those who would
ignore the message and pass on a venereal disease were "worse than the
most cowardly murderer."[649]

Untreated syphilis could progress to the tertiary stage, causing brain
and major artery damage. While there is no way to calculate the exact

Many early public campaigns against venereal disease carried stern warnings.

A syphilitic woman may be as fair as a rose to the glance—

—but more dangerous than a leper.

number of advanced syphilis cases, by the 1930s mental hospitals were crowded with neurosyphilis patients. Other serious complications from syphilis, such as Charcot's joints and aortic aneurysms, were also common. The discovery of antibiotics in the 1940s was a breakthrough in treatment for syphilis as well as gonorrhea. Yet some of the more recently discovered sexually transmitted diseases are incurable (notably AIDS), and undiagnosed and untreated syphilis, gonorrhea, and other venereal infections continue to be a public health concern today.

Tuberculosis

Tuberculosis is an ancient disease woven into the fabric of mankind's history. It is common in places of poverty, crowded and unsanitary living conditions, and inadequate nutrition. It also frequently infects miners and others with damaged lungs. Consumption, as it was once called—also known as the white plague—was contagious, incurable, and often fatal.[650] The development of antibiotics and other therapies have curbed the disease in the United States and Europe, but it still threatens public health today. After years of declining cases, tuberculosis is again on the rise, particularly in developing countries. It was never completely eradicated from areas of the world with crowded, unhygienic living conditions and poor nutrition. Furthermore, it is the leading cause of death among HIV-positive patients. The pandemic of HIV is directly responsible for the recent resurgence of TB. Strains of tubercle bacillus (*Mycobacterium tuberculosis*) are becoming resistant to antibiotics and constitute a potential disaster if they are not isolated and contained.

Tuberculosis is generally transmitted either through the air or, less frequently, in contaminated meat or milk. People infected with the pathogen that causes the disease may develop pulmonary disease if they are susceptible. The onset of pulmonary tuberculosis is slow and insidious with cough, lassitude, loss of weight, fever, and general debility. In advanced cases, expectorated sputum becomes bloody (hemoptysis). Before modern diagnostic methods such as X-rays, hemoptysis was accepted as the definitive symptom. In the case of ingested bacteria from milk or meat, bovine tuberculosis, a condition most common in children, bone and lymph node infections developed. The mortality rate for bovine tuberculosis was over twenty percent.

Well into the twentieth century, many tuberculars came west to ease their condition. It was believed that the cold, dry air of the mountains and High Plains was therapeutic, and it probably was. Among the proponents of the western "cure" was Mark Twain, who wrote in *Roughing It*, "Three months of camp life on Lake Tahoe would restore an Egyptian

The Desert Sanitarium, Tucson, Arizona, circa 1935, now the site of the Tucson Medical Center. Many patients with tuberculosis came to the West in the belief that the high altitude, clean air, and dry climate was curative. —Courtesy Arizona Historical Society

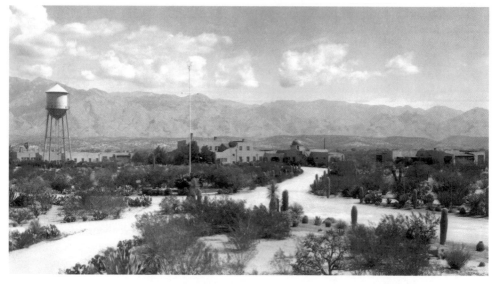

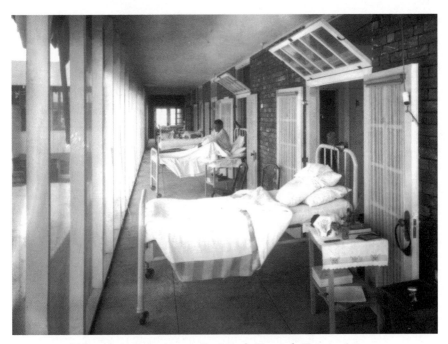

Tuberculosis sanitarium at St. Mary's Hospital, Tucson, Arizona
—Courtesy Arizona Historical Society

mummy to pristine vigor . . . I know a [consumptive] who went there to die but he made a failure of it."[651] In fact, a lot of consumptives who came west survived. Among the most popular relocations were to Albuquerque, Denver, and Tucson. Albuquerque, someone once quipped, had only two industries: the railroad and tuberculosis.

California was also a major destination—so many tuberculars migrated to the Golden State that in 1900 the California Board of Health attempted to ban them from entering.[652] According to some estimates, twenty-five percent of the people who came west were seeking better health, most of them tuberculars.[653] Many hospitals and sanitariums were built out west in the early twentieth century to accommodate tuberculars. Most provided their patients with some kind of outdoor therapy. Sometimes beds would be rolled out onto a sleeping porch when the weather permitted.

Doctors, because of their likelihood of exposure to infection, were often victims of consumption, and many of them joined the exodus west. In December 1912 Dr. Charles B. Penrose came to Wyoming from

Philadelphia to recuperate from tuberculosis. His own program of reha-
bilitation included shoveling dirt with the city engineer of Cheyenne for
two hours every morning, then riding horseback for two or three hours
more—all in the bitter cold Wyoming winter. He ate enormous meals
and took large doses of cod liver oil several times a day. By March of the
next year, he was fully recovered, proving that some people with hardy
constitutions and the will to survive outlived their disease.[654]

Yet the western climate hardly cured everyone. Tuberculosis was epidemic in the early 1900s in many places in the West, particularly mining
towns and Indian reservations. Miners, their lungs weakened by rock
dust, were susceptible to TB, dubbed "miner's con[sumption]," and the
crowded, unsanitary living conditions of many mining towns were breed-
ing grounds for infectious diseases of all kinds. As a center of industriali-
zation, with the state's only tenement housing, the mining city of Butte
was a prime example. As late as 1930, Butte underground miners had an
annual mortality rate from tuberculosis of 661 deaths per 100,000, ten
times the national average.[655]

In spite of these deplorable numbers, the campaign against the spread
of TB in Montana was strewn with obstacles. It was difficult to convince
politicians at the turn of the century to spend money on disease control.
More difficult still was to convince private companies to do so. Both the
mining and the cattle industries resisted taking responsibility for their
roles in the spread of TB, and progress against the disease was slow.

On June 23, 1916, public-spirited people in Butte formed the
Montana Tuberculosis Association, working with the Federal Bureau of
Mines and the United States Public Health Service to find the cause
of "miner's con." With eighty-five dollars in their coffers, the association
hired Dr. Anthony J. Lanza to begin an investigation of the mines and
to establish a clinic for the diagnosis and treatment of tuberculosis in
Butte. Between 1916 and 1918, Dr. Lanza examined 1,018 miners; 432
(42 percent) of them were found to have lung damage, and 63 of the
men with damaged lungs had tuberculosis.[656] After extensive studies in
the underground mines that included more than ten thousand readings
on the amount of dust in the air at different locations, Dr. Lanza and
engineer D. H. Harrington, assigned to the project by the United States
Bureau of Mines, presented their report. It explained the connections between mine dust, lung damage, and tuberculosis and offered concrete and
practical, albeit expensive, recommendations to the Anaconda Mining
Company for protecting their employees. A later, 1921 report clarified

the conditions known as "miner's lung," a form of pneumoconiosis called silicosis that follows prolonged exposure to rock dust, and "miner's con," which is tuberculosis superimposed on miner's lung.

The report stated that miner's lung "is neither contagious nor infectious, develops slowly, and by the production of scar tissue gradually impairs the function of the lungs." The condition "so predisposes a man to various infections of the lungs and bronchial passages that few victims escape such infection. Pneumonia and tuberculosis are especially likely to occur, and the vast majority of miners with considerable dust damage to the lungs contract tuberculosis and ultimately die of it, particularly if exposure to the dust continues."[657] The report asserted that, in the miner with damaged lungs, tuberculosis was much more progressive and dangerous than in other people.

This damning information was never reported by Montana's news media, however. Anyone familiar with the influence of the mining industry in Montana history will know why. The Anaconda Company controlled most of the newspapers in the state and didn't allow anything to be published that might be detrimental to its interests. The rise of unions in the 1930s eventually helped push through legislation that addressed some of these health issues, though it took decades.

The fight against bovine tuberculosis was no easier. The efforts of Montana veterinarians and physicians to control the disease that lurked in the dairy and beef herds would fill a book. Ranchers and farmers furiously resisted having their cattle tested for tuberculosis—they resented government regulations and any other interference in their business. To add to the problem, the process of testing cattle was difficult in itself, and infected animals had to be destroyed. It was estimated that ten percent of the cattle brought into the state were infected with the tubercle bacillus.[658]

The monumental task of identifying bovine tuberculosis in dairy cows fell to Dr. M. E. Knowles, the state veterinarian, beginning in 1911. To test the cows, the veterinarian had to collect six daily rectal temperatures before injecting tuberculin (a solution of killed tubercle bacilli). Then he took six more daily temperatures. If the animal responded with fever, it had to be destroyed. Needless to say, it was a slow and exhausting process. The cattle had to be rounded up, worked through chutes, and inserted with the thermometers. Because the vet's presence was resented, the dairy hands and cowboys seldom helped. The vet had to work in sometimes cold, wet, muddy, and sloppy corrals, in every kind of weather, often with farmers who were, to say the least, uncooperative. By 1916 the testing law included beef cattle, so veterinarians had to apply their thermometer and needle to these even more difficult critters.

Unscrupulous dealers persisted in sending sick cattle to Montana. At least one Chicago dealer was imprisoned for the practice, and in 1913 an entire shipment of fifty-six cattle had to be destroyed.[659] In addition, furtive farmers and ranchers began to transfer ear tags indicating that a cow was not infected to animals that were not yet tested, and the veterinarians were forced to take photographs of each animal they examined. Later, researchers led by Dr. William Welch of the Montana State Agricultural College Experiment Station developed an intradermal test that was far easier and required a lot less cowboying.[660] In the meantime, ranchers and dairymen gradually became more enlightened, and eventually bovine tuberculosis was controlled.

Not everyone was pleased with the progress of the veterinarians. Dr. Tuttle, who had been trying unsuccessfully for several years to get the state of Montana to require that tuberculosis in humans be reported,

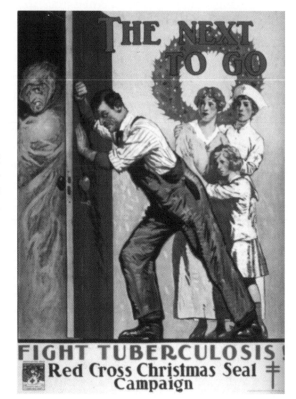

This 1919 Red Cross poster portrays its efforts to combat tuberculosis.

was incensed that more attention had been given to livestock than to people. He said, "Great is Montana, great are her cattle, her sheep, and her mines, but her people are of very little importance according to the present laws for the prevention of disease."[661]

While health advocates battled for better health legislation and enforcement, other efforts focused on TB treatment and on prevention through isolation of the infected. The tuberculosis sanitarium at Galen, Montana, was built in 1913. The hospital, near Warm Springs, satisfied the criteria of the times as ideal for tuberculosis treatment: its elevation was high (4,600 feet), the air was clean and often cold, the surroundings were picturesque, and, as historian Connie Staudohar pointed out, "implied, but not spoken, was the added advantage of isolation."[662] Not only did the public fear this illness and prefer patients be isolated, but the hospital's remoteness made it more difficult for unhappy patients to escape.

Galen grew as a tuberculosis center. Most of the early admissions were patients in a far advanced stage, so recoveries were rare. When Dr. Thomas Tuttle retired from the Montana State Board of Health in 1912, he became the first director of the Galen sanitarium. After he retired in 1915, his successor, Dr. Alexander McDonald, increased the bed capacity. Although McDonald lobbied constantly for an X-ray machine, he died in 1919, the year before this essential equipment was funded. After Dr. McDonald died, Dr. Charles Vidal took over. Originally a Canadian, Dr. Vidal had practiced in Montana for a long time, mostly in mining communities, but he had also worked in France, where he observed the latest developments in the diagnosis and treatment of tuberculosis.

Soon after Vidal arrived at Galen, he took up McDonald's cause for an X-ray machine, and the legislature finally relented. Vidal also made other improvements, and Galen began to have "graduates," patients whose TB was arrested. A tubercular was considered arrested when repeated sputum cultures were found negative for tubercle bacillus. Dr. Vidal even helped former patients find employment after they left the institution. The state health department's biennial report of 1919-20 showed a gradual reduction in the death rate from tuberculosis. Still, Montana did not compare favorably with other northwestern states. Vidal, the Montana Tuberculosis Association, and numerous others carried on in their work to reduce TB and made steady progress into the 1920s and 1930s.

Unfortunately, the efforts to control tuberculosis did not embrace all Montana citizens. Progress lagged behind in prevention and treatment for Native Americans. Children under age five were especially susceptible. On the Indian reservations, tuberculosis accounted for a third of infant deaths. Even though health officials knew of the problem, it was 1926 before preliminary health studies were made and 1930 before any major effort began to control it. By this time, death rates from tuberculosis on the reservations were twenty times those of whites.

In 1926, only 2.4 percent of Montana's population was Indian, but one-fourth of the state's 371 deaths from tuberculosis were Indian.[663] The sanitarium at Galen did not admit Native Americans until 1954, when a separate building was constructed for them. Indians with tuberculosis remained in the home, where they were a potential source of infection to everyone in the household. Furthermore, most sick Indians refused to be hospitalized far away from their home and family. Dr. Arthur C. Knight Jr., medical director at Galen in the 1950s, recalled a young Blackfeet woman with minimal pulmonary involvement. She refused to stay at Galen, returned home, and in a few months came back with advanced tuberculosis and died. She had several children and eventually they were hospitalized with tuberculosis as well.[664]

Though extrapulmonary tuberculosis is not uncommon, Dr. Knight said that in Native American patients, tuberculosis often appeared in unusual locations such as the eyes or tongue, rare in Caucasian tuberculars. There could also be bone involvement. The Crow woman Pretty Shield lost two daughters to tuberculosis. "Sickness came, strange sickness that nobody knew about. . . . My daughter stepped into a horse's track that was deep in the dried clay, and hurt her ankle. I could not heal her: nobody could. The white doctor told me that the same sickness that makes people cough themselves to death was in my daughter's ankle. I did not believe it, and yet she died. . . . Then my other daughter died."[665]

During the 1930s and 1940s, several surgical techniques in the treatment of pulmonary tuberculosis were developed. At Galen Hospital in the early 1930s, after Dr. Vidal's tragic premature death, he was replaced by Dr. Frank I. Terrill, a pioneer bronchoscopist who had trained in these specialized procedures in Europe. Using methods that included pneumoperitoneum, pneumothorax, phrenicotomy, and pulmonary resection, Dr. Terrill effected the arrest of many active cases. Eventually, with these advancements in diagnosis and treatment and with the gradual acceptance of preventive measures among the tribes, Montana's TB mortality rate dropped. In 1916, 521 people died from tuberculosis, but in 1942 the figure had decreased to 195. Proportionally the incidence of the disease in the Indian population had dropped from twenty times that of white people to eight times.[666] Nevertheless, hundreds of new cases were still occurring.

The big breakthrough in treatment came with the discovery of the antibiotic streptomycin, a chemical that specifically inhibited the tubercle bacillus. For the first time, an outright cure for tuberculosis was possible. According to his successor Dr. Knight, Dr. Terrill was so amazed at the response of his patients to streptomycin, which became available in 1946, that "he could not believe his eyes."[667] In 1949 para-aminosalicylic acid (PAS) was added to the drugs that attacked the tubercle bacillus.

Now the hospital at Galen stands empty. Surrounded by cottonwood trees and unkempt lawns, the empty brick structures stand like monuments to the many sufferers who died or were cured there, but they are also memorials to those many, some unnamed, Montanans who saw a goal and reached it. Many frontier physicians, nurses, researchers, politicians, and others played a part in subduing the threat of not only tuberculosis but also typhoid, syphilis, Rocky Mountain spotted fever, influenza, and other diseases. With leaders like Thomas Tuttle, the active and involved Montana State Board of Health saved many lives and prevented considerable suffering.

Polio (Infantile Paralysis)

Infantile paralysis, also known as poliomyelitis, came and went like a ghost, leaving personal tragedy wherever it touched down. At first thought to be restricted to babies, hence the name infantile paralysis, polio was soon discovered to be just as common in older children and young adults. Initial symptoms of this contagious, acute viral illness include fever, sore throat, headache, upset stomach, and muscle stiffness. Polio often left its victims paralyzed, and it was sometimes fatal.

In the summer of 1916, the first, and one of the worst, major epidemic of poliomyelitis spread across America. Six thousand children and young adults died from polio that year, and at least twenty-seven thousand were permanently disabled. Only one percent of polio cases became paralyzed; the total number infected with the virus was in the millions. Of those paralyzed, half later regained normal muscle function, but between two and ten percent died.[668] The epidemics struck mostly in the summer—apparently the virus flourished in warm weather. Several more outbreaks followed the one in 1916, and epidemics continued to occur throughout the first half of the twentieth century, until the Salk vaccine was developed in 1955.

As early as 1793, scientists had noted that the disease was more common in rural settings. In 1916 the Public Health Department of New York City reported 28.5 cases per 100,000; at the same time in sparsely populated Montana, there were 34.2 cases per 100,000.[669] This confirms that populations in rural areas such as Montana were more vulnerable. The explanation? Using our present knowledge about viral infections and immunity, we can surmise that in more populated communities, the few sporadic cases exposed a large number of children to the virus. Many of them ingested enough of the virus to secure their immunity, and others developed subclinical cases that resulted in varying degrees of resistance.

Rural children had developed no such resistance, so polio hit hard in the West. Using Montana as an example, 111 cases of paralytic polio were reported during the fateful summer of 1916, with 24 deaths. During 1920-21 there were 50 victims of poliomyelitis with paralysis in the state. In 1922 another epidemic of polio struck, primarily in Yellowstone County, with 41 cases and 4 deaths. In the terrible summer of 1924, 182 young Montanans were paralyzed by the virus and 23 died.[670] Adding to the difficulty, good medical facilities were scarce on the frontier. But after the first polio epidemics, western communities began to build clinics and treatment centers that eventually rivaled those of larger towns.

Infecting primarily young people, this crippling fever alarmed the public more than any other illness. Further inflaming the "polio panic" were newspaper headlines such as that in the *Helena Independent* on July 9, 1916: "Awful Scourge Creeping West, Baby Paralysis Yet Unchecked." After 1916, for thirty-nine straight summers, American parents lived in daily fear for their children, haunted by visions of paralyzed children on crutches or wheelchairs or confined to gigantic iron lungs. Although polio was a frightful condition, the fear was out of proportion to the risk. In the time before antibiotics and vaccines, children were cursed by many other potentially fatal illnesses, such as scarlet fever, whooping cough, diphtheria, and measles. In the 1920s through the 1940s, the incidence of diphtheria was sometimes more than five times that of polio, tuberculosis struck even more frequently than diphtheria, and scarlet fever and strep throat occurred at least ten times more often than polio.[671] Furthermore, polio was less likely to be fatal than any of these. In spite of these statistics, the crippler polio was the most dreaded of all infectious diseases.

Why the greater worry over poliomyelitis? This emotional reaction was due to the chilling reality of being disabled. As painful as it is for modern readers to contemplate, there was a great stigma in the early decades of the twentieth century toward people in wheelchairs. Disabled children were not allowed to attend school, and some couldn't even go to public places. Cruelest of all, they were often the butt of ridicule. When these children grew up, they would have difficulty getting a job. In the minds of many during that era, to be crippled was worse than death. Nowhere was this feeling stronger than in the West, where everyone was expected to pull his own weight. Most of the work on a farm or ranch was physical, and each family member's contribution was important to the struggling homesteaders' survival. A child with a disability was a painful burden.

After 1916, physicians became inured to panicked parents who rushed their child to the doctor for every sniffle or tummy ache during the summer. At the same time, doctors were hard-pressed to diagnose the first case of a potential epidemic before the disease could spread. With no definitive laboratory tests, doctors relied on physical examination and experience alone. Any summer fever was suspect, since there were numerous subclinical infections that harbored the virus, and not all cases of polio developed the distinguishing symptom of paralysis. By the time symptoms of polio developed, it was often too late for quarantine to do any good.

Health departments tried to curtail polio by standard means, urging parents to instruct their children to wash their hands and to cover their sneezes, admonishing people to dispose of garbage promptly, clean anything that attracted flies, and drink only pasteurized milk. During epidemics, health boards also closed swimming pools and other public places. In Anaconda, Montana, when both daughters of a prominent doctor contracted polio, city officials filled the town's only public swimming pool with dirt. Most people kept their children away from any crowds during the summer. Kids were not allowed to go to the movies, the beach, or the county fair; even Sunday schools were closed during epidemics. While it often seemed a futile exercise, quarantine of polio cases was required by law. The homes of known victims were placarded, and though quarantined families suffered considerable stigma, the public insisted on such measures.

There was no known cure or treatment for poliomyelitis, but doctors could offer help with the complications of paralysis. For paralysis of the breathing muscles (upper neuronal paralysis, or bulbar polio), doctors aspirated the pharynx and the esophagus to prevent obstruction to the airway and used oxygen when available. In extreme cases, surgeons performed a tracheotomy. Skilled nursing care was extremely important, not only for the comfort of the patient but to prevent serious complications such as pneumonia and assorted other secondary infections.

After 1929, the iron lung became available for victims of bulbar polio, and in time it became the heartbreaking symbol of the polio era. Developed at the Harvard School of Medicine, the iron lung was a large rigid cylinder, sealed at each end, that encompassed the patient's torso. Inside, an air pump applied negative and positive pressure at intervals to assist weakened or paralyzed breathing muscles. Later a more sophisticated apparatus evolved, but the principle of alternating air pressure remained the same.

For limb paralysis, doctors and therapists applied various treatments. In fact, treating the effects of polio became an orthopedic specialty in

Iron lung —Courtesy National Library of Medicine, History of Medicine Division

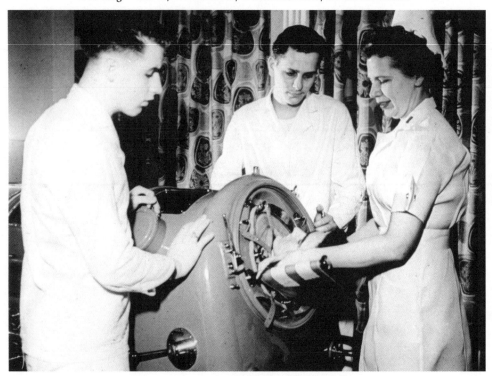

itself. Sedation, applied heat, and splints offset the painful leg cramps, and hydrotherapy was popular in areas of the West with natural hot springs. Orthopedic procedures were developed to stabilize joints in the later stages, allowing patients to sit up in a wheelchair or to use crutches. Most people crippled by the virus regained some muscle strength, and numerous therapies were used in the hope of maximizing recovery.

Around 1940 the Kenny system of physical therapy took America by storm. Developed by Elizabeth Kenny, a charismatic Australian nurse, the method was based on three modes: hot wool packs, passive motion, and reeducation of muscles. The Kenny system was not entirely welcomed by the medical profession, and some still debate its value. Nevertheless, her ideas dominated polio therapy, and because of her influence, the use of splints to immobilize limbs, favored by most physicians, was largely discontinued.[672]

One frontier facility that treated polio in the early days was St. Vincent Hospital and Orthopedic School in Billings, Montana. Dr. Louis Allard, a native of Laurel, Montana, arrived in Billings in 1914. A graduate of Rush Medical College in Chicago, Allard also had postgraduate training in orthopedics. The young, cigar-chomping doctor and Sister Arcadia Lea, of the Sisters of Charity of Leavenworth, formed "an unlikely pair of ministering angels" to hundreds of polio patients.[673] The two instituted a treatment program at St. Vincent Hospital, and by 1922, 467 patients from all over the country had been treated there.

Almost as soon as the polio virus was discovered in 1909, scientists began looking for a vaccine. Early efforts were trial-and-error searches for an antitoxin such as those used for diphtheria and other illnesses. In the early 1950s, gamma globulin injections showed promise in keeping exposed persons from developing polio. Gamma globulin, manufactured from the plasma of multiple blood donors, contains many antibodies. Before antibiotics were developed, it was used for passive immunization in measles, tetanus, and whooping cough.

When the Salk vaccine became available in 1955, there was no more guesswork. The vaccine was made from an inactivated (dead) polio virus that was injected. During the field trials in 1954, over 200,000 children in the United States were injected with the Salk vaccine, with no complications. The next year, vaccination programs were started in earnest. The number of cases in the United States fell from 13.9 per 100,000 in 1954 to 0.5 in 1961.[674] In 1961 the Sabin vaccine, made from an attenuated live virus and administered orally on a sugar cube replaced the Salk vaccine.

With each succeeding year following the institution of these vaccines, the incidence of paralytic poliomyelitis declined.

Infantile paralysis was virtually conquered, a parable of conquest of medical science over contagion. Today, the polio virus is confined to a few cases in underdeveloped countries in southern Asia and western and central Africa. Most physicians alive today who remember the terrible polio epidemics of the 1940s and early 1950s would agree that seeing polio go away was like witnessing a major miracle.

Influenza, the Great Plague of 1918

In 1918, in the midst of the Great War between the Allies and the Kaiser's Germany, "Something new was seeding itself in the throats and lungs of Americans that spring which would bury more human beings than the world war; and, like war, it preferred young adults as victims," historian Alfred W. Crosby Jr. noted.[675] From the spring of 1918 to the spring of 1919, well over twenty million people worldwide died of the Spanish flu. In the U.S., 675,000 Americans, including at least 43,000 servicemen, perished in the epidemic. It was the greatest plague in history.

Wartime censorship prevented the world from knowing the full extent of the epidemic across Europe. Spain, which had no censors, announced that eight million Spaniards had caught the flu during May and June. For no better reason, the killer epidemic was named Spanish influenza. No one had seen a flu of such toxicity. Healthy young men and women were felled suddenly. The disease was so lethal that death within two days was common. The onset of headache, fever, and muscle aches was in many cases followed by impaired breathing, pneumonia, and often death. The sickest had pasty, slate-colored skin, a condition called cyanosis, caused by a lack of oxygen as the lungs filled with fluid. The victim literally drowned in his own juices.

The Spanish flu virus was transmitted by airborne droplets from infected people coughing, sneezing, and spitting. The source of the 1918 pandemic is not known for sure. Historians and epidemiologists are still researching the subject. One theory is that the outbreak began in the United States in the spring of 1918, at an army base in Kansas, and was then carried by American soldiers to Europe. Within months the flu returned to whence it came, in a far more virulent and deadly form, and spread rapidly across the United States from east to west. By mid-September the medical facility at Camp Devens, near Boston, was overwhelmed with thousands of patients, and as many as ninety soldiers died each day. Bodies were "stacked like cordwood" or scattered in confusion around the morgue. In New York, 851 people died in a single day, and 11,000 died in one month in Philadelphia.[676] Meanwhile, soldiers and sailors were also sick and dying at sea and abroad.

As the virus moved west, no one, not even the most isolated people, escaped its wrath. In Kansas, deaths occurred by the hundreds, especially in the army camps. Hospitals and barracks were filled to overflowing, without sufficient cots, bedding, or medicines. Thousands of civilians were infected, too. In Montana, 5,000 citizens perished during the epidemic.[677] The main assault occurred during the fall and winter of 1918, followed by a lesser outbreak in the spring of 1919. The flu struck the state again in 1920, when 267 more deaths were reported.[678] Dr. John C. Docter, the county health officer of Granite County during the epidemic,

Emergency hospital during the World War I influenza epidemic, Camp Funston, Kansas —Courtesy National Museum of Health and Medicine, Armed Forces Institute of Pathology, Washington, D.C.

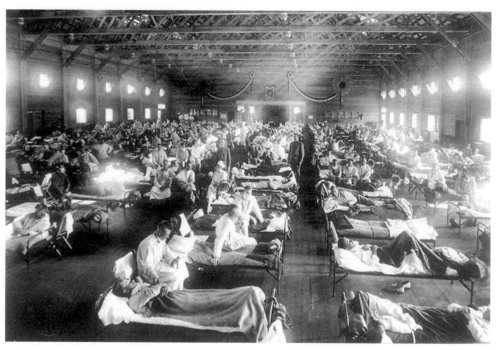

recalled, "Some of my patients died. . . . Mostly it was due to pneumonia. . . . Others died of meningitis. I worked day and night."[679] Louis H. Wolf, who grew up on a homestead near Ryegate, Montana, wrote, "We all came down with the flu . . . . There were so many funerals and no one was able to attend."[680]

Adding to the nation's crisis of extraordinary numbers of patients was a serious shortage of doctors and nurses, since many medical workers were serving in the war and some had succumbed to the flu themselves. Nurses were especially needed, as the flu had no treatment except bed rest and good nursing care. Doctors could do little other than establish the diagnosis. Their limited therapeutic armament consisted mainly of laudanum, whiskey, and mustard or onion plasters on the chest.

Most of the sick depended on volunteers to nurse them. May Anderson Vontver, a young schoolteacher near Lewistown, Montana, who home-steaded 320 acres of land by herself, answered a call from the Red Cross to work in a makeshift hospital in Lewistown. They told her that they hadn't been able to get any volunteers except one trained nurse and said, "Once you get there you will not be able to leave." Vontver remembered, "I had never seen anyone die, but that fall during the time I spent in the flu hospital, I got very well acquainted with death."[681] The matron, a Mrs. Capron, was a trained nurse, and a volunteer nurse known only as Miss Clark assisted her. Tragically Miss Clark contracted the influenza and died, as did the nurse who replaced her. The sickest patients, Vontver said, were the pregnant women, all of whom died.[682] "After a while we even got used to the matron's dog, who invariably would go and lie be-fore the door of the 'dying room' and howl at the event of each passing life."[683]

The little town of Harlowton, Montana, organized a temporary hos-pital, and some of the untrained volunteers helped there. Others, like young Jessie Moore (nee Poindexter), cared for patients in the home. "Sometimes," Moore wrote, "there were two, and once, three funerals in one day. The mortuary became short of caskets." Moore remembered a story of one large family, the Alts. En route to the hospital with carloads of sick Alts, someone noticed that little Joey was nowhere to be found. Moore went back to the house to look for the three-year-old. "I found him on the floor," she reported, "under a table, too ill to whimper."[684] But the story had a happy ending—the whole family recovered.

Montana's health department had experience with epidemics—including the tick-borne rickettsial disease Rocky Mountain spotted fever,

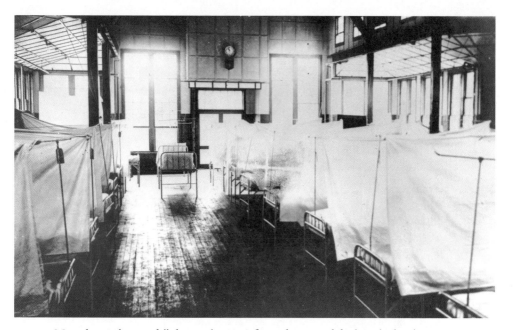

Many hospitals were full during the 1918 flu epidemic, and facilities had to be improvised in other buildings. —Courtesy National Library of Medicine, History of Medicine Division

tuberculosis, and clusters of diphtheria, smallpox, and exanthems—and it was as prepared as it could be for this one. But attempts to establish quarantines and ban public gatherings failed to slow the relentless progress of illness and death, mostly because they were ignored. Measures to curtail group assembly met with stiff resistance from interests as diverse as tavern owners, brothel madams, religious leaders, schoolteachers, parents, theater owners, and sports enthusiasts. These strange bedfellows combined forces to neutralize much of the health department's authority, and some openly defied the restrictions. Health officials in other states had similar experiences.

As governments tried with little success to control the epidemic, families coped with the illness as best they could. Home remedies for the flu abounded. Everyone seemed to have a favorite therapy or preventative. Old family recipes were taken down from kitchen shelves and poured down the gullets of children and adults alike. Tonics of hyssop, dittany, Peruvian bark, orange peel, anise, coriander seed, gentian, yarrow, nutmeg, thyme, rose leaves, and port wine were drunk by the glassful.[685] Most of the remedies were not harmful, and some gave comfort and symptomatic

293

relief. Bags of pungent herbs such as asafetida or camphor strung around the neck were thought to prevent illness. Another agent commonly used for grippe and other respiratory ailments was turpentine. This sometime "worm medicine" was mixed with lard and rubbed on the chest, then covered with a flannel cloth that, according to one Montanan, "drove the medicine right into the lungs."[686] Elmer King of Red Lodge, Montana, believed he knew the secret: "If they'd a' stayed home and eat a bunch a' quinine, I think they'd a been alright."[687]

Even doctors, with few effective options, prescribed medicines of humble or unknown origins. Myra Wilson of Sandpoint, Montana, said that her family avoided the flu with their doctor's prescription, about which she said only that "It was red—and it burned—but it did the trick."[688] Many survivors swore by the whiskey cure, including Louis H. Wolf: "Mother came down [with the flu] . . . and went into double pneumonia. All that Dr. Appleman gave her was whiskey, but this saved her life."[689]

With the public desperately seeking cures, the "patent medicine" industry made millions. Rinsing the mouth with a few drops of Liquid Sozodont in half a glass of water was advertised as a preventative. If you got the disease, "use Men-Tho-Eze and get relief in twenty minutes." Lysol disinfectant and Vicks VapoRub became household names. Horlick's Malted Milk claimed that their product fought the flu, and the Hyomel Inhaler, containing oil of hyomel, would "absolutely destroy germs of influenza."[690]

Homesteaders were not the only people in the West struggling with the deadly epidemic. The flu devastated Native Americans, most of whom lived on or near reservations. Because many of the Indian reserves were set up in desolate, unforgiving places, with unproductive soil and a harsh climate, the tribes were impoverished. With a nearly complete absence of medical facilities in these communities, death was rampant. Under the conditions of the reservations, effective quarantine was impossible,

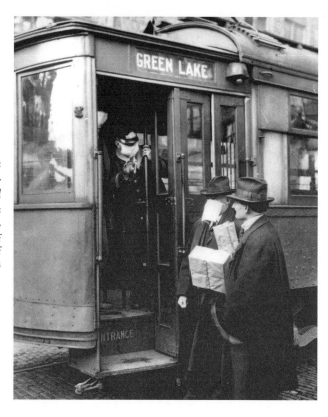

During the influenza epidemic, many communities required citizens to wear masks in public. —Courtesy National Library of Medicine, History of Medicine Division

and flu victims had no access to adequate hospitalization or even decent home care. American Indians were a forgotten people.

The Bureau of Indian Affairs reported that twenty-four percent of reservation Indians caught the flu during the period of October 1, 1918, to March 31, 1919, with an overall mortality rate of nine percent.[691] The Native American mortality in the mountain states of Colorado, Utah, and New Mexico was especially high. The death rate from influenza was twelve percent in Colorado and New Mexico, and sixteen percent in Utah.[692] Alaska had a terrible death toll; natives were "dying by swarms in the dark of the northern nights," as historian Ronald L. Lautaret put it.[693] Hundreds of children were orphaned. In one village, eighty-five percent of the adults died in five days.[694] The epidemic ravaged the coastal areas from Ketchikan to Nome, Cordova to Kodiak, though for unknown reasons it didn't spread inland very far.

On the lower Tongue River in Montana, fifty-three Cheyennes died in two weeks in October 1918.[695] In a 1998 interview, Biscoe Spotted Wolf, chief of the Northern Cheyenne council, described how families waited with their dead in long lines of horse-drawn wagons at the cemetery to hand-dig a place to bury their loved ones. The more traditional members of the tribe carried their dead to the rims overlooking the Tongue River Valley, where under the sandstone ledges they walled each body with small stones to protect it from the ravages of animals and desecrations by white men, who often robbed Indian graves for clothing, weapons, and other items.[696]

Many native people, bewildered by the white man's medicine, refused treatment. At government hospitals, the sick and dying would try to escape their confinement out of fear. The Indians' own tribal treatments were also ineffective. Among the Yavapai, the main shaman therapy was the powwow ceremony, which incorporated elaborate sand paintings. Navajo medicine men used the juice of the Arizona jimsonweed. According to one Indian agent, this juice makes the "pulse run high and causes delirium."[697] Another treatment was horsetail soup. Cheyenne healers treated their flu patients with sweat baths and peyote juice.

In Arizona, which had the largest population of Native Americans, eleven percent of flu victims died. Albert B. Reagan, an employee of the Navajo agency in Tuba City, Arizona, recorded an eyewitness report of the epidemic. He, his wife, and others cared for as many of the sick as they could, moving from place to place across unmarked trails through snowstorms and over treacherous terrain. At the Marsh Pass boarding school, twenty-three children were "frothing at the mouth and delirious," according to Reagan.[698] He listed over one hundred deaths within a radius of twenty-five miles of the school, nearly all of them young adults or children. In one Hopi village, 181 of the 300 inhabitants were sick at one time, suffering without food, water, or shelter. The epidemic caused great panic among the tribes. Inhabitants left for the hills to escape the dreaded disease, abandoning their belongings, including valuable livestock, and leaving their dead unburied. Even family members were left to starve or die from the flu.

This apocalypse of disease waned toward the end of 1918, with a lull in the number of reported cases. By the time the armistice was signed on November 11, 1918, the epidemic had apparently peaked. It was time for a celebration, and people were eager to gather. Armistice Day celebrations brought an effective end to any preventive measures that had been in place. For instance, in Butte, Montana, a community especially hard hit by flu, all rules were broken soon after the armistice. In spite of warnings by health officials, people crowded the streets to celebrate the end of the war and what they perceived as the end of the epidemic. Arrogant city officials reopened schools, churches, and businesses, including most of the drinking and whoring establishments. The illusion of success did not last long, however. During the parades and parties, many citizens who had hitherto avoided the flu were exposed. Not long after the sounds of revelry subsided, more people became sick, causing Dr. Dan Donahue of Butte to say, "World peace could not have come at a worse time."[699]

The second wave of this vicious strain of flu subsided in the spring of 1919, disappearing from the world as fast as it had come. For some reason, the global tragedy of the influenza pandemic is little remembered. Most history texts have ignored this event that compares with the great plagues of Europe. The lack of attention historians have given the pandemic and its impact is amazing. Most schoolchildren are taught about the plagues of the Dark Ages, but very few children or even adults are aware of the greater devastation caused by the 1918 flu. According to author H. L. Mencken, this selective memory is not surprising. "The human mind always tries to expunge the intolerable from memory, just as it tries to conceal it while current."[700]

It should be noted that the epidemiology of the so-called Spanish flu of 1918 is still being studied. It is possible, and some virologists say probable, that the strain that killed millions will return. Fortunately there is constant surveillance around the world for new strains of influenza virus, and as recently as the year 2000, epidemics of avian flu have been recognized and contained. Furthermore, researchers studying the 1918 epidemic have identified DNA fragments from archived autopsy materials, and health workers are hoping to concoct vaccines in case the strain returns.[701] The many advances in virology, immunology, and medical care will no doubt prevent such a great loss of life from influenza in the future. These continuing efforts by scientists around the world should give us a degree of comfort in the twenty-first century. Perhaps by the time the killer virus of that era returns, if it does, science will be prepared.

Medicine in the Third Millennium

Wouldn't it be great if science textbooks spent some time on erroneous past understanding that everybody believed, that the church and the state and the scientists and the philosophers and the schools all taught, and turned out to be completely wrong? Isn't that a very useful lesson?

—Astronomer Carl Sagan, 1996[702]

THROUGH TIME, medical science has ascended a long staircase of knowledge. Progress has been slow and tedious, but inexorably steady. Looking ahead today, we are no more able to predict what the next millennium will bring in the field of medicine than were those alive in the year 1000. Just as early physicians had mistaken beliefs and ineffective treatments, modern medicine may also be the victim of narrow and wrongheaded ideas that the future will clarify. Yet health care in the twenty-first century is undeniably better than ever before. Life expectancy today is extended beyond the dreams of the most optimistic of our forebears.

How did we arrive at this astounding level of medical care? Each new discovery was built on the foundation of work of past scientists. Information about the physiology of the human body steadily accumulated. For example, Antoni van Leeuwenhoek's discoveries with a simple hand lens gave birth to microscopic anatomy. This work eventually allowed for the revolutionary concept of germs, which in turn unlocked further medical mysteries. Each generation of scientists used past intelligence to create new and better treatments and methods.

In addition to the thousands of physicians, chemists, bacteriologists, biologists, physicists, mathematicians, and numerous other scientists who have contributed to the health care we now accept as routine, we owe a debt of gratitude to the shamans of ancient cultures, whose time-tested cures are recently finding their way into the armamentaria of modern doctors. Herbs and other materials in concoctions passed down through the years, ignored by "civilized" medicine for many years, are now being analyzed in chemical laboratories and are being used by clinicians of many different backgrounds.

As it has in the past, medical science will face many more challenges in the future. New illnesses and contagion will confront us. Scientists and doctors continue to struggle to prevent or treat AIDS, SARS (Sudden Acute Respiratory Syndrome), and many other viruses. The potential for bioterrorism is another momentous threat. Fortunately, sanitation, medical research, worldwide surveillance, and continuing education of medical professionals and the public are still priorities in our part of the world, priorities that we should pass on to less-developed societies.

Scientific medicine stands at the threshold of another millenium, a broad horizon in front of us. How we face this unknown future has yet to unfold, to be reported—probably with a mixture of awe and distress—by someone many years hence.

NOTES

Personal Reflections

i. Brewer, *First 100 Years*, 15.

ii. Ferrol Sams, *Run with the Horsemen* (New York and London: Penguin Books, 1983), 90-91.

iii. Brewer, 7-15.

Preface

iv. Published in 1876, *A Century of American Medicine, 1776–1876* was a grim summary of the so-called major achievements of the medical profession during that period. The last sentence in the book, "It is better to have a future than a past," is both prophetic and optimistic. Quoted in Thomas, *Fragile Species*, 8.

v. Turner, "Significance of the Frontier," 1.

Introduction

1. Henry Davidoff, *Pocket Book of Quotations* (New York: Pocket Books, 1942), 65. John Coakley Lettsom was a Quaker physician who, in 1796, founded an institution in Kent, England, for the treatment of children with tuberculosis. Apparently he was also a humorist. See also Cartwright, *Social History of Medicine*, 124.

2. Starr, *Social Transformation*, 42.

3. The term sanguinary is used here in the sense of blood.

4. Sullivan, "Sanguine Practices."

5. Estes and Smith, "*Melancholy Scene*," 7, 9-10, 128.

6. Flexner, *Doctors on Horseback*, 106.

7. Flexner, *Doctors*, 57-120; Hawke, *Benjamin Rush*, 203-223, 320-337.

8. Flexner, *Doctors*, 395-402.

9. Ibid.

10. Ibid.

11. Lipscomb and Bergh, *Writings of Thomas Jefferson*, 242-248.

12. Ibid.

13. Kaufman, *American Medical Education*, 43. See also Groh, "Doctors of the Frontier," 10.

14. Peller, "Walter Reed," 195-211. See also Altman, *Who Goes First?* 129–34.

15. Starr, 97.

16. Gevitz, "Sectarian Medicine."
17. Ibid.
18. Starr, 47-51.
19. McMillan, "Taking the Waters," 8. This work gives the most comprehensive discussion of the "spas" of Montana.
20. Cassedy, *Medicine and American Growth*, 88-93.
21. Kaufman, 45. See also Harvey W. Felter, *History of the Medical Institute* (Cincinnati: n.p., 1902), 41-42.
22. Kaufman, 72.
23. Starr, 100-101.
24. Hansen, "New Images," 629-678
25. Gordon, *Alarming History*, 107.
26. DaCosta, "Methods in Medicine," 409-413.
27. Warner, 472.
28. Reiser, *Medicine*, 157.
29. Magner, *History of Medicine*, 335-44.
30. Osler, "License to Practice," *The [Chicago] Journal*, May 11, 1889.
31. Starr, 40-42. See also Kaufman.
32. Quoted in Kaufman, 111.
33. Rothstein, *American Physicians*, 87-93.
34. In 1848, more than one-fourth of the practicing doctors in Virginia had received only a preceptorship (*Transactions of the American Medical Association*, 359-60).
35. Flexner, *Doctors*, 121-236.
36. Abraham Flexner, *Medical Education*.

Chapter 1

37. St. Pierre and Long Soldier, *Walking in the Sacred Manner*, 19.
38. Dubos, *Man, Medicine, and Environment*, 43-48.
39. Hrdlicka, "Disease."
40. Ibid.; Freeman, "Surgery."
41. Vogel, *American Indian Medicine*, 89.
42. Dunlop, *Doctors*, 14.
43. Vogel, 95.
44. Phillips, *Medicine*, 16.
45. Vogel, 95, 356–57.
46. Cohen, "Native American Medicine."
47. Stone, *American Indian Medicine*, 57.
48. Cohen, 45-57. The Great Mystery goes by many names, such as *Wakan Tanka* to the Lakota Sioux and *Achadadea* to the Crows. The concept, however, is common in virtually all native cultures.
49. Fire and Erdoes, *Lame Deer*, 11-16.
50. Hultkrantz, *Shamanic Healing*, 71-104.
51. Monastersky, "Plumbing Ancient Rituals," A 23.

52. Linderman, *Plenty-Coups*, 28-29.

53. Evers, *Blackfeet*, 162-82.

54. Vogel, 156–57.

55. Denig, *Five Indian Tribes*, 186–87.

56. Vogel, 22-23, says that *shaman* is an Asian term that has come to mean Indian healer. Early observers designated shamans by such terms as healer, sorcerer, seer, educator, and priest. In some tribes, the healer is specialized; some modern students hold that those who practiced herbal medicine were designated medicine men. See also Stone, *American Indian Medicine*, 1-21.

57. Ambrose, *Crazy Horse*, 351-52.

58. Mathes, "Native American Women," 41-48.

59. Hultkrantz, 1-20, 71–104.

60. St. Pierre and Long Soldier, 19.

61. Moorman, "Pioneer Medicine," 795-810.

62. Sigerist, *History of Medicine*, 166-69.

63. Gone, *Seven Visions*, 29-58.

64. Sigerist, *American Medicine*, 166-68.

65. Denig, 73-80.

66. Quoted in McVaugh, "Bedside Manners," 201-23.

67. Sohn, *A Saw*, 40-41.

68. Hart and Moore, *Montana Native Plants*, 67. See also Jeffrey A. Hart, "Ethnobotany."

69. Hart and Moore, 6.

70. Densmore, *How Indians Use Wild Plants*, 322.

71. Hart and Moore, 18-19.

72. Densmore, *How Indians Use Wild Plants*, 352.

73. Vogel, 249-50.

74. Hart and Moore, 27.

75. Hart and Moore, 46.

76. Bill, "Arrow Wounds." For more on bow and arrow wounds, see Steele, "Arrow Wounds and the Military Surgeon."

77. Stone, *American*, 82.

78. Densmore, *Teton Sioux Music*, 253-67.

79. Stone, "Medicine," 73-76.

80. Ibid.

81. Ibid.; T. S. Williamson, in "Dacotas of the Mississippi," 249-55, noted, "During long labor, rattles of the rattlesnake provide a pulverized medicine of much efficacy, possibly because the fetus hears the rattle and hastens to get out of the way."

82. Hart and Moore, 18.

83. Stone, "Medicine," 73-76. Stone bases his information on the observations of "Dr. Feed, U. S. A.," who for six years was in intimate contact with one tribe. Another observer noted only one maternal death in eight hundred deliveries during a four-year residence with the Indians. These informants apparently

noted a difference in the labor of Indian women who carried a half-white infant to term.

84. Denig, 186-87.

85. Riddle, *Eve's Herbs*, 47-48, 54-55.

86. Diamond, *Guns*, 195-214, 354-75.

87. Mann, "1491."

88. Spiess and Spiess, "New England Pandemic of 1616-1622."

89. Mann.

90. Diamond, 195-214; Stone, "Medicine," 27; Black, "Explanation of High Death Rates."

91. Hultkrantz, 13.

92. Diamond, *Guns*, 210. It took approximately fifty years for syphilis to become a chronic condition. Apparently the spirochete evolved in such a way as to keep its victims alive longer.

93. Crosby, *Columbian Exchange*, 122-64.

94. Quoted in Fenn, *Pox Americana*, 198, from Nisbet's *Sources of the River*.

95. Schultz, "Return to the Beloved Mountains," 26-33.

96. Denig, 186.

97. Young, 57-59.

98. Ibid.

99. Crosby, *Columbian Exchange*, 36.

100. Quoted in Stern, *Society and Medical Progress*, 153.

101. Fenn, 195, 208-09.

102. Irving, *Astoria*, 80-81. See also Fenn, 88-90.

103. Denig, 169-70.

104. Ibid., 71-72.

105. Ibid., 71-78.

106. Koch, *Life at Muscleshell*, 296.

107. Winkler, "Drinking on the American Frontier," 413–45.

108. Mancall, *Deadly Medicine*, 75.

109. Ibid., 116-17.

110. Ambrose, *Undaunted Courage*, 179-80.

111. Grinnell, *Fighting Cheyenne*, 94.

112. Abbott and Smith, *We Pointed Them North*, 123-24.

113. Bradley, "Establishment of Fort Piegan."

114. Quoted in Rice, *Black Elk's Story*, 33. See also Drinnon, *Facing West*, 100.

115. Mancall, 170.

116. Garcia, *Tough Trip*, 60-71.

117. Mancall, 69.

118. Bradley, *Contributions* 9.

119. Denig, 54.

120. Ronda, *Lewis and Clark*, 3.

121. Diane D. Edwards, "White Father Medicine and the Blackfeet, 1855-1955: Native American Health and the Department of the Interior," in Hildreth and Moran, *Disease and Medical Care*, 44.

122. Ibid., 41-58.

Chapter 2

123. De Voto, *Journals*, xliv.
124. Jackson, *Letters*, 1: 57–60.
125. De Voto, 489–99.
126. Quoted in Chuinard, *Only One Man Died*, 100.
127. Coues, *History of the Lewis and Clark Expedition*, 1: xx. Coues said, "The most serious defect in the organization of the expedition was the lack of some trained scientist, who should also have been a medical man."
128. Ambrose, *Undaunted*, 110-11. For more on Dr. Patterson, see Chuinard, 171–74.
129. Chuinard, 404.
130. Ambrose, *Undaunted*, 23. See also Chuinard, 106–8.
131. For more on this subject, see Estes and Smith, 119–30. See also Hawke, *Benjamin Rush*.
132. Chuinard, 145–65.
133. Calomel is now recognized as a liver toxin, but it was still used by some physicians until the mid-1930s. Jalap is a strong purgative on its own, derived from a Mexican climbing vine.
134. Quoted in Chuinard, 67.
135. Ibid., 55, 152-53.
136. Quoted in Chuinard, 116.
137. Will, "Lewis and Clark," 2-17.
138. Ibid.
139. For a comprhensive discussion of the Corps' medical equipment and supplies, see Chuinard, 145–65.
140. Loge, "Meriwether Lewis and Malaria," 33–36.
141. Moulton, *Journals*, 2: 81-82.
142. Chuinard, 71.
143. Moulton, 3: 243.
144. Ibid., 3: 281.
145. Ibid., 4: 334.
146. Will, "Lewis and Clark."
147. Moulton, 3: 281.
148. Quoted in Will, "Lewis and Clark." 287.
149. Loge, "Two Dozes of Barks." See also Loge, "Illness at Three Forks: Captain William Clark and the First Recorded Case of Colorado Tick Fever," *Montana, The Magazine of Western History* 50, no. 2: 2-15.
150. Moulton, 2: 306. See also Ambrose, *Undaunted*, 147, 217.
151. See Peck, *Or Perish in the Attempt*, 143–45, 205–6, 208.
152. Ambrose, *Undaunted*, 217.

153. McBride, "British Treatment of Sea Scurvy," 158-77. "Portable soup" was created by the British to prevent scurvy at sea. It was made by combining "the offals of cattle, flavored with salt and vegetables and then evaporating it down to form hard gluelike cakes." Other recipes for this nutritional supplement included mutton, veal, or egg whites.

154. Will, "Medical and Surgical Practice."

155. Fritz, "Meriwether Lewis," 9.

156. Chuinard, 223.

157. DeVoto, *Journals*, 21.

158. Chuinard, 255-58.

159. Ibid., 269-70. Lewis's scientific mind refused to accept the effectiveness of the snake potion without more proof, saying, "I must confess that I want faith as to its efficacy."

160. Ibid., 157-58.

161. Quoted in Will, "Lewis and Clark," 14. See also Ambrose, *Undaunted*, 350.

162. Quoted in Will, "Lewis and Clark," 14.

163. Ambrose, *Undaunted*, 354.

164. Ibid., 355.

165. Chuinard, 376.

166. Quoted in ibid., 368-70. The "string" is the spermatic cord structure, which includes the spermatic artery and veins.

167. Quoted in ibid., 177-80.

168. Ambrose, *Undaunted*, 115.

169. Chuinard, 23–24.

170. Moulton, 5: 125.

171. Quoted in Chuinard, 266.

172. Quoted in Chuinard, 253.

173. Ambrose, *Undaunted*, 380.

174. Ravenholt, "Triumph Then Despair," 366. Embarrassing diseases are seldom recorded in a military officer's record. There was some attempt to get permission to exhume Lewis's body for study, which might have settled the question, but permission was not granted. See also Peck, 295–300.

175. Moulton, 4: 297.

176. Quoted in Chuinard, 289.

177. Will, "Lewis and Clark," 10-11.

178. Fritz, 23.

179. Moulton, 4: 299-302.

180. Chuinard, 289-91. For a comprehensive discussion of the Sulfur Spring water and comments related to Sacagawea's illness, see Loge, "Miracle of Sulphur Spring."

181. Moulton, 4: 302-3.

182. Chuinard, 290.

183. Moulton, 7: 291.

184. Quoted in Chuinard, 389-94.

185. Phillips, "Devoted Botanist," *Bozeman Daily Chronicle*, April 11, 1995.
186. Quoted in Will, "Lewis and Clark," 15.
187. Quoted in Chuinard, 31.

Chapter 3

188. Neihardt, *Song of Jed Smith*. A fictional associate of Jed Smith senses the old trapper's feeling about the country as they sit on their horses looking out at the unspoiled terrain.
189. Neihardt, *Splendid Wayfaring*, 29.
190. Shilton, "Gone Under," 17-24.
191. Oman, "Winter in the Rockies," 34-47.
192. Denig, 9-10.
193. Shilton, 17-24.
194. Neihardt, *Mountain Men*, 109-10.
195. Parkman, *Oregon Trail*, 165.
196. Neihardt, *Splendid Wayfaring*, 49-50.
197. Vestal, *Jim Bridger*, 25-26; Neihardt, *Mountain Men*, 4-28.
198. Moorman, "Pioneer Medicine," 795-809.
199. Erdoes, *Tales from the American Frontier*, 121-27.
200. Osborne Russell, *Journal of a Trapper*, 101-7.
201. Neihardt, *Splendid Wayfaring*, 49-50.
202. Dunlop, *Doctors of the American Frontier*, 13.
203. Ibid., 15.
204. Phillips, 33.
205. Nisbet, *Sources of the River*, 1-7, 128, 158-59, 247, 248-49.
206. Jesse Thompson, "Sagittectomy," 1403-07. Thompson coined the term "sagittectomy" from the Latin word *sagitta*, meaning arrow or arrowhead.
207. Vestal, 91-95, 105-12, 137, 108.
208. Malone, Roeder, and Lange, *Montana*, 41.

Chapter 4

209. Lord, *A Doctor's Gold Rush Journey*, 15. Thus begins Dr. Lord's journey to the goldfields.
210. Ibid., 415.
211. Moorman, 804.
212. DeVoto, *Mark Twain's America*, 19–25.
213. Ibid., 39.
214. Ibid., 109.
215. Ibid., 7.
216. Drury, *Mountains*, 227, 250, 288.
217. DeSmet, *Life, Letters and Travels*, 1475.
218. Palladino, *Anthony Ravalli*, 1-11.
219. Dr. Wilfred P. Schoenberg, S. J., letter to author, June 16, 1994.

220. Small, ed., *Religion in Montana*, 1: 47-76. See also Malone et al., 62-63.

221. Small, 2: 219-54.

222. Thomas J. Wolfe, "Mormons and the Thomsonian Movement in Nineteenth-Century America," in Hildreth and Moran, 18-28.

223. Sohn, *Healers*, 93-105.

224. Root-Bernstein, *Honey, Mud, Maggots*, 119-32.

225. Wolfe; Quebbeman, *Medicine*, 28-30.

226. West, "Golden Dreams."

227. Blair, "The Doctor Gets Some Practice."

228. Ibid.

229. Holmes, *Covered Wagon Women*, introduction to Vol. 4.

230. Ibid., 3: 131-33.

231. Ibid., 1: 42.

232. Ibid., 2: 214-15, 241-42.

233. Dick, *Tales*, 180–81.

234. Quoted in West, *Growing Up*, 218.

235. Lord, 229.

236. Ibid., 430-31. The term "salivated" refers to the side effect of increased salivation from large, toxic doses of calomel.

237. Quebbeman, 32.

238. Moorman, 803–4.

239. Dick, *Tales*.

240. Ibid.

241. Quoted in Dunlop, *Doctors of the American Frontier*, 103-14.

242. Holmes, 10: 267-71.

243. Holmes, 2: 75-76.

Chapter 5

244. Lorenz, "Scurvy in the Gold Rush," 494.

245. Quoted in Read, "Diseases."

246. Lord, 194-95.

247. Ibid., 167.

248. Lorenz, 506.

249. Zhu, "No Need to Rush."

250. Groh, "Doctors of the Frontier," 90.

251. Ibid.

252. Ibid., 35–50.

253. Smith and Brown, *No One Ailing*, 51-66.

254. *Contributions to the Historical Society of Montana*, 2: 111.

255. Riley, *A Place to Grow*, 174.

256. Orestad, *He Named It Powderville.*

257. Seagraves, *Soiled Doves*, x.

258. Luchetti and Olwell, *Women of the West*, 33.

259. Petrik, *No Step Backward*, 48.

260. Petrik, "Bonanza Town," 89. Petrik vividly and extensively covers the subject of frontier prostitution in *No Step Backward*, as does Seagraves in *Soiled Doves*.
261. Quoted in Phillips, 64, from an anonymous source who also said, "She was more sinned against than sinning."
262. Petrik, "Strange Bedfellows," 2-12.
263. Smith and Brown, 10-12.
264. Dunlop, *Doctors of the American Frontier*, 116.
265. Fowler, *Mystic Healers*, 4; Groh, 10.
266. Sohn, *A Saw*, 90.
267. Phillips, 271.
268. Dunlop, *Doctors of the American Frontier*, 127-28.
269. *The Madisonian* (Virginia City, Mont.) December 28, 1878.
270. Ibid.; Phillips, 102-6.
271. Editorial, *New Northwest*, n.d., Montana Historical Society Archives, Helena.
272. Phillips, 90-91.
273. The following is based on Quebbeman, 128–33; Wesson, "George E. Goodfellow"; Trunkey, "Doctor George Goodfellow"; Chaput, *Dr. Goodfellow*; and Dunlop, *Doctors of the American Frontier*, 146–55.
274. Wesson, 238.
275. Quoted in Quebbeman, 128.
276. Groh.
277. This account of the Plummer gang and the vigilantes is based primarily on writings by authors such as N. P. Langford, who was himself a vigilante and thus not entirely credible (Langford, *Vigilante Days*, 148-61; *Montana Post*, February 2, 9, and 23, and November 23, 1867). See also Phillips, 82-86. For a different perspective, see Mather and Boswell, *Hanging the Sheriff* and *Vigilante Victims*.
278. Phillips, 82; Langford, 148-61.
279. Mather and Boswell, *Vigilante Victims*, 145.
280. Ibid., 102.
281. Francis, *Land of Big Snows*, 167-80.
282. Phillips, 210-12.
283. The term "gold mountain" was used by Chinese to indicate a land of opportunity, in this case the American West. See Paul D. Buell, "Chinese Medicine on the 'Gold Mountain': Tradition, Adaptation, and Change," in Hildreth and Moran.
284. Buell, 95-109. See also Petrik, *No Step Backward*, 23, 31, and Malone, *Battle for Butte*, 10, 67.
285. Sohn, *Healers*, 59.
286. Quoted in Phyllis Smith, *Bozeman and the Gallatin Valley*, 128.
287. Sohn, *Healers*, 29–30.
288. Zhu.
289. Shadduck, *Doctors with Buggies*, 153-57.
290. Sohn, *Healers*, 29-30, 91-92.

291. Buell, 95-109.

292. Buell. See also Zhu, 42-57.

293. Buell, 109.

294. Sohn, *Healers*, 59-65.

295. Ibid., 59-64.

Chapter 6

296. Gillett, "U.S. Army Surgeons," 27.

297. Ibid.

298. Wier, "Nineteenth Century Army Doctors," 196.

299. Tate, *Frontier Army*, 174–92.

300. Quoted in Tate, 174-75.

301. Tate, 174–75.

302. Phillips, 397-98.

303. Carmony, "Edgar Mearns," 24.

304. Wengert, "Contract Surgeon."

305. Green, "Neurosurgery on the Frontier."

306. Sohn, "Academic Examinations."

307. Olch, "Medicine in the Indian Fighting Army," 36.

308. Tate, 174-92.

309. Quoted in Wish, *Society and Thought in Early America*, 542.

310. Shryock, *Medicine in America*, 93-95.

311. Tate, 174-92.

312. U.S. Congress, *Report of the Commission*, 1:114, 265. See also Reed et al., *Report on the Origin and Spread of Typhoid Fever*, vol. 1.

313. Olch.

314. Tate, 174–92.

315. Freemon, *Gangrene and Glory*, 38, 142-46, 224.

316. Quebbeman, 2-7, 28-29.

317. Blair, 61.

318. Carpenter, *History of Scurvy*, 222.

319. Duffy, "Medicine in the West," 7-14.

320. Phillips, 41-43.

321. Carpenter, 253.

322. Sohn, *A Saw*, 112.

323. Lowry, *Story the Soldiers Wouldn't Tell*, 104.

324. Ibid.

325. Connell, *Son of the Morning Star*, 155. See also Lawrence R. Murphy, "The Enemy Among Us," 159-265.

326. Olivia, *Fort Larned*, 70–71.

327. Billroth, "Historical Studies."

328. Arthur M. Smith, "Dialing 9-1-1," 49–50.

329. John M. Gibson, *Soldier in White*, 30-32. See also Sternberg, *George M. Sternberg*.

330. Arthur M. Smith, 49–50.

331. Bill, "Arrow Wounds." See also Bill, "Notes on Arrow Wounds," and Steele, "Arrow Wounds and the Military Surgeon of the West."

332. Bill, "Notes."

333. Mays et al., "Treatment of Arrow Wounds."

334. Bill, "Arrow Wounds."

335. Brodhead, "Elliott Coues," 90.

336. Coues, "Some Notes," 323.

337. John M. Gibson. See also Beal, "*I Will Fight No More Forever*," 55-58, and Greene, *Nez Perce Summer*, 88-91, 93-95.

338. Winter, "Medical History of Miles City."

339. Gillett, "U.S. Army Surgeons," 24.

340. Ibid., 20.

341. Connell, 90-92. For more on Col. Guy Henry, see Hallberg and Neal, "For This We Are Soldiers."

342. McGreevy, "Surgeons," 777.

343. Connell, 405.

344. Ibid., 57.

345. Buecker, "Surgeon at the Little Big Horn," 43.

346. Ibid., 46.

347. Twenty-five soldiers were killed, and thirty-four were wounded; six civilians died in the battle, and four received wounds. There are various estimates of Indian casualties, but there were probably between forty-five and one hundred dead and wounded (Greene, 138, 364-65). Most accounts stress the disproportionate number of women and children killed. One estimate listed seventy women and children killed (Beal, 128-43).

348. Beal, 112-27. See also Greene, 117-40.

349. Gibbon had been wounded many times during the Civil War. A debilitating pelvic wound he received at Gettysburg gave him a limp, and he was called "No Hipbone" by the Indians. Bruce Hampton, *Children of Grace*, 155.

350. Beal, 112–27.

351. Bruce Hampton, 173. For an analysis of the medical aspects of the battle, see Steele, "Doctors at the Battle of the Big Hole."

352. Brown, *Flight*, 263.

353. Bruce Hampton, 173. See also Woodruff, "Battle of the Big Hole," 112.

354. Beal, 135, 254-55.

355. Phillips, 189-90. The doctors were Armistead H. Mitchell of Deer Lodge; James Wheelock and O'Dillon B. Whitford of Butte; James C. Merrill of Philipsburg; and William Lee Steele and Thomas Reece of Helena.

356. *Butte Miner*, August 14, 1877.

357. O. O. Howard, *Nez Perce Joseph*, 213.

358. Quoted in Phillips, 189-90.

359. Brown, *Flight*, 265-69.

360. Shields, *Battle of the Big Hole*, 84-85. See also Steele, "Doctors."

361. Raymond Wilson, *Ohiyesa*, 59-62.

362. Gillett, "U.S. Army Surgeons," 84-87.

363. Raymond Wilson, 45-52. Elaine Goodale trained as a teacher and followed a career of service that finally focused on education for the Sioux tribe. The Indian Bureau appointed her supervisor of education in North and South Dakota in 1890. In this capacity she visited Pine Ridge and met her future husband, Charles Eastman.

364. Copeland, *Charles Alexander Eastman*, 7–8. Dr. Eastman attended Beloit College (1876-77), Knox College (1877-80), Dartmouth (1883-87), and Boston University Medical School (1887-90). As a Native American graduate of one of the finest medical schools in the nation, he was exceptional.

365. Eastman, *From the Deep Woods*, 76.

366. Raymond Wilson, 59-62.

367. Eastman, 109-10.

368. Ibid., 111.

369. Quoted in Flood, *Lost Bird of Wounded Knee*, 58-60. In *From the Deep Woods*, 117, Eastman says in summation, "I have tried to make it clear that there was no 'Indian outbreak' in 1890-91, and that such trouble as we had may justly be charged to the dishonest politicians, who through unfit appointees first robbed the Indians, then bullied them and finally in a panic called for troops to suppress them."

370. Lost Bird's poignant story is told in Renee Flood's *Lost Bird of Wounded Knee*.

Chapter 7

371. Alderson, *Bride Goes West*, 205.

372. Swerdlow, *Nature's Medicine*, 9.

373. Fontanarosa and Lundberg, editorial, cited in Swerdlow, 12.

374. Fontanarosa and Lundberg.

375. DeVoto, "Frontier Family Medicine," 3–4.

376. McNeely, "From Untrained Nurses," 72.

377. Sue Hart, *Call to Care*, 11.

378. *Contributions*, vol. 3, 249. See also Schemm, "The Major's Lady"; Ariss, *Historical Sketch*, 15.

379. McNeely, 69-73.

380. Baum and Hollaway, *Broadwater Bygones*, 111. See also Montana Nurses Association, *Nursing in Montana* (1961), 2-4.

381. Vichorek, *Montana's Homestead Era*, 61.

382. Alderson, 202-9.

383. Ibid.

384. Hampsten, *Read This*, 111. See also Peavy and Smith, *Women in Waiting*, 291.

385. Peavy and Smith, *Women in Waiting*, 199-200.

386. Melcher, "Women's Matters," 47-56.

387. Meikle, "Jerks of Montana."

388. Karolevitz, *Doctors of the Old West*, 169-70.

389. Pickard and Buley, *Midwest Pioneer*, 40, 46.

390. Sohn, *Healers*, 93–105.

391. Stillman Jones, personal communication with author. See also Post, ed., *The Cottage Physician*.

392. Jones communication.

393. Shadduck, 310.

394. Root-Bernstein, 4-5.

395. Root-Bernstein. See also D. Blalock, "Grubby Little Secret: Maggots Are Neat at Fighting Infection," *Wall Street Journal*, January 17, 1995.

396. Root-Bernstein, 31-43, 81-97. See also Bauer, *Potions*, 281-83.

Chapter 8

397. *Stitches* 73 (1998): 40–42.

398. McVaugh, "Bedside Manners," 210.

399. Walter A. Brown, "Placebo Effect," 90. A *placebo*, derived from the Latin "I will please," is an inactive substance or a procedure with no intrinsic therapeutic value given or performed to satisfy the patient's symbolic need for therapy.

400. Holbrook, *Golden Age*, 48.

401. Karolevitz, 55.

402. Dick, *Sod House Frontier*, 440-41.

403. Holbrook, 263.

404. Reiling, "Quackery in America."

405. Phillips, 138–39.

406. Carson, *Roguish World*, 32-52, 155-77; McLemee, "Grift, Goats, and Gonads."

407. *Montana Post*, December 24, 1864.

408. Dick, *Sod House Frontier*, 440.

409. *Butte Daily Miner*, June 14, 1885. The word *empiric* in this context refers to the empiric school of medicine, or quackery, as opposed to rational medicine.

410. Ibid.

411. *Butte Daily Miner*, March 27, 1885.

412. Ibid., 410.

413. Quoted in Holbrook, 15.

414. Holbrook, 41.

415. Meikle.

416. Holbrook, 6.

417. Pendergrast, *Coca-Cola*.

418. Quoted in Holbrook, 31.

419. Exhibit at the Museum of Questionable Medical Devices, Minneapolis, Minn.

420. Macklis, "Great Radium Scandal."

421. Fowler, *Mystic Healers*, 5.

422. Holbrook, 196-97.

423. Stratton, *Medicine Man*, 44.

424. Fowler, 5.

425. Fowler, 61-78.

426. Stratton.

427. Holbrook, 31-35.

428. Stratton.

429. Ibid.

430. Ibid., 30.

431. Baum and Hollaway, 134-36.

432. Fowler, 9-10.

433. Sullivan-Fowler, "Doubtful Theories."

434. Ibid, 384–85.

435. Ibid.

436. Clark, "Madstones in North Carolina," 4.

437. Ketner, "Use of Madstones in Oklahoma," 444. See also Clark.

438. Clark, 11.

439. Ketner, 434.

440. Clark, 5.

441. Quebbeman, 218-19.

442. The First Church of Christ, Scientist, was formed in 1879 to "reinstate primitive Christianity and its lost element of healing," according to the Christian Science Publishing Society. The church's founder, Mary Baker Eddy, studied various curative systems for twenty years before she discovered the mental nature of disease.

443. Fowler, 17.

444. Ibid., 15-30.

445. Leffingwell, *Diamonds*, 62.

Chapter 9

446. Vichorek, *Montana's Homestead Era*, 20.

447. William G. Eggleston, "Our Medical Colleges," *The [Chicago] Journal*, May 25, 1889. Eggleston later moved to Montana and was editor of Helena's *Independent & Press* from 1900 to 1902.

448. Joseph Kinsey Howard, *High, Wide, and Handsome*, 196.

449. Spence, *Montana*, 6.

450. Coe, *Frontier Doctor*, 12-13.

451. Shadduck, 309-11.

452. Quoted in McVaugh, 212.

453. Niven, *Manhattan Omnibus*, 103.

454. Annin, *They Gazed*, 1: 326–27.

455. *Butte Miner*, June 11, 1901, quoted in Phillips, 129.

456. Reynolds, *Doctors Reynolds*, 34.

457. Ibid.

458. Quoted in Chapple, *Kayaking the Full Moon*, 106.

459. Chapple, "Doctors of the Wild West," 41. See also Phillips, 392, 398. At the time of his death in 1897, Dr. Chapple was mayor of Billings, and he was active in the planning of St. Vincent's Hospital.

460. Baum and Holloway, 216.

461. Brewer, 18.

462. Baum and Holloway, 215-17.

463. Watson, *Devil Man*, 105.

464. Headwaters Historical Society, *Headwaters Heritage History*, 606.

465. Elaine Mueller and Lindsey M. Baskett, interview with the author, May 1997.

466. Bierman, "Excerpts," 54-55.

467. Brewer, 16-18.

468. Gordon, Lehfeldt, and Morsanny, *Dawn in the Golden Valley*, 57.

469. Dunlop, *Doctors of the American Frontier*, 5, 129.

470. Mueller and Baskett, interview.

471. "Doctor Baskett Fit the Bill of a Small Town Doctor," *Big Timber Pioneer*, March 22-28, 1996.

472. Gordon et al., 68.

473. Hertzler, *Horse and Buggy Doctor*, 116-17.

474. Bridenbaugh, "History of Radiology in Montana."

475. Annin, 326-27.

476. Bridenbaugh.

477. *Ryegate Weekly Reporter*, September 21 and October 5, 1911.

478. Thomas, *Youngest Science*, 13-14.

479. Brewer, 24-25. Camilla May Anderson, M.D., spent her early life in Sidney, Montana. She studied medicine at the University of Oregon, graduating in 1929. She had a thirty-year career in psychiatry, mostly in the eastern United States. See also Vichorek, *Montana's Homestead Era*, 62.

480. Brewer, 19-20.

481. Rutkow, *American Surgery*. 32-33.

482. Hertzler, 214-47.

483. Melcher.

484. Winter.

485. Melcher, 52.

486. Melcher. See also *Great Falls Tribune*, June 6, 1982.

487. Martensen, "For Deliberate Election."

488. Foster, "Successful Case of Cesarean Section."

489. Brewer, 17.

490. Petrik, *No Step Backward*, 82.

491. Leslie J. Reagan, "'About to Meet Her Maker.'"

492. Ibid.

493. Petrik, "Bonanza Town," 256-57, 282.

494. Quoted in Phillips, 203-4, from the collected manuscripts of Judge Llewellyn Link Callaway, circa 1940.

495. Phillips; Petrik, "Bonanza Town."

496. Sohn, *Healers*, 79-82.

497. Winter.

498. Ibid.

499. *Independent Record* (Helena, Mont.), October 17, 1990; Theodora J. Smith (Dr. Benson's daughter), personal papers and communications with the author, May 1996; Dr. Arthur Foeste and Margaret Emmett, interviews with the author. See also Stout, *Montana*.

500. *Independent Record*, October 17, 1990.

501. Genevive Buchanan, tribute read at Benson's memorial service, October 15, 1959.

502. Alma Claus, "Rural Nursing and the Country Doctor," in Montana Nurses Association (1961), 2-3. The author gratefully acknowledges materials sent to him by Jeanne Claus of Bozeman, Mont., Alma's daughter-in-law.

503. Helen Fitzgerald Sanders, *History of Montana*, 2: 898. See also *Progressive Men of the State of Montana*, 2: 1248.

504. Shadduck, 3-5.

505. Shadduck, 309-311.

506. Coe, vii-xviii.

507. Tuchscherer, *Petticoat & Stethoscope*, 26. See also Phillips, 440-43; Dean Sisters and Maria M. Dean Papers.

Chapter 10

508. "History of Montana," Montana Historical Society Archives, photocopy, 1531-32. Helen C. Roberts was the first woman physician in Great Falls. She graduated from Northwestern University in 1888 and was the first female intern at the Cook County Hospital in Chicago. She came to Great Falls in 1891.

509. Magner, *History of Medicine*, 78-79.

510. Ray, "Women and Men," 2.

511. Ibid., 6.

512. Rainbolt, "Jessie Bierman."

513. Remembrance of Ann Whelan Arnold, M.D. (1897-1977), John H. Whelan, personal papers.

514. Peavy and Smith, *Pioneer Women*, 119.

515. Wood, "History of the Practice of Obstetrics in Utah."

516. Ibid.

517. Ibid., 70.

518. Peavy and Smith, 125. See also Wood.

519. Shadduck, 52.

520. Tuchscherer.

521. Phillips, 440–46. See also Tuchscherer, 26-27.

522. "Watershed in American Medicine."

523. Dean Papers.

524. Dr. Arthur C. Knight Jr., interview with the author, September 9, 1997. The patient was Mrs. Augusta Benson of Missoula, age twenty-two. She was in an advanced stage of active tuberculosis and died a short time after admission.

525. Connie Staudohar, "'Food, Rest, and Happyness,'" Part 2, p. 45.

526. Cornell, *Doc Susie*, 1-16.

527. Rowland, *As Long as Life*.

528. The following is based on Staudohar, various newspaper accounts, and unpublished works.

529. *Spokesman-Review* (Spokane, Wash.), March 13, 1955.

530. "Watershed."

531. Margaret Woods and research assistant Jodi Rasker, Museum of the Rockies, Bozeman, Mont., personal letter to author.

532. Cordua, "There's Just One Girl."

533. Ibid.

534. Reynolds.

535. Tuchscherer, v.

536. *Bozeman Daily Chronicle*, June 23, 1997.

Chapter 11

537. *Bozeman Chronicle*, May 13, 1996 (article on historic Bozeman).

538. Starr, 145-79.

539. Quebbeman, 31-32.

540. Sohn, *A Saw*, 51-62, 63-76.

541. U.S. Army Military History Research Collection.

542. Seibel, *Fort Ellis*.

543. Petrik, *No Step Backward*, 3-4.

544. *Montana Radiator*, January 26, 1866, in Malone et al., 69.

545. Phillips, 168-71, 191.

546. Sohn, *Healers*, 23-33.

547. O'Neil, *Muscle, Grit, and Big Dreams*. See also Sam E. Johns, "The Pioneers" (vol. 8), mimeographed manuscript, Flathead County Library, Kalispell, Mont.; a note states that the story was taken from Wildrey, *Whitefish Pilot*, 1941.

548. Pierce C. Mullen, "Frontier Nursing: The Deaconess Experience in Montana, 1890–1960," in Hildreth and Moran, 82–94; McNeeley, 70-76. See also Savitt and Wilms, "Sisters Hospital."

549. Sue Hart, 5-10.

550. Schwidde, *Medicine*, 33-41.

551. Northern Montana Hospital files.

552. *Bozeman Daily Chronicle*, May 13, 1996.

553. Dr. Merrill Burlingame, interview with the author, 1994.

554. http://thechildrenshospital.org/publications/VirtualTour/history/1910.html

555. Ibid.

556. Alfred Lueck, personal communication with author; Dr. Lueck also reported these cases in a Chicago address to the American College of Surgeons and to the Gallatin County Medical Society.

557. Montana Nurses Association, *Nursing in Montana*, 42-46.

558. www.pbs.org/wgbh/amex/nash/timeline/index.html. American Experience Timeline: Treatments for Mental Illness 400 B.C.–1949.

559. Sohn, *Healers*, 32.

560. Ibid., 33.

561. McMillan, "Taking the Waters," 66-70. See also Ed Amberg, *A Century of Service*, for a summary of the history of the Montana State Hospital.

562. Ibid., 69-70.

563. McMillan, "Eldorado,"; Phillips, 102-6, 172-75.

564. Montana State Board of Health, Twenty-Second Biennial Report (1941–42), 11.

565. Ibid., 2-3.

566. "Report of Special Joint Committee," 1-8.

567. Montana State Board of Health, Twenty-Second Biennial Report, 12-13.

568. Ibid., 33-36.

569. Grob, *Mental Illness*, 187-95.

570. Dr. Arthur C. Knight Jr., interview with the author, November 28, 1997.

571. Epstein, "Renal Effects."

572. Root-Bernstein, 44-58. See also Epstein.

573. Magner, 57.

574. McMillan, "Taking the Waters," 23.

575. Ibid.

576. McMillan, "Eldorado."

577. Ibid., 41.

578. Ibid., 58.

579. McMillan, "Taking the Waters," 71-75.

580. Whithorn, *Photo History of Chico Lodge*.

581. Mildred Webb and Phyllis Hillard (Dr. Townsend's nurses), interview with the author, March 1995.

582. Losee, *Doc*, 60.

583. Harry L. Helton Jr., personal communication with the author, April 30, 1997.

584. Brewer, 118-21.

585. Losee, 144-45

586. Brewer, 118-21.

Chapter 12

587. Quoted in Ariss, *Historical Sketch*, 5.

588. Pierce C. Mullen, "Frontier Nursing," in Hildreth and Moran, 82-94.

589. Starr, 154, 155, 159.

590. Baker, *Cyclone in Calico*.

591. *Illustrated History of the Yellowstone Valley*, 592-94.

592. Sarnecky, "Nursing in the American Army."

593. Ibid., 56.

594. Ibid.

595. Ibid.

596. Ibid.

597. Mary D. Munger, "In Tribute to Captain Octavia Bridgewater," in Montana Nurses Association, *Nursing in Montana*, 69-70.

598. Montana Nurses Association (1961), 6-7.

599. McNeely, *From Untrained Nurses to Professional Preparation*, 72.

600. Ariss, 19-21.

601. Rae interview with Montana historian Doris Whithorn, quoted in Tom Lutey, "Pioneering Nurses: Old Stories of Nursing in Montana Hard to Find," *Bozeman Daily Chronicle*, March 1, 1998.

602. Ariss, 19-21.

603. Ibid.

604. Starr, 154–57.

605. Wood, 66–73.

606. Quebbeman, 304.

607. Montana Nurses Association (1961), 64.

608. Mary D. Munger, "Nursing Organizations," in Montana Nurses Association, *Nursing in Montana*, 101-10.

609. Mullen, "Frontier Nursing."

610. Ibid.

611. Montana Nurses Association (1961).

612. Ariss, 5.

Chapter 13

613. Montana State Board of Health, Third Biennial Report (1905-6), 18.

614. Cassedy, *Medicine in America*, 34-35.

615. U.S. Congress, *Report of the Commission*, 1: 114, 265. See also Reed et al., *Report*.

616. Crumbine, *Frontier Doctor*, 132-34.

617. Stratton, 150.

618. Crumbine, 114. In this book Dr. Crumbine honors Dr. Eugene R. Kelley of Washington state and Dr. W. S. Cogswell of Montana for their early efforts to establish health boards: "We need more Kelleys and Cogswells," 95.

619. Montana State Board of Health, Third Biennial Report.

620. Montana State Board of Health, Third Biennial Report, 18.

621. Brewer, 73.

622. Price, *Fighting Tuberculosis*, 11.

623. Mullen and Nelson.

Chapter 14

624. Jessie (Poindexter) Moore, "The 1917-1918 Asiatic Influenza Epidemic," in Harlowton Woman's Club, *Yesteryears and Pioneers*.

625. Hoyt, *Frontier Doctor*, 180-83.

626. Leahy, "'Montana Fever.'"

627. Montana State Board of Health, Second Biennial Report (1903-4), 45.

628. Hertzler, 1-4.

629. Dan Burkhart, "Elkhorn's Cemetery is Grim Reminder of Days of Death," *Billings Gazette*, March 8, 1998.

630. *Madisonian* (Virginia City, Mont.), December 28, 1878.

631. Brewer, 68.

632. Montana State Board of Health, Second Biennial Report, 9, 61.

633. Ibid., 2, 6.

634. Brewer, 13-29.

635. Mullen, "Bitterroot Enigma," 2. See also Phillips, 271.

636. Strain, Family Papers; Phillips, 67.

637. Altman, 134-35.

638. For a thorough discussion, see Victoria A. Harden, *Rocky Mountain Spotted Fever: History of a Twentieth Century Disease* (Baltimore and London: Johns Hopkins University Press, 1990). See also Kalisch, "Rocky Mountain Spotted Fever," and Mullen, "Bitterroot Enigma."

639. "Stalking Mystery Killer of the Bitterroot Valley," *Great Falls Tribune*, March 2, 1952.

640. Altman, 307-8.

641. Malone's draconian treatment is well examined in Judith Walzer Leavitt's *Typhoid: Captive to the Public's Health* (Boston: Beacon Press, 1996).

642. Treacy, "Mountain Fever."

643. Coe, 43-45; Sohn, *A Saw*, 83-85.

644. Brewer, 69-70.

645. Ibid.

646. Jack Docter personal papers, in author's files and used with permission.

647. Brewer, 71; Montana State Board of Health, Second Biennial Bulletin (1903–4), 60-64.

648. Montana State Board of Health, Second Biennial Bulletin, 60-64.

649. Brewer, 71; Montana State Board of Health, Second Biennial Bulletin, 60-64.

650. Consumption was a term that described the way the illness consumed the body. The term tuberculosis was coined after the discovery of the tubercle bacillus in 1882.

651. Quoted in Rothman, *Living in the Shadow*, 137.

652. Staudohar, Part 1, p. 3.

653. Rothman, 3-4, 13.

654. McGreevy, review.

655. Staudohar, Part 1, p. 50.

656. Price, 22.

657. Quoted in Price, 27-33, 24.

658. Price, 15.

659. Ibid., 16.

660. Ibid., 18–19.

661. Quoted in Brewer, 73.

662. Staudohar, Part 2, p. 45.

663. Montana State Board of Health, Thirteenth Biennial Report (1925–26), 19.

664. Dr. Arthur C. Knight Jr., interview with author, Clinton, Montana, September 9, 1997.

665. Linderman, "Pretty Shield," 304.

666. Price, 71.

667. Knight interview.

668. Nathanson and Martin, "Epidemiology of Poliomyelitis."

669. Paul, *History of Poliomyelitis*, 79.

670. Montana State Board of Health, Special Bulletin No. 30, *Epidemic Anterior Poliomyelitis*, November 1925.

671. Daniel J. Wilson, "A Crippling Fear."

672. Pohl, "Kenny Treatment"; Daly, "Early Treatment."

673. Sue Hart, 21-30.

674. Paul, chaps. 39 and 41.

675. Crosby, *Epidemic and Peace*, 20.

676. Ibid., 3–13.

677. For a comprehensive discussion of influenza in Montana, see Mullen and Nelson, "Montanans and 'The Most Peculiar Disease,'" and Steele, "The Flu Epidemic of 1918."

678. Montana State Board of Health, Tenth Biennial Report (1919–20).

679. Docter personal papers.

680. Gordon et al., 60.

681. Vontver, "Reminiscence."

682. William Ian Beveridge and others have also observed that this flu was particularly notorious in pregnant women. They had an increased risk of pneumonia and death, and many suffered premature labor, miscarriage, and stillbirth.

683. Vontver.

684. Jessie Moore.

685. "Reports of the Council on Pharmacy and Chemistry," 1763-64.

686. Myra Wilson, interview with John Terreo, April 1990, OH 1209, Montana Historical Society Archives, Helena.

687. Elmer King, interview with Julie Foster, 1981, OH 368, Montana Historical Society Archives, Helena.

688. Myra Wilson interview.

689. Gordon et al., 60.

690. Mullen and Nelson.

691. Patrias, "American Indian."

692. U.S. Public Health Report, May 9, 1919, p. 1008-9.

693. Lautaret, "Alaska Disaster," 21.

694. Ibid.

695. *Butte Miner*, October 28, 1918.

696. Biscoe Spotted Wolf, interview with author, February 4, 1998, Ashland, Montana. See also Steele, "Flu Epidemic of 1918."

697. Albert B. Reagan, "The 'Flu' among the Navajos," 136.

698. Ibid., 132.

699. *Butte Daily Bulletin*, November 14, 1918.

700. Quoted in Rogers, editorial, 2193.

701. Tracy Hampton, "Clues"; Vastag, "Agencies Prepare"; Hammond et al., "Purulent Bronchitis."

Epilogue

702. Quoted in *U.S. News and World Report*, March 18, 1996, p. 78.

GLOSSARY

ague. An archaic term for a fever with chills, especially malaria. See malaria.

allopathy. In early America, allopathic or "heroic" medicine was based on the theory that disease was caused by toxins that needed to be eliminated from the body through such methods as purging, puking, blistering, and bleeding. Compare homeopathy.

bistoury. A long and narrow knife with two sharp edges for enlarging bullet and arrow tracks in tissue to facilitate extraction of the projectile and enhance drainage.

black measles. A synonym for Rocky Mountain spotted fever.

bleeding. See bloodletting.

blistering. Creating blisters on the skin by applying caustic agents, such as mustard plasters, as a medical treatment. The resulting blisters were then drained.

bloodletting. An archaic form of medical treatment, accomplished by cutting into a vein with a lancet or applying leeches. Bloodletting was a common practice until the Civil War, after which time it fell out of favor. See also cupping.

calomel (mercurous chloride). A toxic purge frequently prescribed for many illnesses. It lost favor in the early twentieth century. See also mercury.

castor oil. Oil of castor beans, a potent laxative popular as a cure-all in the nineteenth and early twentieth centuries, when purging the bowels was considered a panacea.

catarrh. An archaic term for inflammation of the mucous membrane, especially of the nose and air passages.

cathartic. An archaic term for laxative.

chloroform (mythylene trichloride). An inhalation anesthetic. Used less frequently than ether.

cholera. A type of dysentery caused by the bacterium *Vibrio cholerae*, transmitted in human waste. Characterized by severe diarrhea and abdominal cramps. The resulting dehydration was often fatal.

Cinchona bark. See Peruvian bark.

clyster. An archaic term for enema.

colic. Spasmotic pains related to the colon. A common symptom in gastrointestinal infections.

Colorado tick fever. A viral disease transmitted by wood ticks, characterized by fever, fatigue, and generalized muscle aches.

consumption. An archaic term for tuberculosis. See tuberculosis.

cupping. An ancient method of bloodletting in which heated cups are inverted and pressed against the skin over an insision in a vein, creating a vacuum to enhance bleeding. Also used to draw pus from an abscess. A similar technique involved placing cups over the affected body part, such as the chest or back, to relieve pain or congestion. The procedure was thought to draw out toxins and stimulate blood circulation.

diphtheria (croup). A contagious, often fatal throat infection caused by the bacterium *Corynebacterium diphtheriae*. It occurs primarily in children under ten and can cause death by either asphyxiation or heart failure. Characterized by the formation of a membrane in the inflamed throat that may obstruct the windpipe. An antitoxin became available in 1895. See also tracheotomy.

dropsy. An archaic term for heart failure.

dysentery. Any severe diarrheal infection, accompanied by passage of mucus and blood. The condition is usually bacterial and transmitted through contaminated water, milk, or food.

ether (diethyl ether). An inhalation anesthetic, extensively used in the late nineteenth and early twentieth centuries.

gangrene. Death and decay of soft tissue due to lack of blood supply. Can lead to death unless affected area is surgically removed. See also hospital gangrene.

gas gangrene. A gangrenous infection caused by *Clostridium perfringens*, a toxin-producing bacteria. Seen in badly contaminated injuries such as battle wounds.

gonorrhea. A contagious venereal disease characterized by inflammation of the genital mucous membranes and the urethra. Caused by the bacterium *Neisseria gonorrhoeae*.

gout. A form of arthritis (joint inflammation) caused by elevations of uric acid in the blood.

heroic medicine. A label applied to allopathic medical practice, which included bloodletting and the use of purgative drugs. See allopathy.

homeopathy. A sect of medical practice based on the premise that extremely low doses of substances that produced the symptoms of an illness could treat the illness by stimulating the patient's own defense and immune processes. Compare allopathy.

hospital gangrene. Before antisepsis was practiced in wartime field hospitals, wounds and surgeries commonly developed bacterial infections. One of these, known as "hospital gangrene," interfered with blood supply and caused gangrene and usually death.

hydrophobia. A synonym for rabies, so called after the fear of water, one of the symptoms of the disease. See rabies.

hydrotherapy. Immersion in water as a treatment for a variety of illnesses. Often prescribed by homeopathic physicians.

influenza. A common, often serious upper-respiratory infection caused by any one of a large number of viruses.

ipecac. A powder derived from the root of *Cephaelis ipecacuanha*, a Brazilian shrub, used as an emetic (to cause vomiting).

jalap. A strong purgative derived from the root of *Ipomoea purga*, a Mexican climbing vine.

lancet. A surgical knife used to make small incisions.

laudanum. A tincture of opium.

leech. A bloodsucking freshwater invertebrate, used in bloodletting. Used today for limited medical purposes.

locked bowels. An archaic term for peritonitis (inflammation of the abdominal lining), especially from a ruptured appendix.

malaria. A parasitic disease of the red blood cells, characterized by chills and fever. Transmitted by mosquitoes.

mercury. A poisonous metal. Various salts of mercury in different combinations were used for many years as medicine, such as mercurous chloride (calomel). Given orally, in ointments, or in baths. Mercury was a long-standing treatment for syphilis.

mountain fever. A fever of unknown cause that seemed to affect newcomers to the Rocky Mountains. It was probably not an entity but a term applied to a variety of illnesses.

neurasthenia. A condition characterized by fatigue, depression, and psychosomatic symptoms.

neurosyphilis. A complication of tertiary syphilis. See paresis.

nitrous oxide. One of the first inhalation anesthetics; also called laughing gas. Ether and nitrous oxide were popular as recreational drugs before they were used as anesthetics.

paresis (general paresis). A term used to denote the dementia and paralysis that may occur in the late stages of syphilis (tertiary syphilis). A form of neurosyphilis.

Peruvian bark (cinchona bark). The plant bark from which is derived quinine, used to combat fevers, specifically malaria. Early physicians also used the bark for any kind of fever, indigestion, and myriad other complaints, and as a poultice for snakebites.

pesthouse. A hospital for those infected with a contagious disease. See also quarantine.

pleurisy. Inflammation of the lining of the thorax, often with an effusion (collection of fluid). A common complication of pneumonia.

pneumonia. Inflammation of the lung, caused by many types of infection.

poliomyelitis (polio; infantile paralysis). An acute infectious viral disease, sometimes fatal, occurring usually in the summertime and infecting primarily young people, characterized by fever and paralysis. Vaccines against polio were developed in the early 1950s by Jonas Salk and Albert Sabin.

puking. Dosing a patient with emetics to cause vomiting, in order to expel toxins from the body.

purging. Dosing a patient with laxatives as a medical treatment, in order to expel toxins from the body. Enemas were also used. See also puking.

quarantine. Enforced isolation of persons with a contagious illness in order to prevent the spread of the disease. Also applied to vessels containing contagious passengers and to contaminated items.

quinine. A bitter, crystalline medicine made from cinchona bark (Peruvian bark), specific against the malarial parasite. See also Peruvian bark.

rabies. A viral infection of the central nervous system, transmitted in saliva by the bite of an infected domestic or wild animal. Caused by the neurotropic *Lyssavirus*. Universally fatal before vaccine was developed.

rheumatism. A condition characterized by inflammation in the muscles, joints, or connective tissues.

Rocky Mountain spotted fever (black measles). A rickettsial infection transmitted by wood ticks that follows a rapid course and is often fatal. Characterized by flulike symptoms and a red rash that turns dark and mottled.

scarlet fever. An acute, contagious streptococcal infection, occurring mostly in children, characterized by inflammation of the nose, throat, and mouth.

Named for the diffuse scarlet-colored rash that accompanied the illness, it often spread rapidly and had many complications, some fatal.

scurvy. A vitamin C deficiency characterized by spongy gums, loose teeth, and bleeding under the skin. An age-old disease that plagued sailors, soldiers, travelers, and others whose diets lacked vitamin C, untreated scurvy had a high mortality rate.

shaman. A traditional Native American healer.

smallpox (variola). A contagious, acute viral illness, often fatal. Characterized by a two-week incubation period of fever and malaise followed by a pustular eruption all over the body with insufferable itching and an unremitting fever. Easily transmitted by nasopharyngeal secretions or via contaminated items such as clothing or blankets. Eradicated in the twentieth century through vaccination.

syphilis. A chronic venereal disease caused by the bacterium *Treponema pallidum*, characterized by three stages. If untreated, can progress from chancres to a rash to brain and major artery damage.

tertiary syphilis. The late stage of syphilis. See also paresis.

Thomsonianism. A system of herbal medicine practiced by the Church of Jesus Christ of Latter-day Saints during the reign of Brigham Young.

tracheotomy. A surgical incision into the trachea (windpipe) to let in air. Sometimes used to treat obstructions caused by diphtheria.

trachoma. A chronic, contagious eye infection, caused by the bacterium *Chlamydia trachomatis*, that can cause blindness.

trephine. (Noun) A surgical instrument used to cut or bore a hole into the skull. (Verb) To operate with a trephine. Also called trepanning. The procedure was done to relieve pressure on the brain. It is an ancient technique and was used by physicians before recorded history.

tuberculosis (TB; consumption; white plague). A chronic, contagious pulmonary disease characterized by cough, loss of weight, fever, general debility, and bloody sputum (hemoptysis). Spread by droplet infection and by contaminated meat or milk. Caused by the bacteria *Mycobacterium tuberculosis*, TB was a common condition with no known treatment until the discovery of streptomycin in the early 1950s. Because most medical authorities believed that the cold, dry, high-altitude air of the West benefited the condition, tuberculars helped populate some western areas.

typhoid fever. A diarrheal fever caused by the bacterium *Salmonella typhi*, spread through the ingestion of water or food contaminated with infected human feces. May result in severe dehydration, damage to the lining of the small intestine, and sometimes fatal septicemia or peritonitis.

typhus. Any of several rickettsial fevers. Different types are transmitted by lice, fleas, or chiggers. Not to be confused with typhoid fever.

variola. A synonym for smallpox.

venesection. A synonym for bloodletting.

whitlow. Infection of the finger or toe, often under the nail and sometimes extending to the underlying bone.

whooping cough. A contagious bacterial infection of the bronchi and lungs, usually occurring in babies and children, caused by the bacterium *Bordetella pertussis*. Characterized by a spasmodic, intractable cough that often produces a "whooping" sound. May be fatal, especially in infants. Resulting pneumonia was a common cause of death, and fatal brain damage from high fever or hemorrhage could also occur. Vaccine was developed in the 1940s.

yellow fever. An acute, infectious viral disease transmitted by mosquitoes and characterized by exhaustion, fever, blood in the urine, and jaundice. Vaccines were developed in the 1930s.

WORKS CITED

Abbott, E. C., and H. H. Smith. *We Pointed Them North: Recollections of a Cowpuncher.* Norman: University of Oklahoma Press, 1939.

Abram, Ruth J. *Send Us a Lady Physician: Women Doctors in America, 1835-1920.* New York: W. W. Norton & Company, 1985.

Ackerknecht, Erwin H. *A Short History of Medicine.* New York: Ronald Press, 1955.

"AFIP Scientists Discover Clues to 1918 Spanish Flu." *AFIP* (Armed Forces Institute of Pathology) *Letter* 155 (1997): 1, 10.

Alderson, Nannie T. *A Bride Goes West.* New York: Farrar & Rinehart, 1942.

Altman, Lawrence K. *Who Goes First? The Story of Self-Experimentation in Medicine.* Berkeley: University of California Press, 1998.

Alvarez, Walter C. "The Emergence of Modern Medicine from Ancient Folkways." *Annual Report of the Board of Regents of the Smithsonian Institution,* 1938.

Amberg, Ed. *A Century of Service.* Warm Springs: Montana State Hospital, 1977.

Ambrose, Stephen E. *Crazy Horse and Custer: The Parallel Lives of Two American Warriors.* New York: Anchor Books, 1975.

———. *Undaunted Courage.* New York: Simon & Schuster, 1996.

Annin, Jim. *They Gazed on the Beartooths.* Vol. 1. Billings, Mont., 1964.

Ariss, E. Augusta. *The Historical Sketch of the Montana State Association of Registered Nurses and Related Organizations.* Great Falls, Mont., 1936.

Armitage, Susan, and Elizabeth Jameson, eds. *The Woman's West.* Norman: University of Oklahoma Press, 1987.

Baird, W. David. *Medical Education in Arkansas, 1879-1978.* Memphis: Memphis State University Press, 1979.

Baker, Nina Brown. *Cyclone in Calico: The Story of Mary Ann Bickerdyke.* Boston: Little, Brown, 1952.

Bauer, W. W. *Potions, Remedies, and Old Wives' Tales.* Garden City, N. Y.: Doubleday & Company, 1969.

Baum, Barbara R., and Grace Averill Hollaway, eds. *Broadwater Bygones.* Townsend, Mont.: Broadwater County Historical Society, 1977.

Beal, Merrill D. *"I Will Fight No More Forever."* Seattle: University of Washington Press, 1993.

Bettman, Otto L. *A Pictorial History of Medicine.* New York: Charles C. Thomas, 1972.

Beveridge, William Ian. *Influenza: The Last Great Plague.* Rev. ed. New York: Neale Watson Academic Publications, 1977.

Bierman, Henry. "Excerpts from the Journals of Henry Bierman." *Montana, The Magazine of Western History* 11, no. 1 (1961): 38-55.

Bill, J. H. "Arrow Wounds." In *A Report of Surgical Cases Treated in the Army of the United States from 1865-1871.* Ed. George A. Otis. War Department, Surgeon General's Office. Circular no. 3, August 17, 1871. Washington, D.C.: Government Printing Office, 1871.

———. "Notes on Arrow Wounds." *Journal of the Medical Sciences* 44 (September 1852): 365-87.

Billroth, Theodor. "Historical Studies on the Nature and Treatment of Gunshot Wounds from the Fifteenth Century to the Present Time." Trans. C. P. Rhoads. *Yale Journal of Biology and Medicine* 4: 119-47.

Black, Francis L. "An Explanation of High Death Rates among New World Peoples When in Contact with Old World Diseases." *Perspectives in Biology and Medicine* 37, no. 2 (Winter 1994): 292-301.

Blair, Roger P. "The Doctor Gets Some Practice: Cholera and Medicine on the Overland Trails." *Journal of the West* 36 (January 1997): 54-66.

Bodemer, Charles W. "Medicine in Nineteenth-Century Montana." *Rocky Mountain Medical Journal* 1979: 66-71.

Bradley, James. "Lt. James A. Bradley Manuscript." Ed. Robert Campbell. In *Contributions to the Historical Society of Montana.* Vol. 9. Helena: Montana State College, 1923.

———. "Establishment of Fort Piegan as Told Me by James Kipp." In *Contributions to the Historical Society of Montana.* Vol. 8. Helena: Montana State College, 1917.

Brewer, Leonard W., ed. *First One Hundred Years: Being a Review of the Beginnings, Growth and Development of the Montana Medical Association.* Missoula, Mont.: Bitterroot Litho, 1978.

Bridenbaugh, John H. "A History of Radiology in Montana." *Journal Lancet* 85, no. 10 (October 1965): 443.

Bright, William. *A Coyote Reader.* Berkeley: University of California Press, 1993.

Brodhead, Michael J. "Elliott Coues and the Apaches." *Journal of Arizona History* 14, no. 2 (1973): 87-94.

Brown, Mark H. *The Flight of the Nez Perce.* New York: G. P. Putnam's Sons, 1967.

———. *The Plainsmen of the Yellowstone.* Lincoln: University of Nebraska Press, 1961.

Brown, Walter A. "The Placebo Effect." *Scientific American*, January 1998, 90–95.

Buecker, Thomas R. "A Surgeon at the Little Big Horn." *Montana, The Magazine of Western History* 32 (Autumn 1982): 34-49.

Burlingame, Merrill G. *The Montana Frontier*. Bozeman: Montana State University, 1980.

Carmony, Neil. "Edgar Mearns and the Crook Black-Tailed Deer." *Arizona Wildlife Views*, November-December 2002, 24-26.

Carpenter, Kenneth J. *The History of Scurvy and Vitamin C*. Cambridge: Cambridge University Press, 1986.

Carson, Gerald. *The Roguish World of Doctor Brinkley*. Toronto: Clarke, Irwin & Company, 1960.

Cartwright, F. F. *A Social History of Medicine*. London: Longman, 1977.

Cassedy, James H. *Medicine and American Growth*. Madison: University of Wisconsin Press, 1986.

———. *Medicine in America: A Short History*. Baltimore: Johns Hopkins University Press, 1991.

Chapple, Steve. "Doctors of the Wild West." *Hippocrates: Health & Medicine for Physicians*, 1996: 31-41.

———. *Kayaking the Full Moon: A Journey Down the Yellowstone River to the Soul of Montana*. New York: Harper Collins, 1996.

Chaput, Don. *Dr. Goodfellow: Physician to the Gunfighters, Scholar, and Bon Vivant*. Tucson: Westernlore Press, 1996.

Chuinard, E. G. *Only One Man Died: The Medical Aspects of the Lewis and Clark Expedition*. Fairfield, Wash.: Ye Galleon Press, 1989.

Clark, J. D. "Madstones in North Carolina." *North Carolina Folklore Journal* 24, no. 1 (March 1976): 3-40.

Coe, Urling C. *Frontier Doctor: Observations on Central Oregon and the Changing West*. Corvallis: Oregon State University Press, 1996.

Cohen, Ken "Bear Hawk." "Native American Medicine." *Alternative Therapies* 4, no. 6 (November 1998): 45-57.

Connell, Evan S. *Son of the Morning Star*. New York: Harper & Row, 1984.

Contributions to the Historical Society of Montana. Vol. 2. Helena: Montana State College, 1896.

———. Vol. 3. Helena: Montana State College, 1900.

———. Vol. 5. Helena, Mont.: Independent Publishing Company, 1904.

Copeland, Marion W. *Charles Alexander Eastman (Ohiyesa)*. Boise: Boise State University, 1978.

Cordua, Olive. "There's Just One Girl." *Bulletin of the San Diego County Medical Society*, November 1962.

Cornell, Virginia. *Doc Susie*. New York: Ivy Books, 1991.

Coues, Elliott, ed. *The History of the Lewis and Clark Expedition*. 4 vols. Reprint. New York: Dover, 1987.

———. "Some Notes on Arrow Wounds." *Medical and Surgical Reporter* 14 (April 28, 1866).

Courtwright, David T. *Addicts Who Survived: An Oral History of Narcotic Use in America, 1923-1940*. Knoxville: University of Tennessee Press, 1989.

———. *Dark Paradise: Opiate Addiction in America Before 1940*. Cambridge: Harvard University Press, 1982.

———. "Opiate Addiction in America." Ph.D. diss., Rice University, 1979.

Crosby, Alfred W., Jr. *The Columbian Exchange*. Westport, Conn.: Greenwood Press, 1972.

———. *Epidemic and Peace, 1918*. Westport, Conn.: Greenwood Press, 1976.

Crumbine, Samuel J. *Frontier Doctor*. Philadelphia: Dorrance & Company, 1948.

DaCosta, J. M. "The Methods in Medicine in the Near Present." *Medical News* 51 (1887): 409-13.

Daly, Mary M. I. "The Early Treatment of Poliomyelitis, with an Evaluation of the Sister Kenny Treatment." *Journal of the American Medical Association* 118, no. 17 (April 25, 1942): 1428–44.

Dean Sisters and Maria M. Dean Papers. Montana Historical Society, Helena.

Denig, Edwin Thompson. *Five Indian Tribes of the Upper Missouri*. Ed. John C. Ewers. Norman: University of Oklahoma Press, 1989.

Densmore, Frances. *How Indians Use Wild Plants for Food, Medicine and Crafts*. Toronto: General Publishing Co., 1974.

———. *Teton Sioux Music*. Washington, D.C.: Government Printing Office, 1918.

DeSmet, Pierre-Jean. *Life, Letters and Travels of Father Pierre-Jean de Smet, S.J., 1801-1873*. Ed. Hiram Martin Chittenden and Alfred Talbot Richardson. New York: F. P. Harper, 1905.

DeVoto, Bernard. "Frontier Family Medicine." *What's New* 19 (1955): 3-5.

———. *The Journals of Lewis and Clark*. Boston: Houghton Mifflin, 1953.

———. *Mark Twain's America*. Reprint. Lincoln, Neb.: Bison Books, 1997.

Diamond, Jared. *Guns, Germs, and Steel: The Fates of Human Societies*. New York and London: W. W. Norton, 1998.

Dick, Everett. *The Sod House Frontier*. Lincoln, Neb.: Johnsen Publishing Company, 1954.

———. *Tales of the Frontier*. Lincoln: University of Nebraska Press, 1963.

Dillard, Annie. "The Wreck of Time." *Harper's Magazine*, January 1998.

Dorsett, Walter B. "Criminal Abortion in Its Broadest Sense." *Journal of the American Medical Association* 19 (September 1908): 937-61.

Dossey, Larry. "The Trickster: Medicine's Forgotten Character." *Alternative Therapies* 2 (1996): 6-14.

Drinnon, Richard. *Facing West: The Metaphysics of Indian Hating and Empire Building*. New York: New American Library, 1980.

Drury, Clifford Merrill, ed. *The Mountains We Have Crossed: Diaries and Letters of the Oregon Mission, 1838*. Lincoln and London: University of Nebraska Press, 1999.

Dubos, René. *Man, Medicine, and Environment*. New York, Washington, and London: Frederick A. Praeger, 1968.

Duffy, John. "Medicine in the West: An Historical Overview." *Journal of the West* 21, no. 3 (July 1982): 6-13.

Dunlay, Thomas W. "'Battery of Venus': A Clue to the Journal-Keeping Methods of Lewis and Clark." *We Proceeded On* 9 (1983): 6-8.

Dunlop, Richard. *Doctors of the American Frontier*. New York: Doubleday, 1965.

———. "Doctors Who Helped Tame the West." *Today's Health* 41 (1963): 44-47, 66-68.

Dupree, A. Hunter. *Science in the Federal Government: A History of Policies and Activities to 1940*. Cambridge, Mass.: Belknap Press, 1957.

Dykeman, Wilma. *Too Many People, Too Little Love: Edna Rankin McKinnon, Pioneer for Birth Control*. New York: Holt, Rinehart & Winston, 1974.

Eastman, Charles A. (Ohiyesa). *From the Deep Woods to Civilization*. 1916. Reprint, Lincoln and London: University of Nebraska Press, 1977.

Eddy, Mary Baker. *Science and Health*. Boston: First Church of Christ, Scientist, 1906.

Edmunds, Kermit. "Military History of Montana." Montana Historical Society Conference, 1991. OH1293 #1. Montana Historical Society Archives, Helena.

Epstein, Murray. "Renal Effects of Head-Out Water Immersion in Humans: A Fifteen-Year Update." *Journal of the American Physiological Society* 72 (1992): 563-621.

Erdoes, Richard. *Tales from the American Frontier*. New York: Pantheon Books, 1991.

Estes, J. Worth, and Billy G. Smith, eds. *A Melancholy Scene of Devastation: The Public Response to the 1793 Yellow Fever Epidemic*. Philadelphia: Science History Publications, 1997.

Ewald, Paul W. *Evolution of Infectious Disease*. Oxford: Oxford University Press, 1994.

Ewers, John C. *The Blackfeet: Raiders on the Northwest Plains*. Norman: University of Oklahoma Press, 1958.

Fairchild, Amy L. "The Polio Narratives: Dialogues with FDR." *Bulletin of the History of Medicine* 75 (2001): 488-534.

Fenn, Elizabeth A. *Pox Americana: The Great Smallpox Epidemic of 1775-82*. New York: Hill and Wang, 2001.

Fincher, Jack. "America's Deadly Rendezvous with the 'Spanish Lady.'" *Smithsonian* 19 (1989): 131-45.

Fire, John (Lame Deer), and Richard Erdoes. *Lame Deer, Seeker of Visions*. New York: Simon & Schuster, 1972.

Fishbein, Morris. *Frontiers of Medicine*. Baltimore: Williams & Wilkins, 1933.

Fitzgerald, Michael Oren. *Crow Medicine and the Sun Dance Chief*. Norman: University of Oklahoma Press, 1991.

Flexner, Abraham. *Medical Education in the United States and Canada*. New York, 1910.

Flexner, James Thomas. *Doctors on Horseback*. New York: Viking Press, 1937.

———. *Washington: The Indispensable Man*. Boston: Little, Brown, 1969.

Flood, Renee Sansom. *Lost Bird of Wounded Knee: Spirit of the Lakota*. New York: Scribner, 1995.

Fontanarosa, Phil B., and George D. Lundberg. Editorial. *Journal of the American Medical Association* 280 (1998): 1618-19.

Foster, H. W. "Successful Case of Cesarean Section." *American Journal of Obstetrics and Diseases of Women and Children* 28, no. 2 (1893): 39-40.

Fowler, Gene, ed. *Mystic Healers & Medicine Shows*. Santa Fe: Ancient City Press, 1997.

Francis, Bertha A. *Land of Big Snows*. Butte, Mont.: Self-published, 1955.

Frazier, Ian. *The Great Plains*. New York: Farrar Straus Giroux, 1989.

Freeman, Leonard. "Surgery of the Ancient Inhabitants of the Americas." *Art and Archeology* 18 (1924): 21-36.

Freemon, Frank R. *Gangrene and Glory: Medical Care during the American Civil War*. Urbana and Chicago: University of Illinois Press, 2001.

———. "Medical Care during the American Civil War." Ph.D. diss., University of Illinois, Champaign-Urbana, 1992.

Frey, Rodney. *The World of the Crow Indian*. Norman: University of Oklahoma Press, 1987.

Fritz, Harry W. "Meriwether Lewis and William Clark and the Discovery of Montana." *We Proceeded On* 8 (October 1988).

Garcia, Andrew. *Tough Trip Through Paradise, 1878-1879*. Ed. Bennett H. Stein. Boston: Houghton Mifflin, 1967.

Garver, Frank H. "The Story of Sergeant Charles Floyd." *Mississippi Valley Historical Association Proceedings* 2 (1908-09): 76-84, 82-83.

Gee, Margaret, Interview, 1984. OH680. Montana Historical Society Archives, Helena.

Gevitz, Norman. "Sectarian Medicine." *Journal of the American Medical Association* 257 (1987): 1636-40.

Gibbons, Boyd. "Alcohol: The Legal Drug." *National Geographic* 182 (February 1992): 2-35.

Gibson, Arrell M. "Medicine Show." *American West*, 1967.

Gibson, John M. *Soldier in White*. Durham, N.C.: Duke University Press, 1958.

Gillett, Mary. *The Army Medical Department, 1865–1917*. Army Historical Series. Washington, D.C.: Government Printing Office, 1995.

———. "United States Army Surgeons and the Big Horn-Yellowstone Expedition of 1876." *Montana, The Magazine of Western History* 39, no. 1 (1989): 16-27.

Gladwell, Malcolm. "The Dead Zone." *The New Yorker*, September 29, 1997.

Gone, Fred P. *The Seven Visions of Bull Lodge, as Told by His Daughter, Garter Snake*. Ed. George Horse Capture. Ann Arbor: Bear Claw Press, 1980.

Gordon, Albie, Margaret Lehfeldt, and Mary Morsanny. *Dawn in the Golden Valley: A County in Montana*. Ryegate, Mont., 1971.

Gordon, Richard. *The Alarming History of Medicine*. New York: St. Martin's Press, 1993.

Green, John R. "Neurosurgery on the Frontier." *Montana, The Magazine of Western History* 17, no. 3 (1967): 18-29.

Greene, Jerome A. *Nez Perce Summer 1877: The U. S. Army and the Nee-Me-Poo Crisis*. Helena: Montana Historical Society Press, 2000.

Grinnell, George Bird. *The Fighting Cheyenne*. New York: Charles Scribner, 1915.

Grob, Gerold N. *Mental Illness and American Society, 1875-1940*. Princeton, N.J.: Princeton University Press, 1983.

Groh, George. "Doctors of the Frontier." *American Heritage* 14, no. 3 (1963): 10.

Haggard, Howard W. *The Doctor in History*. New York: Dorset Press, 1989.

Hallberg, V. R., and J. B. Neal. "For This We Are Soldiers: Guy V. Henry and a Concept of Duty." *Journal of the West* 43, no. 2 (Spring 2004): 63–71.

Haller, John S., Jr. *American Medicine in Transition*. Champaign-Urbana: University of Illinois Press, 1981.

Hammond, J. A. B., et al. "Purulent Bronchitis." *The Lancet*, July 14, 1917.

Hampsten, Elizabeth. *Read This Only to Yourself: The Private Writings of Midwestern Women, 1880–1910*. Bloomington: Indiana University Press, 1982.

Hampton, Bruce. *Children of Grace: The Nez Perce War of 1877*. New York: Henry Holt, 1994.

Hampton, Tracy. "Clues to the Deadly 1918 Flu Revealed." *Journal of the American Medical Association* 291, no. 13 (April 7, 2004): 1553.

Hansen, Bert. "New Images of a New Medicine: Visual Evidence for the Widespread Popularity of Therapeutic Discoveries in America After 1885." *Bulletin of the History of Medicine* 73, no. 4 (1999): 629-78.

Hardy, Ann. "Tracheotomy Versus Intubation: Surgical Intervention in Diptheria in Europe and the United States, 1825-1930." *Bulletin of the History of Medicine* 66 (1992): 536-59.

Harlowton Woman's Club. *Yesteryears and Pioneers*. Harlowton, Mont.: Western Printing & Lithography, 1972.

Hart, Jeff, and Jacqueline Moore. *Montana Native Plants and Early Peoples*. Helena: Montana Historical Society Press, 1992.

Hart, Jeffrey A. "Ethnobotany of the Northern Cheyenne Indians of Montana." *Journal of Ethnopharmacology* 4 (1981): 1-55.

Hart, Sue. *The Call to Care, 1898-1998: Saint Vincent Hospital and Health Center, The First Hundred Years*. Billings, Mont.: Saint Vincent Hospital and Health Center, 1998.

Hawke, David Freeman. *Benjamin Rush, Revolutionary Gadfly*. Indianapolis and New York: Bobbs-Merrill Company, 1971.

Headwaters Historical Society. *Headwaters Heritage History*. Three Forks, Mont.: Headwaters Historical Society, 1983.

Herrmann, J., P. D. Pallister, and J. M. Opitz. "Tetraectrodactyly and Other Skeletal Manifestations in the Fetal Alcohol Syndrome." *European Journal of Pediatrics* 133 (1980): 221-26.

Hertzler, Arthur E. *The Horse and Buggy Doctor*. 1938. Reprint, Lincoln: University of Nebraska Press, 1970.

Hildreth, Martha L., and Bruce T. Moran, eds. *Disease and Medical Care in the Mountain West: Essays on Region, History, and Practice*. Reno and Las Vegas: University of Nevada Press, 1997.

Holbrook, Stewart H. *The Golden Age of Quackery*. New York: Macmillan, 1959.

Holmes, Kenneth L. *Covered Wagon Women: Diaries & Letters from the Western Trails, 1840-1890*. 11 vols. Spokane: Arthur H. Clark, 1991.

Hoopes, Lorman L. *The Last West*. Miles City, Mont.: Skyhouse Publisher, 1990.

Howard, Helen Addison, and Dan L. McGrath. *War Chief Joseph*. Lincoln: University of Nebraska Press, 1941.

Howard, Joseph Kinsey. *Montana: High, Wide, and Handsome*. Lincoln: University of Nebraska Press, 1988.

Howard, O. O. *Nez Perce Joseph: An Account of His Ancestors, His Lands, His Confederates, His Enemies, His Murders, His War, His Pursuit and Capture*. New York: Lee & Shepard Publishers, 1881.

Hoyt, Henry F. *A Frontier Doctor*. Boston: Houghton Mifflin, 1929.

Hrdlicka, Ales. "Disease, Medicine and Surgery among the American Aborigines." *Journal of the American Medical Association* 99, no. 20 (November 12, 1932): 1661-66.

Hultkrantz, Ake. *Shamanic Healing and Ritual Drama: Health and Medicine in Native North American Religious Traditions*. New York: Crossroad Publishing, 1992.

Hunt, Robert R. "The Blood Meal: Mosquitoes and Agues on the Lewis & Clark Expedition" (2 parts). *We Proceeded On* 18, nos. 2 and 3 (May and August 1992).

Hurwood, Bernhardt J. "Healing and Believing." *Health* 16 (Jun 1984): 15-16.

Hyams, Kenneth C., F. Stephen Wignall, and Robert Roswell. "War Syndromes and Their Evaluation: From the U.S. Civil War to the Persian Gulf War." *Annals of Internal Medicine* 125 (1996): 398-405.

An Illustrated History of the Yellowstone Valley: Biographical Sketches. Spokane: Washington Western Historian Publication Co., 1907.

Irving, Washington. *Astoria*. Ed. Richard Dilworth Rust. Lincoln: University of Nebraska Press, 1982.

Ivey, Thomas N. "Medicine in the Pioneer West." *The New Physician* 26 (September 1960): 51-56.

Jackson, Donald, ed. *Letters of the Lewis and Clark Expedition, with Related Documents: 1783–1854*. Second edition. 2 vols. Urbana: University of Illinois Press, 1978.

Jefferson, Thomas. *The Writings of Thomas Jefferson*. Ed. A. A. Lipscomb and A. E. Bergh. 20 vols. New York: Thomas Jefferson Memorial Association, 1903.

Jepson, Jill. "Medicine Women: Montana's Pioneer Doctors." *Montana Magazine* 129 (January-February 1995): 30-32.

John, T. Jacob. "The Final Stages of the Global Eradication of Polio." Editorial. *New England Journal of Medicine* 343, no. 11 (September 14, 2000): 806–7.

Kalisch, Phillip A. "Rocky Mountain Spotted Fever: The Sickness and the Triumph." *Montana, The Magazine of Western History* 23, no. 2: 45-55.

Karolevitz, Robert F. *Doctors of the Old West: A Pictorial History of Medicine on the Frontier*. Seattle: Superior Publishing, 1967.

Kaufman, Martin. *American Medical Education: The Formative Years, 1765-1910*. Westport, Conn., and London: Greenwood Press, 1976.

Keegan, J. J. "The Prevailing Pandemic of Influenza." *Journal of the American Medical Association* 71 (1918): 1051-58.

Ketner, K. L. "A Study of the Use of Madstones in Oklahoma." *Chronicles of Oklahoma* 46, no. 4 (1968): 433-49.

King, Elmer. Interview, 1981. OH368. Montana Historical Society Archives, Helena.

Kirchner, H. E. "Remedial Properties of Herbs." *Let's Live* 25 (1967): 25.

Knee, Stewart E. *Christian Science in the Age of Mary Baker Eddy.* Westport, Conn.: Greenwood Press, 1994.

Koch, Peter. *Life at Muscleshell [sic] in 1869 and 1870.* Annual Report of the Commissioner of Indian Affairs to the Secretary of the Interior, 1870. Reprinted in *Contributions to the Historical Society of Montana.* Vol. 2. Helena: Montana State College, 1896.

Langford, N. P. *Vigilante Days and Ways.* New York, 1893.

Larsell, O. "Medical Aspects of the Lewis and Clark Expedition." *Surgery, Gynecology, and Obstetrics* 85 (1947): 663-69.

Lautaret, Ronald L. "Alaska Disaster: A Short History of a Tragedy." *Alaska,* November 1999.

Leahy, Ellen. "'Montana Fever': Smallpox and the Montana State Board of Health." *Montana, The Magazine of Western History* 53, no. 2 (Summer 2003): 32-45.

Le Barre, Weston. "Folk Medicine and Folk Science." *Journal of American Folk-Lore,* October-December 1942, 197-205.

Leffingwell, Mary. *Diamonds in the Snow.* Self-published, 1992.

Linderman, Frank B. *Plenty-Coups, Chief of the Crows.* Lincoln: University of Nebraska Press, 1962.

———. "Pretty Shield, Medicine Woman." In *The Last Best Place.* Ed. William Kittridge and Annick Smith. Helena: Montana Historical Society Press, 1989.

Lipscomb, A. A., and A. E. Bergh, eds. *The Writings of Thomas Jefferson.* Vol. 11. New York, 1903.

Loge, Ronald V. "Meriwether Lewis and Malaria: Another View of the 'Ague.'" *We Proceeded On* 28, no. 2 (May 2002): 33–36.

———. "Miracle of Sulphur Spring." <http://lewis-clark.org/>.

———. "Two Dozes of Barks and Opium: Lewis and Clark as Physicians." *We Proceeded On* 23 (1997): 10.

Lord, Israel Shipman Pelton. *A Doctor's Gold Rush Journey to California.* Ed. Necia Dixon Liles. Lincoln and London: University of Nebraska Press, 1995.

Lorenz, Anthony J. "Scurvy in the Gold Rush." *Journal of the History of Medicine,* October 1957, 473-510.

Losee, R. E. *Doc: Then and Now with a Montana Physician.* New York: Lyons & Burford, 1994.

Lowry, Thomas P. *The Story the Soldiers Wouldn't Tell: Sex in the Civil War.* Mechanicsburg, Penn.: Stackpole Books, 1994.

Luchetti, Cathy, and Carol Olwell, *Women of the West.* St. George, Utah: Antelope Island Press, 1982.

Macklis, Roger M. "The Great Radium Scandal." *Scientific American,* August 1993.

Magner, Lois N. *A History of Medicine.* New York: Marcel Dekker, 1992.

Major, Ralph H. *A History of Medicine.* Springfield, Ill.: Charles C. Thomas, 1954.

Malkin, Harold M. *Out of the Mist.* Berkeley, Calif.: Vesalius Books, 1993.

Malone, Michael P. *The Battle for Butte.* Helena: Montana Historical Society Press, 1995.

————, Richard B. Roeder, and William L. Lang. *Montana: A History of Two Centuries.* Revised edition. Seattle: University of Washington Press, 1991.

Mancall, Peter C. *Deadly Medicine: Indians and Alcohol in Early America.* Ithaca, N.Y.: Cornell University Press, 1995.

Mann, Charles C. "1491." *Atlantic Monthly* 289, no. 3 (March 2002): 41-53.

Martensen, Robert L. "For Deliberate Election: Cesarean Sections in the 1890s." *Journal of the American Medical Association* 271 (May 25, 1994): 1557.

Massengill, Samuel Evans. *A Sketch of Medicine and Pharmacy.* Bristol, Tenn.: S. E. Massengill, 1943.

Mather, R. E., and F. E. Boswell. *Hanging the Sheriff: A Biography of Henry Plummer.* Salt Lake City: University of Utah Press, 1987.

————. *Vigilante Victims: Montana's 1864 Hanging Spree.* San Jose, Calif.: History West Publishing, 1991.

Mathes, Valerie Sherer. "Native American Women in Medicine and the Military." *Journal of the West* 21 (1982): 41-48.

Mays, B., et al. "Treatment of Arrow Wounds by Nineteenth Century USA Army Surgeons." *Journal of the Royal Society of Medicine* 87 (February 1994): 102-3.

McBride, David. "British Treatment of Sea Scurvy." *Journal of the History of Medicine* 46 (1991): 158-77.

McDermott, John D. "Custer and the Little Bighorn Story: What It All Means." From *Legacy: New Perspectives on the Battle of the Little Bighorn.* Ed. C. E. Rankin. Helena: Montana Historical Society Press, 1996.

McGreevy, Patrick S. "Amon Barber, Charles Penrose, and the War on the Powder River." *Surgery, Gynecology, and Obstetrics* 136, no. 4 (April 1973): 632–38.

————. "Surgeons at the Little Big Horn." *Surgery, Gynecology, and Obstetrics* 140, no. 5 (May 1975): 774-80.

McLemee, Scott. "Grift, Goats, and Gonads." *Chronicle of Higher Education,* December 13, 2002, A15.

McMillan, Marilyn Johnson. "Eldorado of Ease and Elegance: White Sulphur Springs, 1866-1904." *Montana, The Magazine of Western History* 35, no. 2 (1985): 36-49.

———. "Taking the Waters: Montana's Early Hot Springs Resorts." Master's thesis, Montana State University, 1982.

McNeely, Alma Gretchen. "From Untrained Nurses toward Professional Preparation in Montana, 1912-1987." Ph.D. diss., University of San Diego, 1993.

McVaugh, Michael R. "Bedside Manners in the Middle Ages." Fielding H. Garrison Lecture. *Bulletin of the History of Medicine* 71 (1997): 201-23.

Meikle, Lyndel. "Jerks of Montana: Snake Oil Salesmen." Paper presented at the Montana History Conference, Helena, October 1997.

Melcher, Mary, "Women's Matters." *Montana, The Magazine of Western History* 41-42 (Spring 1991): 47-56.

Minton, Daniel. "Population Control: Butte-Silver Bow County Board of Health and Spanish Influenza of 1918." Butte-Silver Bow County Public Archives, Butte, Mont.

"Minutes of the Silver Bow County Health Department, 1890-1920." Butte-Silver Bow County Public Archives, Butte, Mont.

Monastersky, Richard. "Plumbing Ancient Rituals." *Chronicle of Higher Education*, May 17, 2002, A 23.

Montana Medical Association. "Our Diamond Jubilee Meeting." Pamphlet, meeting of the Montana Medical Association, Billings, September 1953.

Montana Nurses Association. *Nursing in Montana.* Helena: Montana Nurses Association, 1961.

Montana Nurses Association. *Nursing in Montana: The Recent Past (A History of Nursing in Montana, 1962-1992).* Helena: Montana Nurses Association, 1992.

Montana State Board of Health Biennial Bulletins. Montana Historical Society Archives, Helena.

Montana State Board of Health Biennial Reports, 1901–58. Montana Historical Society Archives, Helena.

Moore, Michael. *Medicinal Plants of the Mountain West.* Santa Fe: Museum of New Mexico Press, 1979.

Moorman, Lewis J. "Pioneer Medicine in the Southwest." *Bulletin of the History of Medicine* 2 (1947): 795-810.

Morris, Richard B. *Witnesses at the Creation.* New York: New American Library, 1981.

Moulton, Gary E., ed. *The Journals of the Lewis and Clark Expedition.* 13 Vols. Lincoln: University of Nebraska Press, 1983–2001.

Mullen, Pierce C. "Bitterroot Enigma: Howard Taylor Ricketts and the Early Struggle against Spotted Fever." *Montana, The Magazine of Western History* 32, no. 1 (1982): 2-13.

——. Review of *Petticoat and Stethoscope* by Mabel Tuchscherer. *Montana, The Magazine of Western History* 29, no. 4 (1979): 74-76.

——, and Michael L. Nelson. "Montanans and 'The Most Peculiar Disease': The Influenza Epidemic and Public Health, 1918-1919." *Montana, The Magazine of Western History* 37, no. 2 (Spring 1987): 50-61.

Munn, Fred. "Veteran of Frontier Experiences Remembered the Days He Rode with Miles, Howard and Terry." *Montana, The Magazine of Western History* 16, no. 2 (1966): 50-64.

Murphy, Lawrence R. "The Enemy Among Us: Venereal Disease among Union Soldiers in the Far West, 1861-1865." *Civil War History* 31 (September 1985): 159-265.

Murphy, Mary. *Mining Cultures: Men, Women, and Leisure in Butte, 1914–41.* Urbana: University of Illinois Press, 1997.

Nagler, F. P., C. E. van Rooyen, and J. H. Sturdy. "An Influenza Virus Epidemic at Victoria Island, Northwest Territory, Canada." *Canadian Journal of Public Health* 40 (1953): 457-65.

Nathanson, Neal, and John R. Martin. "The Epidemiology of Poliomyelitis: Enigmas Surrounding Its Appearance, Epidemicity, and Disappearance." *American Journal of Epidemiology* 110 (1979): 672-92.

Neihardt, John G. *The Mountain Men.* Lincoln: University of Nebraska Press, 1953.

——. *The Song of Jed Smith.* Lincoln: University of Nebraska Press, 1971.

——. *The Splendid Wayfaring.* Lincoln: University of Nebraska Press, 1970.

Nisbet, Jack. *Sources of the River: Tracking David Thompson across Western North America.* Seattle: Sasquatch Books, 1994.

Niven, Francis L. *Manhattan Omnibus: Stories of Historical Interest of Manhattan and Its Surrounding Communities.* N.p.: Francis L. Niven, 1989.

North, Henry Ringling. *The Circus Kings.* Garden City, N.Y.: Doubleday, 1959.

Olch, Peter D. "Medicine in the Indian Fighting Army, 1866-1890." *Journal of the West* 21, no. 3 (July 1982): 32-41.

Olivia, Leo E. *Fort Larned on the Santa Fe Trail.* Topeka: Kansas State Historical Society, 1982.

Oman, Kerry R. "Winter in the Rockies: Winter Quarters of the Mountain Men." *Montana, The Magazine of Western History* 52, no. 3 (Spring 2003): 34-47.

O'Neil, Carle F. *Muscle, Grit, and Big Dreams.* Kalispell, Mont.: O'Neil Printers, 1996.

Orestad, Helen B. *He Named It Powderville: A History of Southeastern Montana.* Miles City, Mont.: H. B. Orestad, 1994.

Osler, William. *Aequanimitas.* Ed. Paul Dudley White. New York: W. W. Norton, 1963.

Palladino, Lawrence Benedict. *Anthony Ravalli, S. J., Forty Years a Missionary in the Rocky Mountains.* Helena, Mont.: G. E. Boos & Co., 1884.

Parkman, Francis. *The Oregon Trail.* New York: Airmont Publishing, 1964.

Parshall, Gerald. "Yale's Doctor of Dialogue: Contrarian Stephen Carter Takes the Nation's Moral Temperature." *U.S. News and World Report,* March 18, 1996.

Patrias, Karen, ed. "American Indian and Alaska Native Health." N.d. *Current Bibliographies in Medicine* 96, no. 6. National Library of Medicine, Washington, D.C.

Paul, John R. *A History of Poliomyelitis.* New Haven and London: Yale University Press, 1971.

Peavy, Linda, and Ursula Smith. *Pioneer Women: The Lives of Women on the Frontier.* New York: Smithmark Publishers, 1996.

———. *Women in Waiting.* Norman: University of Oklahoma Press, 1994.

Peck, David J. *Or Perish in the Attempt: Wilderness Medicine in the Lewis and Clark Expedition.* Helena, Mont.: Farcountry Press, 2002.

Peller, Sigismund. "Walter Reed, C. Finlay, and Their Predecessors around 1800." *Bulletin of the History of Medicine* 33, no. 3 (May-June 1959): 195-211.

Pelligrino, Edmund D. "The Metamorphosis of Medical Ethics." *Journal of the American Medical Association* 269 (1993): 1158-62.

Pendergrast, Mark. *For God, Country and Coca-Cola.* New York: Scribners, 1993.

Petrik, Paula Evans. "The Bonanza Town: Women and Family on the Rocky Mountain Mining Frontier, Helena, Montana, 1865-1900." Ph.D. diss., State University of New York, 1981.

———. *No Step Backward: Women and Family on the Rocky Mountain Mining Frontier, Helena, Montana, 1865-1900.* Helena: Montana Historical Society Press, 1987.

———. "Strange Bedfellows: Prostitution, Politicians, and Moral Reform in Helena, 1885-1887." *Montana, The Magazine of Western History* 35 (1985): 3-13.

Phillips, Paul C. *Medicine in the Making of Montana.* Missoula: Montana State University Press, 1962.

Phillips County Historical Society. *Yesteryears.* Havre, Mont.: Griggs Printing & Publishing, 1978.

Pickard, M., and R. C. Buley. *The Midwest Pioneer: His Ills, Cures, and Doctors.* Crawfordsville, Ind.: Banta, 1945.

Pohl, John F. "The Kenny Treatment of Anterior Poliomyelitis (Infantile Paralysis): Report of the First Cases Treated in America." *Journal of the American Medical Association* 118, no. 17 (April 25, 1942): 1428–47.

Porter, Joseph C. "Crazy Horse, Lakota Leadership and the Fort Laramie Treaty." In *Legacy: New Perspectives on the Battle of the Little Bighorn*. Ed. C. E. Rankin. Helena: Montana Historical Society Press, 1996.

Post, George W., ed. *The Cottage Physician*. Springfield, Mass.: King-Richardson Co., 1903.

Presser, Marvin W. *Wolf Point: A City of Destiny*. Billings, Mont.: M Press, 1997.

Price, Esther Gaskins. *Fighting Tuberculosis in the Rockies: A History of the Montana Tuberculosis Association*. Butte: Montana Tuberculosis Association, 1943.

Progressive Men of the State of Montana. 2 vols. Chicago: A. W. Bowen, n.d.

Quebbeman, Frances E. *Medicine in Territorial Arizona*. Phoenix: Arizona Historical Foundation, 1966.

Rainbolt, Jo. "Jessie Bierman: Fifty Years of Medicine and Ahead of Her Time." *Montana Magazine* 12, no. 1 (September 1981): 26-28.

Randall, Willard Sterne. *Jefferson: A Life*. New York: Henry Holt, 1993.

Ravenholt, Reimert Thorolf. "Triumph Then Dispair: The Tragic Death of Meriwether Lewis." *Epidemiology* 5 (1994): 366-79.

Ray, Joyce Marie Butler. "Women and Men in American Medicine 1849-1925." Ph.D. diss., University of Texas, 1992.

Read, Georgia Willis. "Diseases, Drugs, and Doctors on the Oregon-California Trail in the Gold-Rush Years." *Missouri Historical Review* 38 (1944): 260-75.

Reagan, Albert B. "The 'Flu' among the Navajos." *Transactions of the Kansas Academy of Science* 30 (1921): 131-39.

Reagan, Leslie J. "'About to Meet Her Maker': Women, Doctors, Dying Declarations, and the State's Investigation of Abortion, Chicago, 1867-1940." *Journal of American History* 77 (March 1991): 1240-64.

Reed, Walter, Victor C. Vaughan, and Edward O. Shakespeare. *Report on the Origin and Spread of Typhoid Fever in the U. S. Military Camps during the Spanish War of 1898*. 2 vols. Washington, D.C., 1904.

Reiling, Jennifer. "Quackery in America." *Journal of the American Medical Association* 34 (1900): 943-45.

Reiser, Stanley Joel. *Medicine in the Reign of Technology*. Cambridge: Cambridge University Press, 1978.

Reisner, Marc. *Cadillac Desert: The American West and Its Disappearing Water*. New York: Viking-Penguin, 1986.

Report of a Reconnaissance from Carroll, Montana Territory, on the Upper Missouri, to the Yellowstone National Park, and Return Made in the Summer of 1875. Washington, D.C.: Government Printing Office, 1876.

"Report of Special Joint Committee of the Senate and House of Representatives of the Twenty-Eighth Legislative Assembly on the Montana State Hospital." 1942. Archives, Montana State Hospital, Warm Springs.

"Reports of the Council on Pharmacy and Chemistry." *Journal of the American Medical Association* 71, no. 21 (November 23, 1918): 1763-64.

Reynolds, Winifred Braine. *The Doctors Reynolds: Three Generations of the Reynolds Family.* Duluth, Minn.: Elizabeth R. Kerns, 1988.

Rice, Julian. *Black Elk's Story.* Albuquerque: University of New Mexico Press, 1991.

Ricketts, Howard Taylor. *Infection, Immunity, and Serum Therapy.* Chicago: American Medical Association Press, 1908.

———. "The New Cure for Diphtheria, Croup, Etc." *Scientific American*, November 1894, 235-44.

Riddle, John M. *Eve's Herbs.* Cambridge, Mass., and London: Harvard University Press, 1997.

Riley, Glenda. *A Place to Grow: Women in the American West.* Arlington Heights, Ill.: Harlan Davidson, 1992.

Rogers, Fred B. Editorial. *American Journal of Public Health* 58, no. 12 (December 1968): 2192-94.

Ronda, James P. "A Knowledge of Distant Parts: The Shaping of the Lewis and Clark Expedition." *Montana, The Magazine of Western History* 41 (1991): 4-19.

———. *Lewis and Clark Among the Indians.* Lincoln: University of Nebraska Press, 1984.

Root-Bernstein, Robert and Michele. *Honey, Mud, Maggots, and Other Medical Marvels: The Science Behind Folk Remedies and Old Wives' Tales.* Boston and New York: Houghton Mifflin Co., 1998.

Rothman, Sheila M. *Living in the Shadow of Death.* New York: Basic Books, 1994.

Rothstein, William G. *American Physicians in the Nineteenth Century.* Baltimore: Johns Hopkins University Press, 1972.

Rowland, Mary Canaga. *As Long as Life: The Memoirs of a Frontier Woman Doctor.* Ed. F. A. Loomis. New York: Fawcett Crest, 1994.

Rupprecht, C. E., B. Dietzschold, and H. Koprowski, eds. *Lyssaviruses.* New York: Springer-Verlag, 1994.

Russell, Osborne. *Journal of a Trapper.* Ed. Aubrey L. Haines. Lincoln: University of Nebraska Press, 1965.

Russell, Rosanna. *A Pictorial History of the Sun River Valley.* Sun River, Mont.: Sun River Historical Society, 1990-91.

Rutkow, Ira M. *American Surgery.* Philadelphia and New York: Lippincott-Raven Publishers, 1998.

Sacks, Oliver. *The Man Who Mistook His Wife for a Hat.* London: Macmillan General Books, 1985.

St. Pierre, Mark, and Tilda Long Soldier. *Walking in the Sacred Manner: Healers, Dreamers, and Pipe Carriers—Medicine Women of the Plains Indians.* New York: Touchstone, 1995.

Salinsky, Michael. "Early Chapters in the Stethoscopes Evolution." *Journal of the American Medical Association* 264 (1990): 2817.

Sanders, Helen Fitzgerald. *A History of Montana.* Chicago: Lewis Publishing, 1913.

Sanders, Marian K., ed. *The Crisis in American Medicine.* New York: Harper & Brothers, 1961.

Sarnecky, Mary T. "Nursing in the American Army from the Revolution to the Spanish-American War." *Nursing History Review* 5 (1997): 49-69.

Savitt, Todd L., and Janice Willms. "Sisters' Hospital: The Sisters of Providence and St. Patrick Hospital, Missoula, Montana, 1873–1890." *Montana, The Magazine of Western History* 53, no. 1 (spring 2003): 28–43.

Schemm, Mildred Walker. "The Major's Lady: Natawista." *Montana, The Magazine of Western History* 2 (January 1952): 5–15.

Schultz, James Willard. "Return to the Beloved Mountains." *Montana, The Magazine of Western History* 7 (1957): 26-33.

Schwidde, Jess T., ed. *Medicine, The Early Days.* Billings, Mont.: 100th Birthday Medical Committee, 1983.

Seagraves, Anne. *Soiled Doves: Prostitution in the Early West.* Hayden, Idaho: Wesanne Publications, 1994.

Seibel, Dennis. *Fort Ellis, Montana Territory, 1867-1886.* Bozeman, Mont.: Gallatin County Historical Society, 1996.

Shadduck, Louise. *Doctors with Buggies, Snowshoes, and Planes: One Hundred Years and More of Idaho Medicine.* Boise: Tamarack Books, 1993.

Shields, G. O. *The Battle of the Big Hole.* Chicago and New York: Rand, McNally & Company, 1889.

Shilton, Earle A. "Gone Under: A Saga of Mountain Men." *The Westerners Brand Book* 20 (1963): 17-24.

Shryock, Richard Harrison. *Medicine in America in the Nineteenth Century.* Baltimore: Johns Hopkins Press, 1966.

Sigerist, Henry E. *American Medicine.* New York: W. W. Norton, 1934.

———. *A History of Medicine.* New York: Oxford University Press, 1955.

Small, Lawrence F., ed. *Religion in Montana, Pathways to the Present.* 2 vols. Billings, Mont.: Rocky Mountain College in cooperation with Skyhouse Publishers, 1992.

Smith, Arthur M. "When 'Dialing 9-1-1' Just Won't Work." *Marine Corps Gazette,* June 1995.

Smith, Duane A., and Ronald C. Brown. *No One Ailing Except a Physician: Medicine in the Mining West, 1848-1919.* Boulder: University Press of Colorado, 2001.

Smith, Phyllis. *Bozeman and the Gallatin Valley*. Helena, Mont.: Falcon Press Publishing, 1996.

Sohn, Anton P. *Healers of the Nineteenth Century, Nevada*. Reno: Greasewood Press, 1997.

————."Nineteenth-Century Academic Examinations for Physicians in the United States Army Medical Department." *West Journal of Medicine* 160, no. 5 (1994): 472-74.

————. *A Saw, Pocket Instruments, and Two Ounces of Whiskey: Frontier Military Medicine in the Great Basin*. Spokane: Arthur H. Clark, 1998.

Spence, Clark C. *Montana: A Bicentennial History*. New York: Norton, 1978.

Spiess, Arthur E., and Bruce D. Spiess. "New England Pandemic of 1616-1622: Cause and Archaeological Implication." *Man in the Northeast* 34 (1987): 71-83.

Starr, Paul. *The Social Transformation of American Medicine*. New York: Harper Collins, 1982.

Staudohar, Connie. "'Food, Rest, & Happyness,' Limitations and Possibilities in the Early Treatment of Tuberculosis in Montana." *Montana, The Magazine of Western History*. Part 1, vol. 47, no. 4 (Winter 1997): 48-57; Part 2, vol. 48, no. 1 (Spring 1998): 44-55.

Steele, Volney. "Arrow Wounds and the Military Surgeon of the West." *Military History of the West* 30, no. 2 (Fall 2000): 153-70.

————."Doctors at the Battle of the Big Hole." *Military History of the West* 32, no. 1 (Spring 2002): 25–33.

————."The Flu Epidemic of 1918 on the Montana Frontier." *Journal of the West* 42, no. 4: 81-90.

————. "Lewis and Clark: Military Explorers, Scientists, and Physicians." *Military History of the West* 31, no. 1 (Spring 2001): 51–65.

Steffen, Jerome O. "William Clark: A Reappraisal." *Montana, The Magazine of Western History* 25, no. 2 (1952): 52-61.

Stegner, Wallace. *Beyond the Hundredth Meridian*. New York: Penguin, 1981.

Stern, Bernhard F. *Society and Medical Progress*. Princeton: Princeton University Press, 1941.

Sternberg, Martha L. *George Miller Sternberg: A Biography*. Chicago: American Medical Association, 1920.

Stevens, Mark. "Chief Joseph's Revenge." *The New Yorker*, August 8, 1994.

Stockel, H. Henrietta. *The Lightning Stick: Arrows, Wounds, and Indian Legends*. Reno: University of Nevada Press, 1995.

Stone, Eric. *American Indian Medicine*. New York: AMS Press, 1978.

————. "Medicine among the American Indians." In *Clio Medica*. New York: Paul B. Hoeber, 1932.

Stout, Tom, ed. *Montana: Its Story and Biography*. Vol. 11. Chicago and New York, 1921.

Strain, Earl, and Sara Wright. Family Papers, 1889-1953. Collection 249. Montana Historical Society Archives, Helena.

Stratton, Owen Tully. *Medicine Man*. Ed. Owen S. Stratton. Norman: University of Oklahoma Press, 1989.

Stuart-Harris, Charles H., Geoffrey C. Schild, and John S. Oxford. *Influenza: The Viruses and the Disease*. Second edition. London: Edward Arnold, 1985.

Sullivan, Robert B. "Sanguine Practices: A Historical and Historiographic Reconsideration of Heroic Therapy in the Age of Rush." *Bulletin of the History of Medicine* 68 (1994): 211–34.

Sullivan-Fowler, Micaela. "Doubtful Theories, Drastic Therapies." *Journal of the History of Medicine and Allied Sciences* 50 (1995): 364-390.

Swerdlow, Joel L. *Nature's Medicine: Plants That Heal*. Washington, D.C.: National Geographic Society, 2000.

Tate, Michael L. *The Frontier Army in the Settlement of the West*. Norman: University of Oklahoma Press, 1999.

Taubenberger, Jeffrey. Interview, *News Hour with Jim Lehrer*. PBS, March 24, 1997.

Thomas, Lewis. *The Fragile Species*. New York: Charles Scribner's Sons, 1992.

———. *The Youngest Science*. New York: Viking Press, 1983.

Thompson, Erwin N. "Woman, Wife, Mother, Missionary: Narcissa Whitman." *Montana, The Magazine of Western History* 13, no. 4 (1963): 15-27.

Thompson, Jesse E. "Sagittectomy: First Recorded Surgical Procedure in the American Southwest, 1535." *The New England Journal of Medicine* 289, no. 26 (December 27, 1973): 1403-07.

Tkach, John R., ed. *Medicine in Bozeman, Montana, in 1983*. Bozeman, Mont.: Gallatin County Medical Society, 1983.

Transactions of the American Medical Association. Philadelphia, 1848.

Treacy, William. "Mountain Fever." *Times and Register* 21 (1890): 75-78.

Trunkey, Donald D. "Doctor George Goodfellow: The First Civilian Trauma Surgeon." *Surgery, Gynecology & Obstetrics* 141 (July 1975): 97-104.

Tuchscherer, Mabel, with John A. Forssen. *Petticoat & Stethoscope: A Montana Legend*. Missoula, Mont.: Bitterroot Litho, 1978.

Turner, F. J. "The Significance of the Frontier in American History." In *The Turner Thesis Concerning the Role of the Frontier in American History*. Ed. G. R. Taylor. Boston: Heath, 1956.

U.S. Army Military History Research Collection. Circular No. 8. May 1, 1875. War Department, U.S. Surgeon-General's Office, Washington, D.C.

U.S. Congress. *Report of the Commission Appointed by the President to Investigate the Conduct of the War Department in the War with Spain.* 8 vols. 56th Cong., 1st sess., 1900. S. Doc. 221.

Vastag, Brian. "Agencies Prepare Worst-Case Flu Vaccine." *Journal of the American Medical Association* 291, no. 12 (March 2004): 1429.

Vestal, Stanley. *Jim Bridger: Mountain Man.* Lincoln: University of Nebraska Press, 1970.

Vichorek, Daniel N. *Montana's Homestead Era.* Helena, Mont.: American Geographic Publishing, 1987.

———. *The Hi-Line.* Helena, Mont.: American and World Geographic Publishing, 1993.

Vogel, Virgil J. *American Indian Medicine.* Norman: University of Oklahoma Press, 1970.

Vontver, May Anderson. "May Anderson Vontver Reminiscence, 1905-1939." SC 958. Montana Historical Society Archives, Helena.

Walsh, Mary R. *Doctors Wanted: No Women Need Apply.* New Haven: Yale University Press, 1978.

Walter, Dave. *Montana Campfire Tales.* Helena, Mont.: Falcon Press, 1997.

Warner, John Harley. "Ideals of Science and Their Discontents in Late Nineteenth-Century American Medicine." *Isis* 82 (1991): 454-478.

"The Watershed in American Medicine: Educating the Physician in Dr. Caroline McGill's Generation." Pierce C. Mullen, curator. Exhibit at the Museum of the Rockies, Bozeman, Mont., 1998.

Watson, Art. *Devil Man with a Gun.* White Sulphur Springs, Mont.: Meagher County News, 1967.

Webb, Walter Prescott. *The Great Plains.* Lincoln: University of Nebraska Press, 1981.

Webster, Robert. "The Flu Pandemic That Might Have Been." *Science* 277 (1997): 1793.

Wengert, James W. "The Contract Surgeon." *Journal of the West* 36, no. 1 (January 1997): 67-76.

Wesson, Miley B. "George E. Goodfellow, Frontier Surgeon and Soldier." *Annals of Medical History* 5 (1933): 236-245.

West, Elliott. "Golden Dreams." *Montana, The Magazine of Western History* 49, no. 3 (Autumn 1999): 2-11.

———. *Growing Up with the Country: Childhood on the Far Western Frontier.* Albuquerque: University of New Mexico Press, 1997.

Whelan, John H. Personal papers. Private collection.

Whithorn, Bill, and Doris Whithorn. *A Photo History of Aldridge: Coal Camp That Died A-bornin'.* Minneapolis: Acme Printing and Stationary, 1965.

———. *Photo History of Chico Lodge.* Livingston, Mont.: Park County News Publisher, 1972.

Wier, James A. "Nineteenth Century Army Doctors on the Frontier and in Nebraska." *Nebraska History* 61 (Summer 1980): 192-213.

Will, Drake W. "Lewis and Clark: Westering Physicians." *Montana, The Magazine of Western History* 21, no. 4 (1971): 2-17.

———. "The Medical and Surgical Practice of the Lewis and Clark Expedition." *Journal of the History of Medicine and Allied Sciences* 14 (1959): 273-97.

Williamson, T. S. "Dacotas of the Mississippi." In *Historical and Statistical Information Respecting the History, Condition, and Prospects of the Indian Tribes of the United States.* Ed. H. R. Schoolcraft. 6 vols. Philadelphia: Lippincott, Grambo & Co., 1851.

Wilson, Daniel J. "A Crippling Fear: Experiencing Polio in the Era of FDR." *Bulletin of the History of Medicine,* 72 (1998): 464-95.

Wilson, Myra. Interview. OH1209. Montana Historical Society Archives, Helena.

Wilson, Raymond. *Ohiyesa: Charles Eastman, Santee Sioux.* Urbana, Chicago, London: University of Illinois Press, 1983.

Wilson, Samuel M. "On the Matter of Smallpox." *Natural History,* September 1994.

Winkler, Allen M. "Drinking on the American Frontier." *Quarterly Journal of Studies on Alcohol* 29 (1968): 413-445.

Winter, Malcolm D., Jr. "Medical History of Miles City." 1990. Private collection.

Wish, Harvey. *Society and Thought in Early America.* N.p., 1950.

Wood, Eugene. "History of the Practice of Obstetrics in Utah." *Rocky Mountain Medical Journal,* April 1967.

Woodruff, Charles A. "Battle of the Big Hole." In *Contributions to the Montana Historical Society.* Vol. 7. Reprint. Boston: J. S. Canner, 1966.

Young, T. Kue. *The Health of Native Americans: Toward a Biocultural Epidemiology.* New York: Oxford University Press, 1994.

Zhu, Liping. "No Need to Rush." *Montana, The Magazine of Western History* 49, no. 3 (Autumn 1999): 42-57.

Archives, Museums, and Organizations

Gallatin County Historical Society and Pioneer Museum, Bozeman, Mont., www.pioneermuseum.org/

Montana Historical Society, Helena, Mont., www.montanahistoricalsociety.org/

Museum of Questionable Medical Devices, Science Museum of Minnesota, Minneapolis, Minn., www.mtn.org/quack/

Museum of the Rockies, Montana State University, Bozeman, Mont. www.montana.edu/wwwmor

Renne Library, Montana State University, Bozeman, Mont.

St. Vincent Hospital Archives, Helena, Mont.

Shodair Hospital Archives, Billings, Mont.

INDEX

Italicized numerals indicate illustrations.

apprenticeship. *See* training, of doctors

Arapaho Indians, 84

Arapooish (Crow chief), 41

Arcadia Lea, Sister, 289

Arikara Indians, 40, 42, 260

Arizona jimson weed, 296

Ariss, E. Augusta, 246

army medicine, 107–30, 201, 224; nurses and, 241–43. *See also* Civil War; Spanish-American War; World War I

Army Nurse Corps, 243

arrow wounds: 69; extraction tools for, 95–96, 121, *121*; treatment of, 30, 67, 68, 120–22, 125

artemesia. *See* mugwort

arthritis, 6, 36, 106, 143, 230

asafetida, 143, 294

Assiniboine Indians, 36, 38, 260

Atwater, Mary Babcock Moore, 206–07, *207*

August flower bitters, 151

Aupaumut (Mohican), 40

autointoxication theory, 161

Avogadro's Law, xxii

Babbage, Miss. *See* Carruthers, Katherine Babbage

Bailey, William J. A., 158

Baker, Josia, 160

Baldwin, William O., 14

Bancroft, B. F., 103

Bannack (MT), 95, 103, 206

Barton, Benjamin Smith, 49

Baskett, Lindsey, 179, 182

Baskett, Lindsey M. (Mac), 182

Basque folk medicine, 144

Battle of the Big Hole, 125–28

Battle of the Clearwater, 122

Battle of the Little Bighorn, 123, 125

Battle of the Rosebud, 123–24

Battle of White Bird Canyon, 122

Battle of Wounded Knee, 123, 128–30

Beal, George W., 175

bear attacks, 66, 225–26

bear grease, 64

Bear Town (MT), 99

Beaver Tom (trapper), 41

Behring, Emil Adolf von, 13

Bend (OR), 170, 199, 274

Benson, Theodore J., 197–98

Bent, William, 20

Bernstein, Robert and Michele, 145

Berry, J. L., 160

bezoars. *See* madstones

Bickerdyke, Mary Ann, 240–41, *241*

Bierman, Henry, 179

Bierman, Jessie, 203–04

Big Foot, Chief, 128

Big Timber (MT), 182

Bill, Joseph H., 120

Billings (MT): nursing school in, 246; hospitals in, 221, 289; smallpox in, 261–62

Billings, Josh, 162

birth control (contraception), 93, 138–39, 193–96. *See also* abortion

bistoury, 95–96

Bitterroot Mountains, 57

Bitterroot Valley, 77, 268, 269, 270; ticks in, 272

Blackfeet Indians, 68, 70; and measles, 35; medicine bundles of, 24; medicine men of, 26–27; and smallpox, 260; and trachoma, 43; and tuberculosis, 43, 284; and whiskey trade, 40

Blackwell, Elizabeth, 202

Blaud's pills, 185

bleeding (therapy), 1–4, 8, 52, 170, 191; and Benjamin Rush, 3, 48–49, 52; and homeopaths, 5; end of practice, 8, 114; among Mayans, 23; for pleurisy, 53; for smallpox, 39; for wounds, 79, 115

Bliss, Tasker H., 117

blistering, 3–5, 75, 97, 115, 274; in army medicine, 79; and homeopaths, 5

bloodletting. *See* bleeding

blood poisoning, 138, 190

blood pressure: high, 158, 230; measurement of, 9, 12, 172, 246

depression, 60, 229

Derringer, Jacob, *152*

Deseret Hospital, 205; midwives at, 245; nursing school in, 245

DeSmet, Pierre Jean, 221

Devens, Camp (Boston, MA), 291

De Voto, Bernard, 132

diarrhea, 47, 143, 225, 253; dysentery (severe diarrhea), 54 (*see also* cholera; typhoid); from scurvy, 83, 114

Dick, Elisha Cullen, 4

Dickey, Nancy W., 211

digestive disorders: treatments for, 33, 50, 54, 131, 138, 144, 147, 158, 232. *See also* diarrhea; ulcers

digitalis, 7, *7*, 11

diphtheria, 33, 80, 86, 134, 186, 263; death rate from, 8, 267; epidemics of, 90, 109, 258, 263–66, 292; folk treatment for, 143; incidence of, 286; Native American treatment for, 20; quarantine for, 254, 293; sources of, 11–12, 254, 265; symptoms of, 185, 186, *263*; vaccine for, xxi, 11, 264–65, *265*

dislocated joints, 52, 175; treatment for, 52, 183

Dix, Dorothea, 227

Docter, John C., 275, 291–92

Dr. Berry's Mineral Water Salts, 160

Doctor Book, The, 144–45

Donahue, Dan, 297

Drake, Daniel, 14–15

dropsy (heart failure), 7

Drouillard, George, 53

Drummond (MT), 275

Dubois, Camp, 49

Dudley, Benjamin, 4

Du Gauche, Chief, 27

Dunlop, Richard, 20, 68

dysentery. *See under* diarrhea.

dyspepsia. *See* digestive disorders

Eagle Shield (Sioux shaman), 31

earache, 78, 144

Eastman, Charles A., 128–29

Ebola fever, 39

Edgar (MT), 197

Edwards, Diane D., 43

Eggleston, William G., 168

electrolytes, 80, 262

Elkhorn (MT), 210, 264

Elko (NV), 217, 220

Elko County Hospital: and Chinese, 104

emigrant wagon trains, *80, 82, 85;* medical care on, 73–86

empyemas, 182–83, 186; and X-rays, 183

enemas, 3, 61, 78, 161–62, 205, 246–47, 274; in Native American medicine, 19, 20, 23, 28

Ennis (MT): hospital at, 234

epidemics: 259–98; of cholera, 74, 76, 81, 87, 113, 262–63; of diphtheria, 90, 109, 258, 263–66, 292; of polio, 285–87; of scarlet fever, 90, 113, 135, 137, 244, 258, 264; of small-pox, 76, 113, 137, 206, 219, 258, 260–62, 292; of whooping cough, 81, 90, 268

epilepsy, 20, 112, 228, 229

Epstein, Murray, 230

erysipelas, 80, 113

ether, 11, 96, 128, 187

Ewan, Clarence, 218

Excelsior Mineral Waters, 161

faith: role in healing, 25, 136, 142, 150

faith healers, 164–66

Federal Bureau of Mines, 280

Felicie, Jacoba, 202

Fenn, Elizabeth, 36

Fenner, Hiram W., *178*

Ferguson, Ellen B., 205

Fergus County (MT), 275

Ffirth, Stubbins, 5

Field, Joseph, 55

Fink, Mike, 67

Fire, John, 21–22

Firming, Thora. *See* Phalen, Thora Firming

Mitchell, Armistead H., 98–100, *100*, 228
Montana Board of Health, 270
Montana Deaconess Hospital, 246
Montana Development Center, 237. *See also* Montana State School and Hospital
Montana Federation of Women's Clubs, 207
Montana Medical Association, 195
Montana Nurses Association, 226
Montana State Agricultural College, 282
Montana State Board of Health, 256–58, 268, 283, 285
Montana State College, 209, 272
Montana State Hospital, 228–30
Montana State Hospital for the Insane. *See* Montana State Hospital
Montana State School and Hospital, 234–38
Montana State University, 234
Montana Tuberculosis Association, 207, 280, 283
Moore, Jessie Poindexter, 292
Moore, S. P., 109
Mormons: medical practices of, 77–82, 205; and women doctors, 204–05
Mormon Battalion, 79
mountain men, 65; medical practices of, 63–71
Movius, A. J., 221
mugwort, 33, 131, *132*
Mullan, James A., 115–16
Mullen, Pierce, 209, 239
Murray Hospital (Butte, MT), 210; nursing school at, 246
Museum of the Rockies, 210
Mussigbrod, Charles, 228
mustard plasters, 2, 138, 143, 144

Nampa (ID), 170
Native American medicine, 19–33; false, 6; shamans in, 24–27, *25*, *26*, 31, 149
Navajo Indians, 296
Neihardt, John, 68

neurasthenia, 233
Nevada Hospital for the Indigent Insane/Nevada Hospital for Mental Diseases, 227–28
New York: cholera in, 79; diphtheria in, 8; flu epidemic in, 291; Public Health Department of, 286
Nez Perce Indians, 30, 32, 126; and Lewis and Clark Expedition, 56, 57–58
Nez Perce War of 1877, 122–23, 125–28
Nightingale, Florence, 133, 239–40, *240*, 242
nitrous oxide, *10*, 11
Niven, Francis, 174
Northern Montana Hospital, 222
nurses, 215, *217*, *223*, *224*, 239–49, *247*, *248*; African American, 242–43; and childbirth, 190; homestead women as, 132–38; male, 74; with military, 127–29 *passim*, 239–43; nuns as, 127, 220–22; training of, 245–49
nursing (breastfeeding), 30

Oliver, N. T. "Nevada Ned," 159
ophthalmoscope, 12, 97, 172
opium, 7, 60, 80; and Chinese, 106; in patent medicines, 156; and prostitutes, 93. *See also* laudanum
Oregon grape, 29, 32
orthopedics 234–36
Osler, William, 13, 270
otoscope, 172

Paiute Indians, 27
Palladino, Laurence B., 221
Pallister, Phillip D. 235–38, *236*
para-aminosalicylic acid, 285
paralysis: from polio 235, 285, 286, 287, 289; from rabies, 162; treatment for, 232, 289;
Parberry, William 232
Parker, Ralph R., 272–73
Parker, Samuel, 74

360

Parkman, Francis, 67
Parsons, Lucena, 81
Pasteur, Louis, xxii, 13; rabies vaccine of, 10, 162, 164
Pasteur Institute, 265
patent medicines, 138–43, *141, 142,* 154–61, *155, 157*
Patterson, William Ewing, 47
Pattie, James Ohio, 64
Paulding, Holmes O., 125
Peavy, Linda, 204
pemmican, 30, 57
penicillin, xxiii. *See also* antibiotics
pennyroyal, 138, *139*
Penrose, Charles B., 279–80
Pepper, William, 204
peritonitis, 56, 113, 184
Peruvian bark (quinine). *See* cinchona bark
pessaries, 93, 138
Petrik, Paula, 93, 94, 218
Phalen, Thora Firming, 244–45
phenobarbital, 229
Phillips, Paul C., 69
Phillips Milk of Magnesia, 147
Philipsburg (MT), 94
Phoenix (AZ): nursing school in, 245
Pierce's Pleasant Pellets, 161
Pine Ridge (SD), 128, 129
Pinkham, Lydia, 142
placenta praevia, 191
Placerville (CA), 95
plague, 254, 259; and Native Americans, 33
plague, white. *See* tuberculosis
Plato, 6
pleurisy, 53, 143
Plummer, Henry, 103
Plymouth Colony, 34
pneumonia, 38, 89, 145, 182–83, 220, 281; and influenza, 290; treatment of, 173; and whooping cough, 268; and X-rays, 183
pneumonia jacket, 174, 246
Pococke, L. Rodney, 90, *90*

Point, Nicholas, 75, 134
Pointer, Samuel, 163
polio, 285–90; bulbar, 288; epidemics of, 258, 260, 285–87; quarantine for, 254, 287–88; treatments for, 288, 288–89; vaccines for, xxi, 289–90
Pompey. *See* Charbonneau, Jean Baptiste
Pope, Elijah, Sr., 163
Porro section, 192
Porter, Henry Renaldo, 125
Potts, Daniel T., 66
poultices, 8, 28, 50, 55, 61, 143, 241
Pratt, Romania Bunnell, 205
pregnancy, 136, 189–90, 201, 204; and influenza, 292; Native Americans and, 31; unwanted (*see* abortion, birth control). *See also* childbirth, miscarriage
Pretty Shield, 284
prostatectomies, 249
prostitution: in mining camps, *91,* 91–94, 276; and Chinese, 104; and U.S. Army, 116–17
Pryor (MT), 197
Pryor, Nathaniel, 52
puking. *See* vomiting
pulmonary edema, 226
Pure Food and Drug Act, 157
purgatives. *See* enemas; laxatives; purging; vomiting
purging, 1–4, 161–62; and Lewis and Clark Expedition 48, 51–52; for measles, 70; among Native Americans, 23 (*see also* enemas); opposition to, 5, 15, 114; and Benjamin Rush, 2–3, 48, 52; for smallpox, 39; for syphilis, 5; for wounds, 34, 115
Putio, Aino Hamalainen, 191

quack doctors, 150–54
quarantine, 12, 251, 254–55, 259, 268, 287–89, 293
Queen Anne's lace, 138, *139*
quinine, 7, 50, 114, 294

for, 97, 108; in mining camps, 95–104, 99; among mountain men, 66–71; among Native Americans, 19–20, 30–31; by nurses, 221; by quack doctor, 153; for polio, 288; for tuberculosis, 284

Swamp Root (medicine), 159

sweat baths, 57, 64, 296. See also hydrotherapy

sweat lodges 19, 22, 22–23, 134

syphilis, xxiii, 33, 34, 51–52, 58–60, 59, 92–93, 276–77; and mental illness, 228, 229–30; among soldiers, 112, 116, 216–17; treatments for, 11, 59, 232

syringes: enema, 20, 50; hypodermic, 11; penile, 50, 59

Talbott, Nellie, 94

tapeworms. See worms

tartar emetic, 51, 114

Taylor, Susie King, 241

Terrill, Frank I., 284–85

tetanus, 120, 289; vaccine for, xxi

thermometer, 12, 50, 97, 171; veterinary, 281

Thomas, Lewis, 185

Thompson, David, 69–70

Thomson, Samuel, 78

Thomsonian medicine, 77–78, 205

Three Forks (MT): hospital in, 223

thunderclappers, 42, 52, 53, 54

tick fevers: Colorado tick fever, 54, 185; Rocky Mountain spotted fever, 254, 255, 285, 292; Texas fever, 270

Tombstone (AZ), 100–102

tonsils: and diphtheria, 264; diseased, 3, 61; surgical removal of, 197

Toston (MT), 134

tourniquets, 50, 170

Townsend (MT), 134, 178

Townsend, G. A., 233

tracheotomy, 186–87, 186, 264

trachoma, 43

training of doctors, 13–16, 150–54, 168, 191; by apprenticeship, 13–14;

in army, 110–11; women and, 202–04, 211. See also licensing of doctors

training of midwives, 245

training of nurses, 245–49

Treacy, William, 274

trephine, 19–20, 111

Tuba City (AZ), 296

tuberculosis, 277–85; bovine, 281–83; climate as beneficial to, 168, 207, 278–80; miner's consumption, 280–81; in mining towns, 90, 209, 280–81; and Native Americans, 33, 36, 284–85; quarantine for, 254; sanitariums and hospitals for, 278–79, 278, 279, 283–85; transmission of, 11–12, 254, 278

Tubman, Harriet, 241

Tuchscherer, Mabel, 211

Tucson (AZ): tuberculosis sanitariums in, 278, 278, 279

Turner, Anna, 242

turpentine, 294

Tuttle, Thomas D.: 206, 256, 270–71, 275; and Galen State Hospital, 283–84; and Montana Board of Health, 206, 256–58, 275, 283, 285; and tuberculosis, 282–83

Twain, Mark, 278–79

typhoid, 11–12, 113, 273–76; epidemics of, 80, 153, 273–74; houseflies as carriers of, 273, 274, 275; and Native Americans, 27, 33

Typhoid Mary, 273

typhus, 271

ulcers, 113, 145, 147, 188

United States National Formulary, 28

United States Public Health Service, 280

urine: medicinal use of, 78–79

vaccination, xxi, 258; for diphtheria, 11, 264–65; for measles, 268; for polio, 289–90; for rabies, 10, 162, 164; for Rocky Mountain spotted fever, 255,

272–73; for smallpox, xxi, 47, 48,
75, 109, 258, 260, 262; for whooping cough, 268
venereal diseases, 91–94, 116–17,
276–77. See also gonorrhea; syphilis
Vesalius, Andreas, xxi
Vicks Vaporub, 295
Vidal, Charles, 283–84
Virginia City (MT), 100, 103, 153,
220, 264, 265; hospitals in, 221
Virginia City (NV), 220
vitamins: A, 115; B, 12, 30; C, xxii, 30,
54, 83, 105, 116; D, 30
Vogel, Virgil J., 24
vomiting: as purge, 2, 7, 34, 51, 78,
114, 274; as symptom, 179 (see also
digestive disorders)
Vontver, May Anderson, 292

wagon trains, 80, 82, 85; medical care
on, 73–86
Waiilatpu (WA), 74
Walker, Dora E., 206
Walker, Mary E., 202, 203
Walla Walla Indians, 57
Warm Springs State Hospital for
Mental Diseases. See Montana State
Hospital
Warner's Safe Kidney Cure, 142
Washington, George, 3–4
Wasserman test, 276
water sanitation, 251–54, 257, 275. See
also cholera; typhoid
Watkins, C. F., 183
Watson's Mill (NV), 219
Weeks, Oscar Dalton, 161
Welch, William, 282
Wells, Horace, 11
West, Elliott, 79
White Bird, Chief, 126
White Sulphur Springs (MT), 178,
183, 232
whitlows, 53

Whitman, Marcus, 35, 71, 74–75
Whitwell, William, 199
whooping cough, 138, 268, 289; death
rate from, 267, 268; epidemics of,
81, 90, 268; folk treatment for, 143;
and Native Americans, 35; quarantine for, 254; vaccine for, xxi, 268
William of Saliceto, 171
Willis, Edward, 95
Willis, George C., 102
Willow Creek (MT), 179
willow bark, 28
Wilson, Myra, 294
Wolf, Louis H., 292, 294
Woods, Margaret, 210
Worden, Tyler, 272
World War I, 221, 297; flu epidemic
during, 290–98; hospital gangrene
during, 120; medical knowledge
gained during, 179; noncombat casualties in, 111; nurses in, 242, 243
worms: earthworms as curative, 143;
patent medicine for infestation of,
160; prescription to treat infestation of, 173; roundworms, 70, 160;
screwworms, 117; tapeworms, 11

X-rays, 12, 13, 183, 223, 278, 283;
equipment, 184

yarrow, 28, 29, 293
Yavapai Indians, 296
Yellowstone National Park, 223–26
Yellowstone Park Hospital, 224,
224–26, 225
yellow fever, 3, 55
York (of Lewis and Clark Expedition),
45, 53
Young, Brigham, 77, 204–05
Yount, George C., 66

zinc sulfate, 56, 93

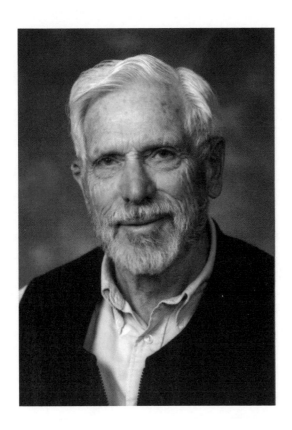

ABOUT THE AUTHOR

Volney Steele was born in a small town in northwest Arkansas in 1922, the son of the town's only physician and its only schoolteacher. After spending two years as a general practitioner in Meeker, Colorado, Dr. Steele practiced pathology in Bozeman, Montana, from 1959 to 1986. After retiring he served for several years overseas with Project HOPE and Pathologists Overseas. A passionate student of the history of medicine, he has published several articles on the subject. The Volney Steele Endowment to the Montana State University Foundation has helped support the Medical History of the West Conference in Bozeman since 2000. Dr. Steele received an honorary doctorate from Montana State University in the spring of 2005, in recognition of his contributions in conservation, medicine, history, and public service.

In addition to *Bleed, Blister, and Purge: A History of Medicine on the American Frontier*, Mountain Press Publishing Company publishes a series of Roadside Geology guides, Roadside History guides, full-color plant and bird guides, outdoor guides, horse books, and a wide selection of western Americana titles, as well as The Tumbleweed Series—reprints of classic cowboy short stories and novels by the famed artist and storyteller Will James.

For more information about our books, please give us a call at 800-234-5308 or mail us your address and we will happily send you a catalog. If you have a friend who would like to receive our catalog, simply include his or her name and address. Thank you for your interest in our titles and for supporting an independent press devoted to providing high-quality books to readers interested in the world around them.

Name _____

Address_____

City _____

State_____ Zip_____

MOUNTAIN PRESS PUBLISHING CO.
P.O. Box 2399 / Missoula, Montana 59806
Phone: 406-728-1900 / Fax: 406-728-1635
TOLL FREE: 1-800-234-5308
E-mail: info@mtnpress.com
Web site: www.mountain-press.com